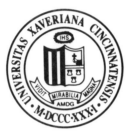

Nutrition and Aging

Bristol-Myers

Nutrition

Symposia

Series Editor
JERRY L. MOORE
Nutritional Division
Mead Johnson & Company

Nutrition and Aging

Edited by

MARTHA L. HUTCHINSON
Department of Pathology
Tufts New England Medical Center
Boston, Massachusetts

HAMISH N. MUNRO
USDA Human Nutrition Research Center on Aging at Tufts
Boston, Massachusetts

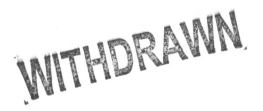

ACADEMIC PRESS, INC.
Harcourt Brace Jovanovich, Publishers
San Diego   New York   Berkeley   Boston
London   Sydney   Tokyo   Toronto

ACADEMIC PRESS, INC.
1250 Sixth Avenue, San Diego, California 92101

United Kingdom Edition published by
ACADEMIC PRESS INC. (LONDON) LTD.
24–28 Oval Road, London NWI 7DX

Library of Congress Cataloging in Publication Data

Nutrition and aging.

   (Bristol-Myers nutrition symposia ; v. 5)
   Papers presented at the Fifth Bristol-Myers
Symposium on Nutrition Research, held in Boston on
Oct. 31 and Nov. 1, 1985.
   Includes index.
   1. Aging—Nutritional aspects—Congresses.
2. Aged—Nutrition—Congresses. I. Hutchinson,
Martha L. II. Munro, Hamish N. (Hamish Nisbet)
III. Bristol-Myers Symposium on Nutrition Research
(5th : 1985 : Boston, Mass.) IV. Series. [DNLM:
1. Aging—congresses. 2. Nutrition—in old age—
congresses. W3 BR323F v.5 / QU 145 N9701 1985]
QP86.N83 1986   612'.67   86-14005
ISBN 0–12–362875–X (alk. paper)

PRINTED IN THE UNITED STATES OF AMERICA

88 89   9 8 7 6 5 4 3 2

Contents

1   Aging and Nutrition: A Multifaceted Problem

HAMISH N. MUNRO

2   Physiologic Interface of Aging and Nutrition

JOHN W. ROWE

3 Nutrition and Organ Function in a Cohort of Aging Men

JORDAN TOBIN

4 Impact of Aging and Nutrition on Human Skin: Studies at the Cellular Level

BARBARA A. GILCHREST
AND PHILIP R. GORDON

5 Vitamin D Synthesis by the Aging Skin

MICHAEL F. HOLICK

6 Implications of Gastric Atrophy for Vitamin and Mineral Nutriture

ROBERT M. RUSSELL

7 Trace Elements and the Needs of the Elderly

WALTER MERTZ

8   Role of Dietary Antioxidants in Aging

JEFFREY B. BLUMBERG
AND SIMIN NIKBIN MEYDANI

9   Aging Animal Models for the Study of Drug–Nutrient Interactions

PAUL M. NEWBERNE

13   Exercise and Muscle Metabolism in the Elderly

WILLIAM J. EVANS

14   Aging of Rats: The Roles of Food Restriction and Exercise

JOHN O. HOLLOSZY AND E. KAYE SMITH

15   Nutritional Factors in Age-Related Osteoporosis

B. LAWRENCE RIGGS

16 Significance of Vitamin D in Age-Related Bone Disease

HECTOR F. DeLUCA

17 Diet, Immunity, and Longevity

ROBERT A. GOOD AND AMAR J. GAJJAR

18 Nutrition and the Aging Hematopoietic System

DAVID A. LIPSCHITZ

19 Nutrition and the Aging Cardiovascular System

ROBERT B. McGANDY

Contributors

Numbers in parentheses indicate the pages on which the authors' contributions begin.

Jeffrey B. Blumberg (85), Nutrition Immunology and Toxicology Laboratory, USDA Human Nutrition Research Center on Aging at Tufts, Boston, Massachusetts 02111

Hector F. DeLuca (217), Department of Biochemistry, College of Agricultural and Life Sciences, University of Wisconsin—Madison, Madison, Wisconsin 53706

William J. Evans (179), USDA Human Nutrition Research Center on Aging at Tufts, Boston, Massachusetts 02111

Amar J. Gajjar (235), University of South Florida, Department of Pediatrics/St. Petersburg, All Children's Hospital, St. Petersburg, Florida 33731-8920

Philip J. Garry (117), Department of Pathology, Clinical Nutrition Laboratory, University of New Mexico School of Medicine, Albuquerque, New Mexico 87131

Barbara A. Gilchrest (35), USDA Human Nutrition Research Center on Aging at Tufts, Boston, Massachusetts 02111, and Boston University School of Medicine, Boston, Massachusetts 02118

Robert A. Good (235), University of South Florida, Department of Pediatrics/St. Petersburg, All Children's Hospital, St. Petersburg, Florida 33731-8920

Philip R. Gordon (35), USDA Human Nutrition Research Center on Aging at Tufts, Boston, Massachusetts 02111, and Boston University School of Medicine, Boston, Massachusetts 02118

Michael F. Holick (45), USDA Human Nutrition Research Center on Aging at Tufts, and Departments of Physiology and Nutrition, Tufts University, Boston, Massachusetts 02111

John O. Holloszy (193), Department of Medicine, and Office of Laboratory Animal Care, Washington University School of Medicine, St. Louis, Missouri 63110

William C. Hunt (117), Department of Pathology, Clinical Nutrition Laboratory, University of New Mexico School of Medicine, Albuquerque, New Mexico 87131

Frank L. Iber[1] (169), University of Maryland School of Medicine, and Baltimore Veterans Administration Medical Center, Baltimore, Maryland 21218

Mary Bess Kohrs (139), Department of Community Health Sciences, University of Illinois at Chicago, Chicago, Illinois 60612

David A. Lipschitz (251), Division of Hematology/Oncology and Division on Aging, University of Arkansas for Medical Sciences, and John L. McClellan Veterans Administration Hospital, Little Rock, Arkansas 72205

Robert B. McGandy (263), Tufts University Schools of Medicine and Nutrition, and USDA Human Nutrition Research Center on Aging at Tufts, Boston, Massachusetts 02111

Walter Mertz (71), USDA Human Nutrition Research Center, Beltsville, Maryland 20705

Simin Nikbin Meydani (85), Nutrition Immunology and Toxicology Laboratory, USDA Human Nutrition Research Center on Aging at Tufts, Boston, Massachusetts 02111

Hamish N. Munro (1), USDA Human Nutrition Research Center on Aging at Tufts, Boston, Massachusetts 02111

Paul M. Newberne (99), Department of Pathology, Boston University School of Medicine, Boston, Massachusetts 02118

B. Lawrence Riggs (207), Endocrine Research Unit, Mayo Clinic and Foundation, Rochester, Minnesota 55905

John W. Rowe (11), Division on Aging, Harvard Medical School, Boston, Massachusetts 02215

Robert M. Russell (59), USDA Human Nutrition Research Center on Aging at Tufts, Boston, Massachusetts 02111

E. Kaye Smith (193), Department of Medicine, and Office of Laboratory Animal Care, Washington University School of Medicine, St. Louis, Missouri 63110

Jordan Tobin (23), Gerontology Research Center, NIA, Francis Scott Key Medical Center, Baltimore, Maryland 21224

---

[1] Present address: Department of Gastrointestinal Disease, Hines Veterans Administration Hospital, and Stritch College of Medicine, Hines, Illinois 60141.

Editor's Foreword

In the United States and the world at large, the average age of the population is increasing. Breakthroughs in preventive medicine and clinical science are contributing significantly to this trend. It seems reasonable to project only a few years hence that 60-year-olds in many parts of the world can expect almost another quarter century of healthy, active living. In spite of the encouraging trends, however, our knowledge of the aging process and of what environmental factors contribute to longer, healthier, and more productive later years remains limited.

To address one of the environmental factors that has a significant influence on aging, the fifth annual Bristol-Myers Symposium on Nutrition Research was held in Boston, Massachusetts, October 31 to November 1, 1985. This conference, on "Nutrition and Aging," afforded scientists the opportunity to present and discuss findings that included the effects of the aging process on the body's physiological functions, the effects of nutrient intake on organ function, and the gap between the documented nutrient intake and nutrient needs of the elderly as it may influence the aging process. The conference was held under the auspices of Tufts University School of Medicine and was organized by Drs. Stanley N. Gershoff, Martha L. Hutchinson, and Hamish N. Munro. These proceedings were also completed under the guidance of Drs. Hutchinson and Munro.

On behalf of the sponsor, Bristol-Myers Company, as well as all of us who look forward to active and healthy golden years, I extend thanks to Drs. Gershoff, Hutchinson, and Munro and all the other contributors for a job well done.

Jerry L. Moore
Series Editor

Foreword

More than ten percent of all Americans are over 65 years of age, and that percentage is expected to double within the next three decades. Other countries around the world are experiencing similar trends, yet surprisingly little systematic study has been made of the special nutritional needs of this large and rapidly growing segment of the world's population.

The fifth annual Bristol-Myers Symposium on Nutrition Research, organized by Tufts University School of Medicine, brought scientists from around the world together to focus on "Nutrition and Aging." The resulting body of scientific and clinical information is contained in this volume.

The papers gathered here represent a significant contribution to our knowledge of the role of nutrition in preventing and limiting the physical, mental, and emotional problems associated with the aging process.

In addition to funding the Bristol-Myers nutrition symposia series, we have committed nearly $3 million over the past five years in unrestricted grants supporting nutrition research at major institutions in the United States and other countries. I am pleased to note that, in 1985, we added two new institutions to the program—the University of California, Davis, and the University of Toronto.

Another important element of the program is the annual Bristol-Myers Award for Distinguished Achievement in Nutrition Research, an annual prize of $25,000 to an individual scientist. The 1985 award was presented to Dr. Clement A. Finch, professor of medicine at the University of Washington, for his work on iron metabolism and anemia.

Through our Mead Johnson subsidiary, Bristol-Myers' commitment to clinical research in nutrition dates back to the early years of this century. For more than 70 years, Mead Johnson has pioneered in developing products to meet the nutritional needs of infants, children, and adults. We expect that commitment to remain strong in the years ahead.

It is our hope that symposia such as the one reported here will continue to stimulate the exchange of ideas and information regarding the latest developments in nutrition research and its growing importance in the prevention and treatment of disease.

Richard L. Gelb
Chairman of the Board
Bristol-Myers Company

Preface

The papers collected in this volume were presented in Boston on October 31 and November 1, 1985, as the fifth Bristol-Myers Symposium on Nutrition Research. This year's international symposium dealt with "Nutrition and Aging" and provided a picture of the many facets of nutrition in its relationship to the aging process and to the maintenance of the health of the elderly. It is thus anticipated that the publication of the proceedings will provide the reader with a conspectus of the various ways in which nutrition is a significant environmental factor in aging.

This volume begins with a general overview. Thereafter the other eighteen chapters represent four areas of research. Chapters 2–5 deal with the relationship of nutrition to changes in physiological function during the aging process. In Chapters 6–10, factors influencing the nutrient needs of the elderly are discussed, while Chapters 11–14 examine socioenvironmental aspects affecting the nutritional status of the elderly. The final chapters (15–19) cover the impact of nutrition in the etiology of age-related degenerative diseases.

The process of editing this volume in the series has been both an education and a pleasure for us, and we wish to express our thanks to the participants for their contributions. The editors' only regret is that they were unable to capture and include the lively discussion that took place after each presentation, in which the audience participated vigorously with penetrating questions and observations from medical practitioners as well as from laboratory scientists.

Lastly, it is a pleasure to acknowledge the generosity of the Bristol-Myers Company and its subsidiary, the Mead Johnson Company, in supporting this symposium and in providing support for nutrition research through their grants program. Our task as editors has been greatly facilitated by the continuous and skilled help of Ann Wyant and

Ralph Weaver of the Bristol-Myers Company and Jerry Moore of the Mead Johnson Company throughout the symposium and subsequently in the course of preparing the manuscripts for publication.

Martha L. Hutchinson
Hamish N. Munro

Nutrition and Aging

Aging and Nutrition: A Multifaceted Problem

Hamish N. Munro

USDA Human Nutrition Research Center on Aging at Tufts
Boston, Massachusetts

I. INTRODUCTION

Interest in geriatric medicine is increasing with the growing awareness of the progressively larger number of adults in this category and their need for medical care (Rowe, 1985). The proportion of people 65 years of age and older currently varies from 5% or less in some underdeveloped countries with a high birth rate to 16% or more in some areas of Western Europe. Statistical data from the United States collected by Brody and Brock (1985) demonstrate that senior citizens have increased from 4% of the population in 1900 to 11% in 1978 and are projected to approach 14% by the year 2000. The implications of this for health care and for Social Security are obvious.

This introduction to the Bristol-Myers Symposium on Nu-

1

trition and Aging emphasizes the variety of problems that have to be resolved in determining the role of nutrition in aging. To introduce some order into surveying the role of nutrition in aging, it is profitable to divide the area into three sections. In discussing these, it will become apparent that senior citizenship is the terminal portion of a continuous process of change in tissue function, disease patterns, and nutrient intake which can be identified earlier in adult life when preventative measures may be most effective.

First, many organ functions and metabolic parameters decrease progressively throughout adult life. At the same time, intakes of most nutrients also decline, and this phenomenon may be a factor contributing to the functional losses associated with aging. Second, the incidence of many chronic diseases becomes more frequent as age advances. In a number of these conditions (e.g., cancer, heart disease, hypertension), there is reason to suspect long-term nutritional habits to be contributing factors. Third, the amounts of individual nutrients needed in the diet of old people in order to sustain their health have been inadequately documented. The reduced intake of nutrients noted among middle-aged people as they grow older becomes accelerated in the elderly so that many old people consume smaller amounts of individual nutrients than are recommended for young adults. In most cases, it is not yet possible to demonstrate that such reduced levels of intake increase the age-related loss of tissue function or other aspects of aging among senior citizens. Perhaps more important is whether improved nutrient intakes of the elderly will reduce further loss of tissue function or delay onset of age-related diseases.

II. AGE-RELATED CHANGES IN BODY COMPOSITION AND METABOLISM

As Rowe points out in Chapter 2 of this volume, advancing age is accompanied by progressive physiological changes in the functions of most major organs as well as the accumulation of diseases. Furthermore, the severity and clinical manifestations of these physiological and pathological changes are modifed by changes in body composition, diet, exercise, and other environmental factors that include smoking and alcohol consumption.

Studies of the effect of aging on body composition are quite extensive and show that there is a progressive loss of lean body mass throughout middle age and old age, with some tendency for the rate of loss to increase in later life (Forbes, 1976). For example, Swedish men lose about 1 kg lean body mass between the ages of 70 and 75 years (Steen *et al.*, 1979). This loss of lean body mass is largely accounted for by skeletal muscle, which can shrink as much as 40% between the ages of 20 and 80 years (Cohn *et al.*, 1980). This is confirmed by the reduced output of creatinine and of 3-methylhistidine in the urine of elderly people (Munro and Young, 1978) and by other evidence such as a reduced number of contractile fibers in the muscles of old people (Lexell *et al.*, 1983). A striking and important example of age-related change in body composition is osteoporosis, which begins in middle age or earlier (Riggs, Chapter 15).

Metabolic changes occurring with aging are also well documented. In many cases, the alteration in metabolism is best seen in response to a challenge. Thus the fasting blood sugar level is little affected by age, but the response to a standard dose of glucose is impaired to an increasing extent as individuals grow older (Rowe, Chapter 2). Similarly, aging reduces the capacity to metabolize lipids (Kritchevsky, 1979). Protein metabolism is also affected by aging. Albumin synthesis rate was measured by us (Gersovitz *et al.*, 1980) on young and elderly adults at two levels of protein intake. When dietary protein was raised from a low to an adequate level, synthesis rate in the young adults increased, but not in the case of the elderly.

III. AGING AND TISSUE FUNCTION

The most extensive and comprehensive studies of the effect of age on tissue and organ function in man come from the Baltimore Longitudinal Study on Aging, in which more than 1000 men of various ages have been studied for periods of up to 25 years. This unique cohort thus provides both cross-sectional and longitudinal data on the effects of aging on many physiological functions. The major findings have recently been assembled in book form (Shock *et al.*, 1984). Shock (1972) concludes that the functions of different organs erode progressively throughout adult life at different rates. Thus between the ages of 30 and 80 years, nerve conduction declines 15%, cardiac output by 30%, renal blood flow by 50%, etc., in the average adult man. A second edition of the *Handbook of the Biology of Aging* (Finch and Schneider, 1985) contains several chapters summarizing changes in nervous system function with aging. The immune system also decreases in functional efficiency with age (Hausman and Weksler, 1985).

Animal models provide the most extensive evidence of dietary effects on the rate of aging of tissues and organs (for review, see Guigoz and Munro, 1985). It has been repeatedly confirmed that rats that are growth-retarded from an early age by caloric restriction live longer, an effect that is still evident if food restriction is imposed on young adult rats. In addition to better survival, almost all tissue functions are better retained as the underfed rat or mouse ages. Skeletal muscle is better preserved, responses of tissues to hormones decline much later due to extended conservation of hormone receptors, and T-cell-dependent immunological responses are better maintained. Some of these benefits of dietary restriction also occur when the aging rodent is exercised (Goodrick *et al.*, 1983; Holloszy and Smith, Chapter 14).

In addition to the benefits of caloric restriction in preserving function, the incidence of a number of chronic diseases of aging rats is reduced and the time of their onset is delayed by caloric restriction. For example, chronic nephritis, periarteritis, myocardial degeneration, and a variety of tumors are frequent in the older *ad libitum*-fed rat and mouse, but are less significant in the calorie-restricted rodent (Good and Gajjar, Chapter 17). This supplements the evidence, gathered from human experiments and epidemiological studies, showing that dietary factors are relevant to the incidence of these conditions in man (McGandy, Chapter 19).

These studies raise the question of the potential benefits of nutrition, exercise, and other environmental variables in diminishing the incidence of chronic age-related diseases and in attaining the maximum human life span. Fries (1980) has proposed that life span is determined by two factors. One is the occurrence of chronic disease which shortens the "natural" life span of the individual. He regards such chronic illnesses as susceptible to some degree of prevention by better life-styles, of which nutrition is an important component. The second factor restricting life span is classified by Fries as "natural aging," by which he recognizes progressive and inevitable loss of function. Thus, as we learn to eliminate the chronic diseases, the normal life span of human survival according to Fries will continue until about 80 years of age, after which most people will die from inevitable failure of organ functions at some time between 80 and 90 years of age.

This picture seems incompatible with other evidence on morbidity and mortality. Thus Katz *et al.* (1983) have applied the life table technique to assess the fate of senior citizens in Massachusetts in two ways: first, how many years they are able to operate independently without help, then how long they survive in a dependent state, which is defined as needing help in rising from bed, bathing, dressing, and/or eating. Thus, as shown in Table I, men and women aged 65–69 years of age function in an active state for about the same period of time (9.3 years for men and 10.6 years for women). Thereafter, the men survive in a dependent state for a further 3.8 years but the women continue in dependency for 8.9 years, thus accounting for most of the difference in the total life

TABLE I

Active and Total Life Expectancy of the Elderly[a]

	Men (years)	Women (years)
Age group	60–69	60–69
Life expectancy		
Total	13.1	19.5
Active	9.3	10.6
Dependent[b]	3.8	8.9

[a] Adapted from Katz et al. (1983).
[b] For rising, bathing, dressing, or eating.

span of men and women. The criteria for identifying the onset of the dependent phase listed above all relate to the ability to deploy neuro-muscular coordination and thus indicate deterioration of the nervous system. On the other hand, statistical studies show that two-thirds of deaths occurring between 80 and 84 years of age and 70% from 85 years onward are due to cardiovascular events, that is, heart disease, cerebro-vascular disease, and arteriosclerosis (Brody and Brock, 1985). The longer survival of women is probably attributable to their slower development of cardiovascular disease.

IV. NUTRIENT NEEDS AND INTAKES OF THE ELDERLY

Estimates of the nutrient needs of elderly adults are largely extrapolations of the needs of young adults, supplemented by a limited amount of direct experimentation on old people. Actual intakes of nutrients by the elderly have been assessed in various surveys, mostly by recollection of food consumed. The precision of these estimates depends on the care exercised in such studies and, importantly, on having an accurate knowledge of the nutrient composition of the foods consumed. For example, the second Health and Nutrition Examination Survey (Abraham et al., 1982) provides a valuable view of recent nutrient intakes and nutritional status of a balanced sample of the American population, except that it stops at 74 years, thus excluding the nutrition picture for the older segment most at risk.

There is general agreement that the energy intake of adults diminishes throughout adulthood. Thus, in the Baltimore Longitudinal Study of

Aging, cross-sectional data of energy intake showed total daily energy intakes by the men in the survey to diminish steadily from 2700 kcal at age 30 years to 2100 kcal at age 80 years (Shock, 1972). One-third of this decline of 600 kcal per day can be accounted for by the reduced basal metabolism resulting from the shrinking lean body mass of older people. The remaining two-thirds represented a progressive reduction in physical activity. This picture is confirmed by longitudinal studies on the same group (Tobin, Chapter 3) and by a number of published studies reviewed elsewhere (Munro et al., 1987). The Recommended Dietary Allowances (National Academy of Sciences, 1980) of energy for adult men of different ages are in good agreement with intakes observed in the HANES surveys, but the recommended allowances for adult women of all ages are several hundred calories greater than have been observed to be consumed in these surveys. The low energy consumption of women has been confirmed by direct calorimetry and by using $^3H_2^{18}O$ dissociation, the latter method being potentially a good direct index of energy expenditure over the whole 24 hours (Prentice et al., 1985).

Since food is consumed in response to a desire for enough energy, the amounts of nutrients associated with various energy sources in the diet are likely to be reduced in proportion to the diminishing energy consumption of aging adults. This is borne out by nutrient consumption data. Thus the intakes of protein (Munro, 1964) and of zinc (Sandstead et al., 1982) are proportional to the caloric intakes of adults. The data of Exton-Smith and Stanton (1965) show that this phenomenon can obtain for old people even over a single decade during which energy intake is falling. They report nutrient intakes of women between the ages of 70 and 80 years living alone; the data show that, over this decade, total energy intake was reduced by 19%, protein by 24%, calcium by 18%, iron by 29%, and ascorbic acid by 31%. What we do not know is whether these reductions place the elderly consumer in jeopardy of insufficiency great enough to impair tissue function.

The complexity of deciding on nutrient needs for the elderly is illustrated by the case of folic acid (Munro, 1987). The Recommended Dietary Allowance (National Academy of Sciences, 1980) for folic acid is 400 μg daily for adults of all ages. However, this has been challenged as being too generous. A survey made in Canada (National Health and Welfare, 1977) showed that elderly men consumed an average of 150 μg folate daily, while women received 130 μg, data that are almost identical to those of a Swedish survey (Jagerstad and Westesson, 1979). These low intakes did not result in megaloblastic anemia or in low blood folate levels. In a survey of elderly in New Mexico (Garry and Hunt, Chapter 10), diet contributed less than 200 μg folate to the average daily intake of this vitamin. Other factors contribute to the assessment of the folate status of the elderly. Thus, achlorhydria, which affects about 20% of the elderly, reduces acidity in the proximal part of the small intestine and thus impairs folate absorption; however, overgrowth of intestinal bacteria due to the absence of acidity may compensate by providing additional folate (Russell, Chapter 6). Availability of dietary folate is also impaired by consumption of ethanol and by certain drugs commonly consumed by the elderly.

A major area reflecting the complexity of nutrient needs is the role of nutrition in osteoporosis leading to fracture. The onset of this loss of bone density occurs early in adult life (20–40 years) and in many women accelerates after the menopause, so that they show a higher frequency of fracture than occurs in men of comparable age (Table II). Thus a process starting in early or middle adult life becomes the cause of disease in the elderly, implying that nutrients and other measures applied during the early stages may be most effective in reducing the impact of this important degenerative condition. Factors thought to be involved in promoting bone loss include too little dietary calcium, phosphorus, and vitamin D, along with too much protein, phytate, and dietary fiber. In addition, insufficient exercise contributes to loss of bone density. The relative merits of these nutrients are discussed in this volume by Holick (Chapter 5), Riggs (Chapter 15), and DeLuca (Chapter 16), and are also reviewed by Munro (1987). Interventions designed to reduce bone loss could include raising the intake of calcium by fortifying the food chain, which is already enriched in the United States by the addition of vitamin D_2 or D_3 to milk and margarine. The use of estrogens to retard postmenopausal loss of bone salts and treatment with 1,25-dihydroxyvitamin D are more appropriate for individuals under medical supervision.

TABLE II

Incidence of Osteoporosis and Fracture by 80 Years of Age[a]

Measurement	Men (%)	Women (%)
Average reduction in bone density	12	25
Cumulative fractures		
Wrist	4	14
Vertebra	4	8
Femur	1.5	5

[a] Adapted from Nordin (1980).

V. FACTORS IN THE NUTRITIONAL STATUS OF
THE ELDERLY

The elderly provide a more varied spectrum of nutritional status than is encountered in younger groups of adults. This occurs because of social and functional factors affecting the older person. A typical picture of a group at risk for malnutrition is the elderly widow living on a restricted income. She is often socially isolated and may be house-bound by osteoarthritis or other crippling disabilities. Old men living alone are commonly ignorant of the need for a balanced diet and are liable to show evidence of mild deficiencies. In addition to these primary factors that increase the risk of malnutrition, secondary causes of malnutrition in the older population include malabsorption due to a variety of causes, including achlorhydria (Russell, Chapter 6), alcoholism with its substitution of ethanol calories for foods containing important nutrients (Iber, Chapter 12), and the extensive use of therapeutic drugs which interfere with nutrient utilization in various ways (Roe, 1985). In the case of drugs, it may be desirable for the physician to use supplements in order to raise the intakes of certain vitamins whose utilization is impaired by the medicament.

All these risk factors make it desirable for the physician to include them in an assessment of the health of their elderly patients. Prendergast (1984) provides an extensive program for examining elderly people that includes many of the risk factors described above.

Preventive measures against malnutrition among the elderly include self-administration of vitamin and mineral supplements, a common practice in most communities. For example, in a population of elderly in New Mexico, Garry et al. (1982) found that 57% of men and 61% of women were taking supplements, resulting in raising intakes of certain vitamins to several times the Recommended Dietary Allowances. A more rational approach is represented by nutrition intervention programs that provide home-delivered meals or congregate feeding. Kohrs (Chapter 11) has evaluated the impact of such programs, which are not limited to nutritional benefits but also provide psychological stimulation, notably for those participating in congregate meals.

REFERENCES

Abraham, S., Carroll, M. D., Dresser, C. M., and Johnson, C. L. (1982). "Dietary Intake Findings, United States 1976–1980." Natl. Cent. Health Stat., U.S. Dep. Health Hum. Serv., Hyatsville, Maryland.

Brody, J. A., and Brock, D. W. (1985). *In* "Handbook of the Biology of Aging" (C. E. Finch and E. L. Schneider, eds.), 2nd ed., pp. 3–26. Van Nostrand-Reinhold, Princeton, New Jersey.

Cohn, S. H., Vartsky, D., Yasmura, S., Sawitsky, A., Zanzi, I., Vaswani, A., and Ellis, K. J. (1980). *Am. J. Physiol.* **239**, E524–E530.

Exton-Smith, A. N., and Stanton, B. R. (1965). "Report of an Investigation into the Dietary of Elderly Women Living Alone." King Edward's Hospital Fund, London.

Finch, C. E., and Schneider, E. L., eds. (1985). "Handbook of the Biology of Aging," 2nd ed. Van Nostrand-Reinhold, Princeton, New Jersey.

Forbes, G. B. (1976). *Hum. Biol.* **48**, 161–173.

Fries, J. F. (1980). *N. Engl. J. Med.* **303**, 130–135.

Garry, P. J., Goodwin, J. S., Hunt, W. C., Hooper, E. M., and Leonard, A. G. (1982). *Am. J. Clin. Nutr.* **36**, 319–331.

Gersovitz, M., Munro, H. N., Udall, J., and Young, V. R. (1980). *Metab., Clin. Exp.* **29**, 1075–1086.

Goodrick, C. L., Ingram, D. K., Reynolds, M. A., Freeman, J. R., and Cider, N. L. (1983). *Exp. Aging Res.* **9**, 203–209.

Guigoz, Y., and Munro, H. N. (1985). *In* "Handbook of the Biology of Aging" (C. E. Finch and E. L. Schneider, eds.), 2nd ed., pp. 878–893. Van Nostrand-Reinhold, Princeton, New Jersey.

Hausman, P. B., and Weksler, M. E. (1985). *In* "Handbook of the Biology of Aging" (C. E. Finch and E. L. Schneider, eds.), 2nd ed., pp. 414–432. Van Nostrand-Reinhold, Princeton, New Jersey.

Jagerstad, M., and Westesson, E.-K. (1979). *Scand. J. Gastroenterol.* **14**, Suppl. 52, 196–202.

Katz, S., Branch, L. G., Branson, M. H., Papsidero, J. A., Beck, J. C., and Greer, D. S. (1983). *N. Engl. J. Med.* **309**, 1218–1224.

Kritchevsky, D. (1979). *Fed. Proc., Fed Am. Soc. Exp. Biol.* **38**, 2001–2006.

Lexell, J., Henriksson-Larsson, K., and Sjöström, M. (1983). *Acta Physiol. Scand.* **117**, 115–122.

Munro, H. N. (1964). *In* "Mammalian Protein Metabolism" (H. N. Munro and J. B. Allison, eds.), Vol. 2, pp. 3–39. Academic Press, New York.

Munro, H. N. (1987). *In* "Nutrition and Metabolism in Patient Care" (J. M. Kinney, K. N. Jeejeebhoy, G. L. Hill, and O. E. Owen, eds.). Saunders, Philadelphia, Pennsylvania (in press).

Munro, H. N., and Young, V. R. (1978). *Am. J. Clin. Nutr.* **31**, 1608–1614.

Munro, H. N., Suter, P., and Russell, R. M. (1987). *Annu. Rev. Nutr.* (in press).

National Academy of Sciences (1980). "Recommended Dietary Allowances," 9th rev. ed. NAS, Washington, D.C.

National Health and Welfare (1977). "Nutrition Canada: Food Consumption Patterns Report." Natl. Health and Welfare, Ottawa, Canada.

Nordin, B. E. C. (1980). *In* "Metabolic and Nutritional Disorders in the Elderly" (A. N. Exton-Smith and F. I. Caird, eds.), pp. 123–145. Wright, Bristol, England.

Prendergast, J. M. (1984). *In* "Nutritional Intervention in the Aging Process" (H. J. Armbrecht, J. M. Prendergast, and R. M. Coe, eds.), pp. 289–292. Springer-Verlag, Berlin and New York.

Prentice, A. M., Davies, H. L., Coward, A. W., Murgatroyd, P. R., Black, A. E., Goldberg, G. R., Ashford, J., Sawyer, M., and Whitehead, R. (1985). *Lancet* **1**, 1419–1422.

Roe, D. A. (1985). *Drug–nutrient Interactions*, **4**, 117–135.

Rowe, J. W. (1985). *New Engl. J. Med.* **312**, 827–835.

Sandstead, H. H., Henriksen, L. K., Greger, J. L., Prasad, A. D., and Good, R. (1982). *Am. J. Clin. Nutr.* **36,** 1046–1059.

Shock, N. W. (1972). *In* "Nutrition in Old Age" (L. A. Carlson, ed.), pp. 12–23. Almqvist & Wiksell, Stockholm.

Shock, N. W., Greulich, R. C., Andres, R., Arenberg, D., Costa, P. T., Lakatta, E. G., and Tobin, J. D. (1984). "Normal Human Aging: The Baltimore Longitudinal Study of Aging," NIH Publ. No. 84–2450. Natl. Inst. Health, Washington, D.C.

Steen, G. B., Isaksson, B., and Svanberg, A. (1979). *J. Clin. Exp. Gerontol.* **1,** 185–200.

2

Physiologic Interface of Aging and Nutrition

John W. Rowe

Division on Aging
Harvard Medical School
Boston, Massachusetts

I. INTRODUCTION

The normal aging process has a varied and important clinical impact, which has the potential for important modification by nutritional factors. A thorough knowledge of age-related physiologic changes that occur in man, in the absence of disease, is critical to a proper understanding of disease in

11

Nutrition and Aging

old age. It is the interaction of normal age-related physiologic changes with a variety of pathologic abnormalities that provides clinical geriatric medicine with many of the special aspects that differentiate it from health care of younger adults (Rowe, 1977). The clinical study of aging might be likened to an onion in which the true age effects are found at the center with cofactors and confounding co-variables representing the concentric layers surrounding this center. Over the past couple of decades we have striven to assiduously dissociate the effects of disease from those of "normal aging." In removing this first outside layer of the onion, in which the diseases are found, we have advanced far beyond the initial clinical studies when healthy young individuals were compared to frail institutionalized elders (Rowe, 1977). However, removal of this disease layer does not isolate aging effects but leaves several concentric layers of other co-variables that are more difficult to identify and more subtle in their effects than the diseases common in old age. These confounding variables include medication use, diet, exercise, anthropometric changes, and psychosocial factors. This chapter will review the basic principles of gerontologic physiology as they apply to clinical medicine and discuss ways in which nutritional factors may influence the clinical impact of the physiology of aging.

Before discussing the interaction of normal aging with disease states it is appropriate to emphasize three major factors which may play important roles in the expression of disease in the elderly: the *variability* of age-related changes, their *plasticity*, and the importance of a concept of *exposure over time*. Nutritional considerations play an important role in our understanding of the ways in which each of these "principles" influences clinical care.

II. FACTORS AFFECTING EXPRESSION OF DISEASE IN THE ELDERLY

A. Variability

A major factor dominating the expression of disease in late life is the marked variability that characterizes physiologic changes with age (Gordon and Shurtleff, 1973). Decades of study of normal and abnormal aging have shown, perhaps more clearly than anything else, that as people get older they become less like each other, not more like each other. The marked variability in the clinical manifestation of disease in the elderly is due, in part, to (1) variability in underlying physiologic changes, (2) other diseases that the individual has accumulated over time, (3) the pattern of response to illness and interaction with health care professionals that is characteristic of the elderly, and (4) the varying degrees of severity of pathophysiologic processes.

The variability between elderly individuals in physiologic capacity may be importantly influenced by nutrition in several ways. There may be direct nutritional influences, such as differing intakes of micro- or macronutrients, or indirect influences, such as diet-induced alterations in body composition. The importance of considering cofactors of aging such as personal habits, diet, body composition, and activity can be seen in the studies of Vestal *et al.* (1975), who evaluated the differences between 307 subjects aged 18 to 92 years in the clearance of antipyrine, a model drug eliminated almost entirely by the liver. These studies excluded subjects with abnormal liver function or those taking medications; in addition, tobacco, alcohol, and coffee use varied markedly among the subjects. While there was a statistically significant inverse relationship between age and antipyrine clearance, the variability in the data was great (Fig. 1). When the relative contributions of age and other factors to the variance in the data were analyzed, cigarette smoking was found to be related to antipyrine clearance. The data indicated that smoking status, which was adversely proportional to age, was a better predictor than age of plasma drug clearance, describing 12% of the vari-

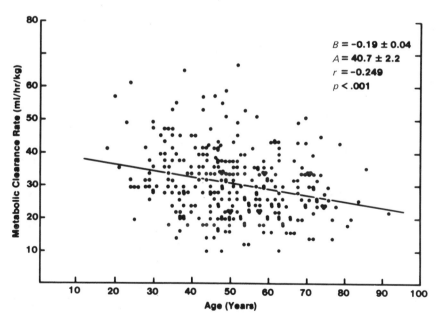

Fig. 1. Decline in metabolic clearance rate of antipyrine with age. (From Vestal *et al.*, 1975.)

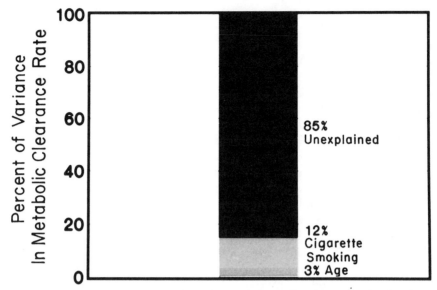

Fig. 2. Contributions of age and smoking to the overall variance of antipyrine clearance in healthy men across the adult age range. (From Vestal *et al.*, 1975.)

ance as opposed to 3% predicted by age (Fig. 2). Thus, an apparent age-related difference in drug kinetics may not be related to the physiologic effects of age but may simply reflect age-associated differences in habits or other variables.

B. Plasticity

For many years, it was felt that age-related changes were irreversible. Few clinicians approached their elderly patients with a view that much benefit could be derived from modifying lifelong life-style or dietary habits. This view is changing rapidly as we come to recognize the marked plasticity or modifiability of many age-related changes previously considered to be fixed. One recent report of old age and smoking (Jajich *et al.*, 1984) demonstrated that elderly smokers had a 52% higher risk for mortality from coronary disease than nonsmokers and that quitting smoking late in life was associated with a rapid and sustained reduction in mortality from coronary disease. This provides support for efforts to reduce smoking in elderly long-term smokers and has substantially brightened the picture for the emergence of preventive strategies in geriatrics. Similar cause for optimism regarding prevention in the

elderly is found in studies showing that treatment of sustained elevations of systolic and diastolic blood pressure in the elderly is associated
with a substantial reduction in mortality and morbidity (Veterans Administration Cooperative Study Group, 1972; Hypertension Detection
Follow-up Program, 1979).

A final example of the plasticity of aging relates to the potential value
of physical exercise to retard age-related losses in bone mass in the
elderly. Several studies suggest that retardation of age-related bone loss
may occur in response to moderate exercise in older people, including
the very elderly. Thus, Aloia and colleagues (1978) evaluated the effect
of one hour of exercise three times weekly for one year on total and
regional bone mass in a group of women who had undergone menopause an average of four years earlier. They found that the level of total
body calcium increased significantly in the exercise group, suggesting
that exercise had a beneficial effect in retarding involutional blood loss.
This also applies to much older women. In another prospective controlled study, Smith and Reddan (1976) found that 30 minutes of exercise three times weekly over a three-year period resulted in a significant
increase in bone mineral content (4.2%) in elderly nursing home residents, while a control group had a 2.5% reduction. In a follow-up investigation (Smith *et al.*, 1981), these same investigators studied four groups
of elderly nursing home residents: a control group, a group receiving
dietary supplements of calcium and vitamin D, a group enrolled in a
physical activity program, and a group engaging in exercise as well as
receiving calcium and vitamin D supplementation. The moderate exercise regimen, which was accomplished while the subject was sitting in a
chair, consisted of 30 minutes of physical activities three times a week.
Over a three-year period, exercise induced significant increases in bone
mineral content as compared with that in controls. Surprisingly, however, exercise combined with calcium and vitamin D supplementation
yielded an intermediate effect.

C. Exposure over Time

The increased time that elderly individuals have been alive predis-
poses them to certain diseases or losses of function apart from the biological or physiologic changes of age per se. Several specific examples
can be cited. Polycystic kidney disease represents a heritable condition
in which the clinical manifestations are frequently not expressed until
the sixth decade of life. The aging process itself has no influence, as far
as is known, on the development of cysts in kidneys. It is clear, how-

ever, that these individuals must live until at least the sixth decade of life before they show the manifestations of this inherited disease, due to the combination of the disease and age-related loss of kidney function. A second class of abnormalities that appears to be more related to the passage of time than to changes associated with age are disorders due to accumulated exposure to environmental or dietary toxins. Cutaneous cancers secondary to sun exposure in individuals with fair skin are likely to be more prevalent in older individuals than in younger individuals because older individuals have greater cumulative exposure to the ultraviolet radiation in sunlight (Gilchrist et al., 1979). Similarly, individuals who smoke cigarettes are more likely to develop pulmonary carcinoma in middle or late life than during younger adulthood because of the time required to accumulate exposure to a carcinogenic dose of cigarette tobacco (Doll and Peto, 1976) and the time lag from initiation to detection of disease. A final example of a disorder with a long latency period and increased prevalence with advancing age can be seen in the development of mesothelioma after exposure to asbestos. Peto (1979) has shown in three different age cohorts that the apparent increase with age in mesothelioma risk is not related to age per se but rather to the time since exposure to asbestos.

In a nutritional context, it may be that lifelong exposures to certain dietary constituents play an important role in the development of apparent age-related patterns of nutritionally related diseases and that modification of these patterns would result in much greater reductions in the incidence of certain diseases, such as atherosclerosis, in the elderly than has generally been thought possible or likely.

III. PHYSIOLOGIC CHANGES OCCURRING WITH ADVANCING AGE

With these principles of variability, plasticity, and exposure over time in mind, we now turn to a review of the major types of physiologic changes that occur with advancing age and the possible impact that nutritional factors may have on their clinical expression. Four types of clinical changes will be discussed, i.e., factors that do not change with age, physiologic changes that increase the likelihood or severity of disease, physiologic changes that have a direct clinical impact, and, last, physiologic changes that have a strong nutritional component and mimic specific disease states. In the latter instance, the carbohydrate intolerance of aging will be discussed as a prime example of an apparent age-related factor with a major nutritional component.

A. Variables Which Do Not Change with Age

From a clinical standpoint, one important type of change that occurs with age is no change at all. Too frequently, clinicians are apt to ascribe a disability or abnormal physical or laboratory finding to "old age" when the actual cause is a specific disease process. An example of this lack of change may be seen in the hematocrit. Elderly persons with lower hematocrit levels may be incorrectly categorized as having "anemia of old age." Physicians may fail to investigate the basis of an anemia thus found in elderly individuals and conclude that either no treatment or iron supplementation of the diet is warranted. However, data from the Framingham Study (Gordon and Shurtleff, 1973) indicate that in healthy individuals living in the community there is no change in the hematocrit with age. Thus a lower hematocrit level in an elderly person cannot be ascribed to anemia of old age and requires proper investigation and treatment.

B. Physiologic Changes Which Increase the Likelihood or Severity of a Disease

This category encompasses age-related reductions in the function of numerous organs that place the elderly person at special risk of increased morbidity from diseases in those organs. Studies in carefully screened subjects across the adult age range indicate that advancing age is accompanied by inevitable changes that are separable from the effects of diseases. Advancing age after adulthood is associated with progressive age-related reduction in the function of many organs, including major losses in renal, pulmonary and immune functions (Rowe, 1977). Simultaneous linear reductions in homeostatic capabilities in these organs result in geometric reductions in the total homeostatic capability of the organism—and age-related "homeostenosis." When coupled with the functional impairments associated with disease states, this constricted homeostatis is responsible for the markedly increased vulnerability of the elderly to morbidity during acute illness or trauma, such as burns, major surgery, or the administration of medications (Fig. 3).

C. Physiologic Changes with a Direct Clinical Impact

Although age is not a disease but a normal process, some age-related physiologic changes clearly have adverse clinical sequelae and normal aging should thus not be considered harmless. Perhaps the use of the

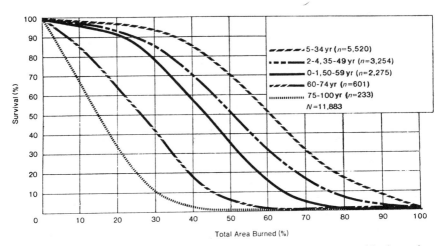

Fig. 3. Survival of patients as a function of the total percentage of body surface burned and age. (From Feller *et al.*, 1976.)

terms "normal" or "normative" aging has been deleterious since it does imply that these changes have no attributable risk. More widespread use of the term "usual aging" instead of normal aging might more clearly indicate the possibility that these age-related changes might be associated with risk for increased morbidity and thus should be the target of potential studies to modify their effects.

The "normal" age-related changes that may have direct clinical impact, and which are clearly influence by nutritional factors, include menopause, osteoporosis, atherosclerosis, arteriosclerosis, and development of cataract. In the case of cataract, posttranslational nonenzymatic modifications of central lens proteins (Tripathi and Tripathi, 1983) occur with advancing age in normal individuals and to a much more rapid extent in individuals with diabetes mellitus. It is possible that normal age-related increases in ambient sugar levels, to be discussed in detail below, play an important role in these apparent age-related changes and that dietary modifications in the elderly, which result in less wide excursions in blood sugar, either directly because of modifications in carbohydrate intake or indirectly through alterations in body composition, might potentially have a beneficial effect on the development of "senile cataract."

D. Physiologic Changes which Mimic Specific Disease—Carbohydrate Intolerance

For over 60 years it has been known that advancing age is associated with progressive decrements in glucose tolerance. Many clinical studies indicate a very slight, approximately 1 mg/dl per decade, age-related increase after maturity in fasting blood sugar levels in healthy humans. This change is not affected by gender and is only slightly enhanced by cortisone administration (Davidson, 1979; Andres and Tobin, 1977). This modest age-related increase in fasting blood glucose levels is accompanied by rather striking increases in blood sugar responses after oral or intravenous glucose challenge of elderly subjects. Lack of consideration of the age effect on glucose tolerance will result in an erroneous diagnosis of impaired carbohydrate tolerance or diabetes in many healthy elderly. In an extensive review of the English literature, Davidson (1979) found that the average postglucose challenge increase in blood sugar with advancing age was 9.5 mg/dl per decade at one hour and 5.3 mg/dl per decade at two hours. The higher postprandial glucose levels seen with aging are also reflected in increased levels of glycosylated hemoglobin A_{1C} with age (Graf *et al.*, 1978), a factor which suggests that "senescent hyperglycemia" might potentially play a role, as noted previously, in the nonenzymatic modification of proteins and their subsequent deleterious effects such as the development of cataract.

Alterations in glucose absorption associated with aging are unlikely to play an important role in these findings since similar results are found on both oral and intravenous glucose testing. Distribution of blood glucose levels at one and two hours after glucose challenge in the elderly is unimodal, which suggests that the change does not reflect the increasing prevalence of a second population of diabetics who are skewing the data.

It is clear that marked limitation of physical activity as well as administration of diets low in carbohydrate will impair glucose tolerance. Evidence that age-associated changes in body composition may play an important role in determining age effects in carbohydrate metabolism, even under basal conditions, has been developed by Elahi and colleagues (1982) in a study of fasting levels of glucose, insulin, glucagon, and growth hormone in normal male volunteers ranging in age from 23 to 93 years. In these studies, fatness was associated with increases in basal insulin, glucagon, and fasting glucose, while basal fasting levels of these main gluco-regulatory hormones were not influenced by aging per se. While the apparent age-related impairment in glucose metabolism is less after this careful screening of the elderly subjects, an age effect persists in postchallenge glucose levels (Reaven and Reaven, 1980). Thus, carbohydrate economy is an excellent example of the "peeled-onion" approach to development of gerontological investigation. At first, the carbohydrate intolerance of aging was contaminated by increase with age in the incidence of diabetes mellitus. After diabetic individuals were excluded from study groups, it was noted that the older individuals persisted with modest levels of hyperglycemia compared to their younger counterparts. Studies then went on to show that dietary abnormalities or changes in body composition were important contributors, as well as perhaps reduction in exercise, to this age-related hyperglycemia. Nonetheless, after accounting for the contributions of these co-variables, a substantial effect of "aging" remained.

Subsequent physiologic studies of the mechanisms of the effect of aging on glucose balance have shown that circulating levels of insulin are not impaired with age after glucose challenge and that the sensitivity of the old liver to suppression of glucose production by insulin also remains intact. Several studies (Rowe *et al.*, 1983; Fink *et al.*, 1983a; DeFronzo, 1979) have shown that advancing age is associated with a progressive impairment in the sensitivity of peripheral tissues to insulin, without modification of the affinity or number of insulin receptors. After correction for differences between age groups in lean body mass, age-related effects of insulin action persisted in these studies (Rowe *et al.*, 1983; Fink *et al.*, 1983b). Subsequent studies of *in vitro* insulin action on isolated adipocytes have shown age-related impairment in glucose transport, which may be the rate-limiting step in glucose metabolism in the elderly. Studies employing modern molecular biological techniques can now be performed to evaluate the specific mechanisms of the age effects on glucose transport. Such studies will also form the basis for evaluation of the exact mechanisms of age-related confounding factors such as diet and body composition so that a broad-based elucidation of the molecular mechanism and relative contributions of the various aging and age-related effects can be developed.

The carbohydrate intolerance of aging represents an excellent example of the importance of clarification of age versus age-related factors. The remaining chapters in this volume deal with some of the specific points of interface between gerontology and nutrition and provide in-depth examples of the importance of variability, plasticity, exposure over time, and the value of dissociating age effects from those of age-related confounding factors.

IV. SUMMARY

Just as children are not simply young adults, the elderly are not just old adults, but represent a group with special characteristics and needs. The physiologic changes that accompany normal aging serve as the substrate for the influence of age in the presentation of diseases, their response to treatment, and the complications that ensue. Increasing evidence indicates that this age–disease interaction may be strongly influenced by nutritional factors and deficiencies. Further understanding of this complex age–nutrition–disease interaction will permit the design of interventions to prolong health as well as life.

ACKNOWLEDGMENTS

Supported by grants from the National Institutes of Health (AG00599 and AG04390), the Veterans Administration, the Commonwealth Fund, the John A. Hartford Foundation, and the John D. and Catherine T. MacArthur Foundation.

REFERENCES

Aloia, J. F., Cohn, S. H., Ostuni, J. A., Cane, R., and Ellis, K. (1978). *Ann. Intern. Med.* **89,** 356–358.

Andres, R., and Tobin, J. D. (1977). "The Biology of Aging," pp. 357–358. Van Nostrand-Reinhold, Princeton, New Jersey.

Davidson, M. B. (1979). *Metab., Clin. Exp.* **28,** 688–705.

DeFronzo, R. A. (1979). *Diabetes* **28,** 1095–1101.

Doll, R., and Peto, R. (1976). *Br. Med. J.* **2,** 1525–1536.

Elahi, D., Muller, D., Tzonkhoff, D., Andres, R., and Tobin, J. D. (1982). *J. Gerontol.* **37,** 385–391.

Feller, I., Flora, J. D., Jr., and Bawol, R. (1976). *JAMA, J. Am. Med. Assoc.* **236,** 1943–1947.

Fink, R. I., Kolterman, O. G., Kao, M., and Olefsky, J. M. (1983a). *J. Clin. Endocrinol. Metab.* **58,** 721–725.

Fink, R. I., Kolterman, O. G., Green, J., and Olefsky, J. M. (1983b). *J. Clin. Invest.* **71,** 1523–1535.

Gilchrist, B. A., Blog, F. B., and Szabo, G. (1979). *J. Invest. Dermatol.* **73,** 219.

Gordon, T., and Shurtleff, D. (1973). "The Framingham Study: Epidemiologic Investigation of Cardiovascular Disease," HEW Publ. No. NIH 74–478. U.S. Department of Health, Education and Welfare, Washington, D.C.

Graf, R. J., Halter, J. B., and Porte, D. (1978). *Diabetes* **27,** 834–839.

Hypertension Detection Follow-Up Program (1979). *JAMA, J. Am. Med. Assoc.* **242,** 2572.

Jajich, C. L., Ostfeld, A. M., and Freeman, D. H. (1984). *JAMA, J. Am. Med. Assoc.* **252,** 2831–2834.

Peto, J. (1979). *Ann. N. Y. Acad. Sci.* **330,** 195–203.

Reaven, G. M., and Reaven, E. P. (1980). *Mol. Cell. Biochem.* **31,** 37–47.

Rowe, J. W. (1977). *N. Engl. J. Med.* **297,** 1332–1336.

Rowe, J. W., Minaker, K. L., Pallotta, J. A., and Flier, J. S. (1983). *J. Clin. Invest.* **71,** 1581–1587.

Smith, E. L., and Reddan, W. (1976). *AJR. Am. J. Roentgenol.* **126,** 1297.

Smith, E. L., Reddan, W., and Smith, P. E. (1981). *Med. Sci. Sports Exercise* **13,** 60–64.

Tripathi, R. C., and Tripathi, B. J. (1983). *J. Gerontol.* **38,** 258–270.

Vestal, R. E., Norris, A. H., Tobin, J. D., Cohen, B. H., and Shueh, N. W. (1975). *J. Pharmacol. Exp. Ther.* **18,** 425–432.

Veterans Administration Cooperative Study Group (1972). *Circulation* **45,** 991–1004.

3

Nutrition and Organ Function in a Cohort of Aging Men

Jordan Tobin

Gerontology Research Center, NIA
Francis Scott Key Medical Center
Baltimore, Maryland

I. INTRODUCTION

We instinctively realize that the food we eat must have something to do with the way we feel and how healthy we are. We extrapolate from our everyday heartburn and indigestion to the search for the diet that even if it is not a prescription for immortality perhaps will add both years to our life and life to our years. And why not. We recognize the marked influence malnutrition and vitamin deficiencies have on health, we recognize the relationship of diet to specific diseases such as diabetes, and more recently we have been exposed to the relationship of dietary intake to heart disease

23

and cancer, the two leading causes of death in Western societies. We couple this with the ever present search for immortality and remember Ponce de León's Fountain of Youth and Metchnikoff's *Lactobacillus bulgaricus* (now ever present on the TV ads as yogurt), and we think perhaps that there is something to diet and aging. Perhaps the aging process is affected by what we eat, and if we only knew enough to eat the "right" foods our chances of survival would improve.

The thought that dietary intake might be an important determinant of how fast we age is particularly attractive. In contrast to the immutable nature of our genetic makeup (as exemplified by the sage advice "choose long-lived parents") our diet is under our control and is amenable to change. When investigating the relationships of diet to aging, organ function, and disease states, however, it is important to recognize that diet is not only under an individual's voluntary conscious control but it is also influenced by subconscious decisions as we respond to advertising, advice, and fads, and to secular factors known and unknown that are beyond our control as technological and manufacturing changes occur.

The dietary intakes of the volunteers of the Baltimore Longitudinal Study of Aging (BLSA) will be used to illustrate true aging changes in intakes, apparent age changes that are really effects of secular changes, and the relationships of these changes and levels to physiological functions including serum cholesterol levels, kidney function as estimated by creatinine clearances, and metabolic activity as estimated by glucose tolerance tests.

II. THE BALTIMORE LONGITUDINAL STUDY OF AGING

A. Subjects

The Baltimore Longitudinal Study of Aging is a longitudinal study of the physiological, psychological, and sociological changes that occur with aging in a cohort of human volunteers. It was started in 1958 by Dr. Nathan Shock as an effort to determine what changes occur in normal humans as they age and has continued as an intramural effort of the National Institute on Aging. Full details of the study, as well as reprints of all the longitudinal papers published from the study, are presented in a recent book (Shock *et al.*, 1984). The volunteers customarily return to the Gerontology Research Center (GRC) for a $2\frac{1}{2}$-day reexamination at one- to two-year intervals. Since 1958, 1142 men ranging in age from 17 to 102 have been seen at least once, and by 1981 667 of them had made at least five visits. Females were added to the study in 1978 and at present over 400 have been seen at least once, but since no dietary information is available in this cohort they are not included in this report. The cohort is predominantly a self-recruited, highly educated (70% college educated and 40% with advanced degrees), upper-middle socioeconomic class (84% managerial, technical, or professional occupations), and considers itself healthy (94% self-rate their health as good to excellent).

On each visit they get a thorough medical history and physical examination and undergo over 40 physiological, psychological, and sociological examinations. Included in these tests are measurements of kidney function (creatinine clearance determinations), serum cholesterol, and tests of glucose metabolism (oral glucose tolerance tests). From 1961 to 1965 and from 1968 to 1975 seven-day dietary diaries were obtained on 845 men at least once and on 489 of these men at least three times.

B. Dietary Evaluations

1. Method

At the time of their visit to the Center, the volunteers were instructed in keeping a dietary diary. When discharged they were given a seven-day diary and asked to fill it out at home during a "normal" week. It was sent back to the dietician, reviewed, any questions clarified, and then coded and subsequently analyzed by a computer program developed by the Heart Disease Control Program, USPHS. Cross-sectional results of the first panel of dietary diaries were presented (McGandy et al., 1966) and provided valuable information of the dietary intakes of community-dwelling normal volunteers. The volunteers continued to submit dietary information on their subsequent visits to the GRC, and in 1983 Elahi et al. presented a longitudinal evaluation of the dietary changes over these years. In addition to presenting the cross-sectional and longitudinal analysis of the data, the study was designed to evaluate, on a cohort sample, any effects of cohort differences or secular changes.

2. Epoch Analysis

The study was divided into three 5-year epochs of time: 1961–1965, 1966–1970, and 1971–1975. Subjects were chosen for inclusion in the study if they had at least one diary in each of the three epochs and had graduated into the next 5-year age group at the time of the second diary. The age distribution of the 180 men who met the criteria for selection is shown in Fig. 1. The number of subjects in each 5-year age group in each

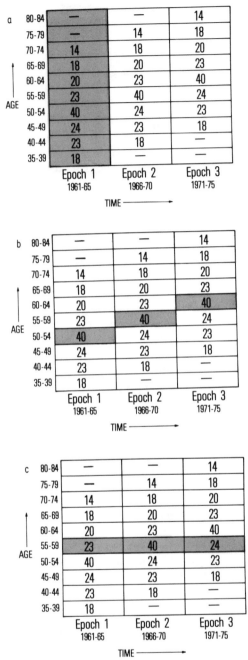

Fig. 1. Number of subjects in each age group, in each epoch. (a) The cross-sectional approach, (b) the longitudinal approach, and (c) the time-series approach. Data from Elahi *et al.* (1983).

epoch is in each cell. Three classical cross-sectional studies are possible, one in each of the three epochs, as demonstrated in Fig. 1a. In contrast, a longitudinal evaluation of each of the eight cohorts is demonstrated by the hatched shading in Fig. 1b that highlights the 40 individuals who were 50–54 in Epoch I, 55–59 in Epoch II, and 60–64 in Epoch III. Finally, a time series analysis evaluates the results at one age across the three epochs. This is illustrated in Fig. 1c, where the shading highlights the 55- to 59-year-old age groups. There were 23 individuals who were 55–59 years old in Epoch I, 40 who were 55–59 in Epoch II, and 24 who were 55–59 in Epoch III. Analysis of the data from these different groups of subjects, all the same age but at different epochs, examines the effect of secular changes.

3. *Polyunsaturated/Saturated Fatty Acid Ratio—A Secular Phenomenon*

This approach, as discussed in more detail in the original paper, permits the evaluation of each variable from the three perspectives: cross-sectional, longitudinal, and time-series, an examination which is necessary before one can attribute differences or changes to a true aging effect. The ratio of the intake of polyunsaturated to saturated fatty acids (P/S ratio) is an important example of this phenomenon and is shown in Fig. 2. The three cross-sectional curves in Fig. 2a each demonstrate that there is no difference in the P/S ratio between the young and the old subjects. They also show that at each age there is a marked secular effect with the ratio being higher in Epoch II than in Epoch I, and higher still in Epoch III than in Epoch I. Thus from 1961 to 1975 the diets of the American males changed. The men in each age group ate more polyun-

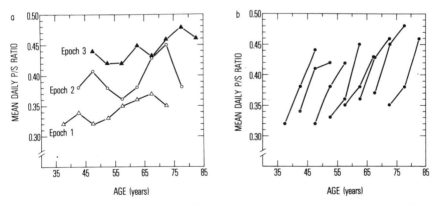

Fig. 2. Age versus P/S intake. (a) The cross-sectional curves derived from each of the three epochs and (b) the longitudinal curves from each of the eight cohorts.

saturated fat while they were decreasing their intake of saturated fat, with a resulting increase in their P/S ratio. The same data points are connected, not cross-sectionally in each epoch, but longitudinally in each cohort in Fig. 2b. Each cohort has a marked increase in the P/S ratio which, since it represents the changes in an individual followed over time, might be considered an effect of aging. In fact, this is not an effect of age, but rather a marked secular effect which overrides any age effect which might be present.

Similar analyses were performed for the macronutrients as recorded in the diaries and a true aging effect was found in the intake of calories, fat, and saturated fatty acids. A time-series effect was found in carbohydrate intake and P/S ratio, and a mixed effect of time and age in the intake of cholesterol.

III. PHYSIOLOGICAL FUNCTIONS

A. Serum Cholesterol

1. Secular Changes

Part of the reason for the interest in nutritional variables revolves around their relationships to physiological variables or to disease states. The epidemiological evidence linking heart disease to serum cholesterol levels and in turn serum levels to the dietary intake of both cholesterol and to the P/S ratio is an example of the importance of diet. The serum cholesterol levels of the volunteers of the BLSA were examined in a report by Hershcopf *et al.* in 1982. After an extensive clinical evaluation to remove diseases, drugs, and other artifacts from consideration, there were 783 normal males who had at least one serum cholesterol measured for cross-sectional studies. These studies demonstrated the typical cross-sectional results with levels higher in middle-aged men than in the young and lower in old men than in the middle-aged. More detailed examination of the data, however, demonstrated that there was a pronounced secular effect in serum cholesterol levels with a marked drop in average levels occurring in 1972 (Fig. 3). There were two distinct eras of cholesterol measurement: Era I from 1963 to 1971 and Era II from 1971 to 1977. At each age the values in Era I were higher than those in ERA II.

Extensive methodological and statistical investigations ruled out artifact or method changes as an explanation of these differences, and correlations with other important variables which are related to cholesterol levels were examined. Primary among these were changes in diet and

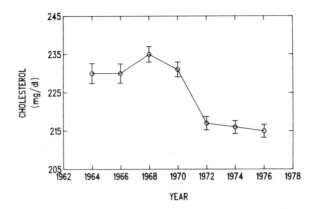

Fig. 3. Mean serum cholesterol values for each 2-year period of the study.

obesity. The studies of Elahi *et al.* (1983) had demonstrated a marked secular change in the diets of the BLSA participants at the same time that the changes in serum levels were occurring.

2. *Relationship to Dietary Changes*

A reasonable hypothesis was that the public health advice that the health professions and the lay press had been giving for years about the danger of cholesterol and saturated fats in the diet was having an effect. Perhaps we had heeded the advice, changed our diet, and lowered our cholesterol. If this hypothesis were operable, we would expect that those individuals who had had the largest change in dietary intakes would be the same individuals who would have the largest decrease in serum levels, and that those who had had the least change in diet (or even a change in the opposite direction) would have the least decrease (or even an increase) in serum cholesterol. This hypothesis was not supported. There was no significant correlation between change in dietary intake of cholesterol or change in P/S ratio and change in serum cholesterol. Figure 4 shows the scatter plot of the change in P/S intake between Era I and Era II plotted against the change in serum cholesterol over the same time period for the 309 volunteers who had cholesterol measured in each era. Those who had increased their P/S ratio the most were *not* the ones who changed their serum cholesterol the most.

Additional evidence against the hypothesis is the calculation of how much change in serum cholesterol might be expected from the magnitude of change in dietary P/S ratio in the BLSA. The estimates range from 2.7 to 5.5 mg/dl decrease secondary to the dietary changes, far short of the 11.4 mg/dl change observed (Hershcopf *et al.*, 1982).

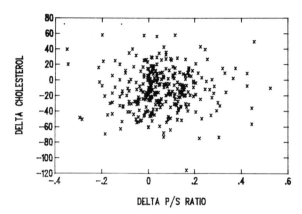

Fig. 4. Change of P/S intake between Era 1 and Era 2 versus change in serum cholesterol levels between Era 1 and Era 2.

B. Creatinine Clearance

1. Age Effect

The change of creatinine clearance, a measure of kidney function,
with age has been well documented both cross-sectionally and longitudinally (Rowe *et al.*, 1976). This decrease in renal function occurs across
the age span, and is seen in normal individuals who have been extensively screened to rule out diseases or medications as causative factors.
This significant decline in function is an average response and there are
individuals whose rate of change (slope) of creatinine clearance, analyzed longitudinally, does not fall with age, and some who in fact show
an increase in performance (Shock *et al.*, 1979; Lindeman *et al.*, 1985).
Attempts have been made to relate this measure of kidney performance
to other physiological variables such as blood pressure (Lindeman *et al.*,
1984), and a recent provocative concept questions the relationship to the
dietary intake of protein (Brenner *et al.*, 1982). The hypothesis suggests
that high intake of protein presents the renal system with a load that will
eventually overwork the kidney and lead to decreased function.

2. Relationship to Dietary Protein Intake

Of the 256 males with five or more observations of kidney function
who made up the normal group in the study of blood pressure 191 had
had dietary diaries collected. There was no significant correlation between grams of protein ingested or percentage of calories that came
from protein and contemporaneous creatinine clearance measurements.
Since the hypothesis suggests that there may be a time lag before the

excess load has an effect on renal function, the 80 individuals who had had a dietary assessment at least 10 years prior to a creatinine clearance measurement were examined. Again there was no significant correlation between dietary protein 10 years earlier and creatinine clearance. The subjects who had ingested the most protein were not those who had the poorest kidney function, nor were those who had ingested the least protein the ones who had the best function.

It should be emphasized that this is a free-living normal population. While there was a range of protein intakes from 45 to 185 g/day there were no subjects with malnutrition nor were there subjects with inordinately high protein intakes. Perhaps such abnormal extremes would be necessary to show significant correlations.

C. Glucose Tolerance

1. Age Effect

The area of glucose metabolism is one in which the importance of dietary intake has been well documented. The extreme of glucose intolerance, the disease diabetes mellitus, has as one of the mainstays of treatment control of diet. Coupled with this is the recognition of the importance of obesity and physical activity, both as treatments for the disease state and as contributors to the impairment of glucose metabolism associated with the disease. There is a profound effect of age on glucose metabolism (Andres, 1971) and it is important to determine how much of the decrease in glucose metabolism is due to a primary effect of age and how much is secondary to changes in other variables that also change with age, i.e., obesity, physical activity, and dietary intake of carbohydrate (Tobin, 1984).

2. Relationship to Diet, Obesity, and Activity

There were 336 normal individuals who had oral glucose tolerance tests (glucose dose = 1.75 g/kg), estimates of customary carbohydrate intake from dietary diaries, estimates of physical activity from activity questionnaires, and Body Mass Index (BMI) as estimates of obesity. Individual bivariate correlations between these variables showed that increasing age and obesity were associated with a decrease in performance on a glucose tolerance test while increased carbohydrate intake and increased physical activity were associated with improved performance. Since these variables also change with age (carbohydrate intake as g/day and physical activity decrease with age, and BMI has a quadratic relationship, increasing to middle age, plateauing, and then decreasing), a stepwise multiple regression analysis was used to determine the combined effect of these four variables on glucose performance. The regression equations and correlation coefficients at each step are presented in Fig. 5.

Age was the most significant variable, accounting for most of the variance (12%), and appeared first in the stepwise procedure. Obesity as measured by BMI or as BMI squared to account for the quadratic nature of the variable appeared next and accounted for an additional 2.0% of the variance. Grams of carbohydrate appeared next as a negative coefficient since increased carbohydrate lowered the two-hour glucose value and accounted for an additional 1.1% of the variance. When these three variables were included in the equation the fourth variable, physical activity, did not add any further information and was not included in the final equation.

Thus age, obesity, and carbohydrate content of the diet all have independent effects on glucose metabolism, and it is not correct to assume that their effects are mediated only as secondary phenomena. Age was the most significant variable from a statistical point of view and therefore appeared in the equation as the first variable. It is valuable, however, to recognize the strength of each of these coefficients in terms of the expected impact they would have on the two-hour glucose value given their expected ranges of values. The age might be considered to go from 20 to 80 years, a range of 60 years. Since the two-hour glucose value increases 1.0 mg/dl for each additional year of life (slope = 1.0), this would change the glucose value by 1.0 × 60 or 60 mg/dl over the entire age range. An expected range for BMI would be from a lean person of 20.0 to an obese person with a BMI of 30.0. The slope for BMI squared was 0.035, which would result in a maximum difference in the two-hour glucose of 17.5 mg/dl. Carbohydrate content in the diet might be expected to range from 150 to 300 g and, with a slope of −0.07, this would result in a 10.5 mg/dl decrease in glucose. Thus, all of these coefficients are statistically significant, but the magnitude of their effect

$$\text{GLUCOSE} = 97 + 1.02 \times \text{AGE} \qquad\qquad \begin{array}{c}\text{R}\\0.364\end{array}$$

$$= 70 + 1.01 \times \text{AGE} + 0.04 \times \text{BMI}^2 \qquad 0.390$$

$$= 93 + 0.99 \times \text{AGE} + 0.03 \times \text{BMI}^2 - 0.07 \times \text{CARB} \qquad 0.404$$

Fig. 5. Stepwise multiple regression analysis of the two-hour serum glucose value (oral glucose tolerance test) and age, body mass index squared (BMI^2), and carbohydrate intake (Carb). Each independent variable is added in turn, and the equation and correlation coefficient is shown for one, two, and all three variables.

on glucose tolerance is large for age and relatively smaller for both obesity and diet once age has been taken into account.

IV. CONCLUSIONS

Seven-day dietary diaries from the volunteers of the Baltimore Longitudinal Study of Aging were used to examine nutrition and organ function in aging men. The complexities of the analysis of variables from the viewpoint of aging, cohort effects, and secular effects were apparent, and a marked secular effect was demonstrated for the P/S ratio. Attempts to relate dietary intakes, or changes in intakes, to physiological functions revealed another layer of complexity.

A marked secular effect on serum cholesterol could not be correlated with the marked secular effect on dietary P/S ratio. Kidney function, as estimated by the creatinine clearance, was not related to contemporaneous levels of protein intake, nor was it related to protein intakes 10 years previously. The effect of carbohydrate intake on glucose tolerance was demonstrable, but not impressive when compared to the effects of age and obesity. Thus hypotheses generated in laboratory animals or in populations with extreme ranges of intakes, functions, or diseases could not be borne out, or they assume less importance, when examined in a healthy normal aging population.

The study of the relationships and interrelationships of diet, aging, physiological function, and disease is complicated. The same reasons that make diet so interesting and important to study, its variability and potential for change, make interpretation of results complex. There are personal and societal factors that influence what we eat, there are many pathways, both direct and indirect, whereby diet may exert its effect, and there are relationships that may be circular rather than causative. All of these caveats should serve not to frighten away the intrepid investigators but rather to warn them of the hazards ahead and underscore the importance of the work.

REFERENCES

Andres, R. (1971). *Med. Clin. North Am.* **55**, 835–846.
Brenner, B. M., Meyer, T. W., and Hostetter, T. H. (1982). *N. Engl. J. Med.* **307**, 652–659.
Elahi, V. K., Elahi, D., Andres, R. A., Tobin, J. D., Butler, M. G., and Norris, A. H. (1983). *J. Gerontol.* **38**, 162–180.
Hershcopf, R. J., Elahi, D., Andres, R., Baldwin, H. L., Raizes, G. S., Schocken, D. D., and Tobin, J. D. (1982). *J. Chronic Dis.* **35**, 101–114.

Lindeman, R. D., Tobin, J. D., and Shock, N. W. (1984). *Kidney Int.* **26,** 861–868.

Lindeman, R. D., Tobin, J. D., and Shock, N. W. (1985). *J. Am. Geriatr. Soc.* **33,** 278–285.

McGandy, R. B., Barrows, C. H., Jr., Spanas, A., Meredith, A., Stone, J. L., and Norris, A. H. (1966). *J. Gerontol.* **21,** 581–587.

Rowe, J. W., Andres, R., Tobin, J. D., Norris, A. H., and Shock, N. W. (1976). *J. Gerontol.* **31,** 155–163.

Shock, N. W., Andres, R., Norris, A. H., and Tobin, J. D. (1979). *Proc. Int. Congr. Gerontol., 11th, 1979,* pp. 525–527.

Shock, N. W., Greulich, R. C., Andres, R. A., Arenberg, D., Costa, P. T., Jr., Lakatta, E. G., and Tobin, J. D. (1984). "Normal Human Aging: The Baltimore Longitudinal Study of Aging." U. S. Govt. Printing Office, Washington, D.C.

Tobin, J. D. (1984). *In* "Altered Endocrine Status during Aging" (V. J. Cristofalo, G. T. Baker, III, R. C. Adelman, and J. Roberts eds.), pp. 115–124. Liss, New York.

Impact of Aging and
Nutrition on Human Skin:
Studies at the Cellular Level

Barbara A. Gilchrest and
Philip R. Gordon
USDA Human Nutrition Research Center on Aging at Tufts
Boston, Massachusetts and
Boston University School of Medicine
Boston, Massachusetts

I. INTRODUCTION

Until recently, aging in the skin was widely viewed as an unfortunate aesthetic event, but one without physiologic consequence and without prospect of effective intervention beyond cosmetics or plastic surgery. A large literature now documents in the skin of healthy adults both morphologic and physiologic age-associated changes, many of which directly predispose the elderly to cutaneous injury or disease. Those elderly individuals suffering from disorders such as diabetes, hypothyroidism, or malnutrition are at yet greater risk of cu-

Nutrition and Aging

taneous morbidity. Overall, a national survey reveals that approximately 40% of noninstitutionalized Americans aged 65 to 74 years suffer from a skin problem sufficiently severe to warrant medical attention and that the average individual has 1.5 such disorders (Johnson and Roberts, 1977). The very elderly and those unable to live independently can safely be assumed to experience an even higher prevalence of skin disorders.

We do not presently know the extent to which age-associated functional losses in the skin might result from lifelong dietary deficiencies or excesses, or the extent to which established losses, regardless of pathogenesis, might be favorably influenced by nutritional factors. However, overwhelming epidemiologic and laboratory-based evidence indicates that another environmental factor, ultraviolet light exposure from the sun, has major long-term consequences (Gilchrest, 1984). Indeed, "photoaging" is directly responsbile for perhaps 90% of all skin cancers and a similar proportion of such familiar cosmetic changes as wrinkling, coarseness, and irregular pigmentation, characteristic of old skin. By analogy, specific dietary patterns may influence the perceived aging process in skin and other body tissues by modifying the immediate cellular environment.

The following discussion summarizes the major age-associated functional losses identified in skin, then describes one approach to quantifying and correcting such losses at the cellular level, with emphasis on the probable role of nutritional factors.

II. CLINICAL ASPECTS OF SKIN AGING

The major changes in the skin's appearance attributable to aging itself are "dryness" (by which is meant roughness), fine wrinkling, laxity, and a tendency to form benign neoplasms (Gilchrest, 1984; Tindall and Smith, 1963).

Table I lists the more striking functional losses recognized in old skin. Supporting data, associated anatomic changes, and presumed clinical consequences of such losses are reviewed elsewhere (Gilchrest, 1984; Kligman et al., 1985). When quantified, most of these cutaneous functions have been found to decline by approximately half during adulthood from the maximal value observed in healthy young adults, a pattern previously noted for function capacity in other body organs such as heart, lungs, and kidneys (Mildvan and Strehler, 1960).

Of special relevance to the present discussion, wound healing and proliferative capacity in the skin have been shown to decline with age by several criteria in healthy non-sun-damaged adult skin. A decrease in

TABLE I

Functional Losses in Old Skin

Cell replacement	Immune responsiveness
Wound healing	Vascular responsiveness
Barrier function	Thermoregulation
Chemical clearance	Sweat production
Sensory perception	Sebum production
Mechanical protection	Vitamin D production

epidermal turnover rate of approximately 50% between the third and eighth decades has been determined in 100 volunteers aged 18–80 years by measuring desquamation rates for corneocytes (cells of the stratum corneum or outer barrier layer), confirming earlier measurements (Grove and Kligman, 1983). Similarly, the thymidine labeling index of intact human epidermis has been reported to decline from 5.1% in 19- to 25-year-olds to 2.8% in 69- to 85-year-olds (Kligman, 1979). Repair rate for injured skin likewise declines with age in man, whether measured as time for complete healing of facial abrasions (Orentreich and Selmanowitz, 1969), development of wound tensile strength (Sandblum et al., 1953), rate of collagen deposition (Viljanto, 1969), or regeneration of excised blister roofs (Grove, 1982).

III. *IN VITRO* STUDIES OF SKIN AGING AND NUTRITIONAL REQUIREMENTS

The evolution of "conventional" nutrition research has several interesting parallels to the now rapidly expanding field of cellular growth regulation. At the turn of the century, early attempts to maintain experimental animals on "chemically simplified" diets containing all the compounds then believed to be physiologically significant resulted in the animals' rapid decline and death (McCollum, 1957a) and led some years later to the identification and purification of several vitamins and other essential nutrients. Analogously, it was not possible to cultivate "fastidious" human cells such as the keratinocytes discussed below during the first 60–70 years of *in vitro* investigation; success was achieved only with the recognition that such cells required specific substances not provided by standard nutrient media and serum supplements (Ham, 1974; Gospodarowicz and Moran, 1976; Serrero et al., 1979).

As in the early nutrition work, in which certain vitamins were first defined functionally as "growth-promoting factors" for the experimental animal species (McCollum, 1957a), the cellular growth control literature is presently replete with "growth factors" initially named in most instances for the principal target cell. Some but certainly not all of these growth factors have been fully characterized and purified. In some instances, such as vitamin D, well-defined "nutrients" (Omdahl and DeLuca, 1973) are being found to serve as hormones (Norman, 1980) and/or growth regulators (MacLaughlin *et al.*, 1985) at least *in vitro*, further blurring current distinctions between these classes of compounds.

Work now under way in the Cutaneous Gerontology Laboratory at the USDA Human Nutrition Research Center on Aging at Tufts University seeks to advance our understanding of nutrition and aging at the cellular level by pursuing three interrelated problems: (1) nutritional and/or growth factor requirements for individual cell types in the skin, (2) the influence of donor age on these requirements, and (3) the possible role of nutrients in modifying age-associated or age-accelerating injuries to the skin. Selected studies in these areas are discussed below.

A. Keratinocyte Growth Factor

The past decade has witnessed a substantial increase in our understanding of the factors influencing growth and differentiation of human keratinocytes, the constantly self-renewing cell population which comprises the epidermis and forms the skin's outer barrier layer. Hydrocortisone (Rheinwald and Green, 1975), epidermal growth factor of EGF (Rheinwald and Green, 1977), and a variety of agents that stimulate cyclic AMP (Green, 1978) have all been shown to increase growth rate and prolong culture life span; vitamin A (Fuchs and Green, 1981) and calcium ion concentration (Rice and Green, 1978; Boyce and Ham, 1983) are known to exert strong influences on the differentiation program. However, poorly defined factors derived from fetal bovine serum and murine 3T3 "feeder" cells (Rheinwald and Green, 1975), human fibroblasts and keratinocytes (Gilchrest *et al.*, 1983), bovine hypothalamus (Maciag *et al.*, 1981) or pituitary (Peehl and Ham, 1980; Boyce and Ham, 1983), and human placenta (O'Keefe *et al.*, 1985) under appropriate culture conditions have been shown to have far more striking beneficial effects on human keratinocytes *in vitro* than have the well-characterized factors originally identified by their activity for intact tissues or other cell types.

The above dichotomy suggests that major nutrient and growth factor requirements for the keratinocyte remain to be identified. One possible example is the keratinocyte growth-promoting activity in human and bovine hypothalamus. Ongoing experiments utilizing sensitive serum-free systems are consistent with the presence of a single low molecular weight factor which we have termed keratinocyte growth factor or KGF (Gilchrest, 1984). Whether KGF is more properly classified as a "growth factor" or "nutrient" cannot be resolved prior to its complete characterization.

B. Age-Associated Loss of Growth Factor Responsiveness

To explore the major clinical problem of impaired wound healing in old skin, cultures of normal epidermal keratinocytes and dermal fibroblasts were established from skin fragments of healthy newborns and adults obtained during elective surgical procedures (Gilchrest, 1983; Plisko and Gilchrest, 1983). The cultures were maintained in serum-free hormone-supplemented media under conditions expected to support good growth, and cell yield was determined after predetermined growth periods (4–10 days). Newborn keratinocytes and fibroblasts consistently yielded strikingly better growth than did adult cells plated at equal density and maintained under identical conditions. Moreover, the dose response to either serum mitogens or more defined growth factors was severely blunted in the adult-derived cultures. These differences were clearly attributable to reduced growth rates as opposed to attachment rates for the adult-derived cells, since the proportion of cells that firmly attached to the dish within 24 hours, permitting subsequent growth, did not vary with donor age.

However, these studies compared immature to mature donors (rather than young mature to old mature donors) and cell donor site was different in the two age groups (newborn foreskin versus adult truncal skin). To assure that the decreased proliferation was truly related to aging, similar studies were undertaken using skin biopsy specimens derived from the upper medial arm of 20 healthy adults aged 22–27 years and 60–82 years (B. M. Praeger and Gilchrest, 1986). Under serum-free conditions, keratinocyte cultures derived from young adults showed an eightfold increase in cell yield over the tested dose range of KGF, the strongest mitogen in this system, while cultures derived from old adults showed a fourfold increase. Growth obtained under optimal conditions was three- to fivefold greater for younger adult than for old adult cultures, a statistically significant age-associated loss despite the expectedly large interdonor variation. Parallel changes were observed for dermal fibroblast responsiveness to EGF, a well-studied major mitogen for this cell type.

These results are consistent with published studies of WI-38 cells (fetal lung fibroblasts widely used in gerontologic research) demonstrating a loss of responsiveness to EGF and other growth factors during *in vitro* aging (Phillips *et al.*, 1984) and with the report of Harley *et al.* (1981) that fibroblast cultures derived from young adult skin require a lower concentration of an insulin-like preparation to stimulate 50% and 95% maximal DNA synthesis than do cultures derived from old adult skin.

Loss of growth factor responsiveness during *in vitro* aging has been related in some instances to decreased number of specific binding sites (Cristofalo and Rosner, 1979) and in others to lack of protein phosphorylation following growth factor–receptor binding (Carlin *et al.*, 1983). However, other lines of investigation suggest an alternative explanation. Using defined culture conditions, it has been shown that the growth rate of normal cells varies with the concentration of individual nutrients in the medium (McKeehan and McKeehan, 1981; McKeehan *et al.*, 1981) and that mitogens, in the form of serum or certain well-characterized growth factors, enhance cell growth under limiting conditions by specifically reducing the requirements for selected nutrients (Lechner and Kaighn, 1979; McKeehan and McKeehan, 1980). In this framework, age-associated loss of growth factor responsiveness might result from an increase in nutrient requirements that can no longer be satisfied by standard culture media even in the presence of otherwise potent mitogen-modulators.

Age-associated nutrient insensitivity is further suggested by work in our laboratory regarding the effect of calcium ion concentration ($[Ca^{2+}]$) on confluent density or, equivalently, on density-dependent growth inhibition of human dermal fibroblasts (F. C. Praeger and Gilchrest, 1986). Based on the observation that elevated $[Ca^{2+}]$ increases confluent density of both mouse BALB/c 3T3 cells (Dulbecco and Elkington, 1975) and human WI-38 fibroblasts (Praeger and Cristofalo, 1980), experiments were undertaken to examine this effect using dermal fibroblasts obtained from upper medial arm biopsies of healthy adults and from newborn foreskins. Early passage fibroblasts were grown to confluence in serum-supplemented nutrient medium containing approximately 2.0 mM Ca^{2+} and in this medium containing an additional 1.5–5.0 mM Ca^{2+}. Compared to controls in basal medium, newborn-derived fibroblasts exposed to additional Ca^{2+} had a 110–450% increased cell yield, attributable to a prolongation of exponential growth phase and associated with an altered cell morphology. Comparison of cultures from five donors aged 22–27 years to cultures from five donors aged 66–83 years revealed that addition of 2 mM Ca^{2+} stimulated confluent density of young adult-derived fibroblasts by an average of 210%, while old adult-derived fibroblasts were stimulated by 29%, a highly significant difference suggesting a relative refractoriness to extracellular calcium ion concentration with age.

C. Protection of Keratinocytes by Carotenoids

Carotene has long been recognized as a vitamin A precursor (McCollum, 1957b), but other roles for dietary carotenoids may exist (Simpson and Chichester, 1981). Epidemiologic evidence suggests that diets rich in β-carotene may protect against the development of cancer in man (Peto *et al.*, 1981), and dietary carotenoids have been reported to reduce the tumorigenicity of both UV and chemical carcinogens in mice (Mathews-Roth, 1982; Mathews-Roth and Krinsky, 1984).

In view of the "photoaging" phenomenon discussed earlier and the recognized ability of carotenoids to scavenge free radicals and photooxidation products (Krinsky, 1982; Krinsky and Deneke, 1982), experiments were undertaken to examine the possible UV-protective effect of β-carotene on human keratinocytes *in vitro* (P. R. Gordon, N. I. Krinsky, and B. A. Gilchrest, unpublished observations). First passage epidermal cells were plated in serum-free medium containing an emulsion of β-carotene, the emulsion vehicle alone, or no additive. After 2 days, paired cultures were exposed to a variable physiologic dose of UV, then allowed to grow an additional 6 days in their respective media. Unirradiated control cultures were not affected by the presence of β-carotene or the vehicle and achieved good growth over the 8-day period. Unsupplemented or vehicle-supplemented irradiated cultures showed an approximately 50% decrease in cell yield, while UV-irradiated cultures supplemented with β-carotene equalled or exceeded the unirradiated controls at all but the highest UV dose, at which this protective effect was lost. These preliminary data suggest that the presence of β-carotene in the immediate cellular environment modifies an otherwise deleterious effect of UV on keratinocyte proliferation and life span *in vitro*.

By extrapolation, tissue concentration of carotenoids or other dietary antioxidants may influence the rate of photoaging or even oxidant-mediated "intrinsic" aging in the skin.

IV. CONCLUSIONS

Nutrition research is currently crossing a threshold from conventional animal studies to studies of nutrient requirements and functions at the cellular level. Rapid technical and conceptual advances in cell biology should guarantee findings of clinical relevance to the skin and other body organs compromised by the aging process.

REFERENCES

Boyce, S. T., and Ham, R. G. (1983). *J. Invest. Dermatol.* **81,** 335–405.

Carlin, C. R., Phillips, P. D., Knowles, B. B., and Cristofalo, V. J. (1983). *Nature (London)* **306,** 617–620.

Cristofalo, V. J., and Rosner, B. (1979). *Fed. Proc., Fed. Am. Soc. Exp. Biol.* **38,** 1851–1856.

Dulbecco, R., and Elkington, J. (1975). *Proc. Natl. Acad. Sci. U.S.A.* **72,** 1584–1588.

Fuchs, E., and Green, H. (1981). *Cell* **25,** 617–625.

Gilchrest, B. A. (1983). *J. Invest. Dermatol.* **81,** 184s–189s.

Gilchrest, B. A. (1984). "Skin and Aging Process." CRC Press, Boca Raton, Florida.

Gilchrest, B. A., Karassik, R. L., Wilkins, L. M., Vrabel, M. A., and Maciag, T. (1983). *J. Cell. Physiol.* **117,** 235–240.

Gospodarowicz, D., and Moran, J. S. (1976). *Annu. Rev. Biochem.* **45,** 531–558.

Green, H. (1978). *Cell* **51,** 801–811.

Grove, G. L. (1982). *Arch. Dermatol. Res.* **272,** 381–385.

Grove, G. L., and Kligman, A. M. (1983). *J. Gerontol.* **38,** 137–142.

Ham, R. G. (1974). *In Vitro* **10,** 119–129.

Harley, C. B., Goldstein, S., Posner, B. I., and Guyda, H. (1981). *J. Clin. Invest.* **68,** 988–994.

Johnson, M. L. T., and Roberts, J. (1977). "U.S. Advance Data" No. 4. U.S. Department of Health, Education and Welfare, Washington, D.C.

Kligman, A. M. (1979). *J. Invest. Dermatol.* **73,** 39–46.

Kligman, A. M., Grove, G. L., and Balin, A. K. (1985). *In* "Handbook of the Biology of Aging" (C. E. Finch and E. L. Schneider, eds.), pp. 820–841. Van Nostrand-Reinhold, Princeton, New Jersey.

Krinsky, N. I. (1982) *In* "The Science of Photomedicine" (J. D. Regan and J. A. Parrish, eds.), pp. 397–407. Plenum, New York.

Krinsky, N. I., and Deneke, S. M. (1982). *JNCI, J. Natl. Cancer Inst.* **69,** 205–209.

Lechner, J. F., and Kaighn, M. E. (1979). *Exp. Cell Res.* **121,** 432–435.

McCollum, E. V. (1957a). "A History of Nutrition," p. 451. Houghton Mifflin, Boston, Massachusetts.

McCollum, E. V. (1957b). "A History of Nutrition," pp. 234–236. Riverside Press, Cambridge, Massachusetts.

Maciag, T., Nemore, R. E., Weinstein R., and Gilchrest B. A. (1981). *Science* **211,** 1454.

McKeehan, W. L., and McKeehan, K. A. (1980). *Proc. Natl. Acad. Sci. U.S.A.* **77,** 3417–3421.

McKeehan, W. L., and McKeehan, K. A. (1981). *J. Supramol. Struct. Cell. Biochem.* **15,** 83–110.

McKeehan, W. L., McKeehan, K. A., and Calkins, D. (1981). *J. Biol. Chem.* **256,** 2973–2981.

MacLaughlin, J. A., Gange, W., Taylor, P., Smith, E., and Holick, M. F. (1985). *Proc. Natl. Acad. Sci. U.S.A.* **82,** 5409–5412.

Mathews-Roth, M. M. (1982). *Oncology* **39,** 33–37.

Mathews-Roth, M. M., and Krinsky, N. I. (1984). *Photochem. Photobiol.* **40,** 671–673.

Mildvan, A. S., and Strehler, B. L. (1960). *In* "The Biology of Aging" (B. L. Strehler, J. D. Ebert, H. B. Glass, and N. W. Shock, eds.), pp. 216–235. Waverly Press, Baltimore, Maryland.

Norman, A. W. (1980). *In* "Vitamin D Molecular and Clinical Nutrition" (A. W. Norman, ed.), pp. 197–250. Dekker, New York.

O'Keefe, E. J., Payne, R. E., and Russell, N. (1985). *J. Cell. Physiol.* **124,** 439–445.

Omdahl, J. C., and DeLuca, H. F. (1973). *Physiol. Rev.* **53,** 327–372.

Orentreich, N., and Selmanowitz, V. J. (1969). *Trans. N.Y. Acad. Sci., Ser. B* **31,** 992–1012.

Peehl, D. M., and Ham, R. G. (1980). *In Vitro* **16,** 516–526.

Peto, R., Doll, R. P., Buckley, J. D., and Sporn, M. B. (1981). *Nature (London)* **290,** 201–208.

Phillips, P. D., Kaji, K., and Cristofalo, V. J. (1984). *J. Gerontol.* **36,** 11–17.

Plisko, A., and Gilchrest, B. A. (1983). *J. Gerontol.* **38,** 513–518.

Praeger, B. M., and Gilchrest, B. A. (1986). *Mech. Ageing Dev.* (in press).

Praeger, F. C., and Cristofalo, V. J. (1980). *In Vitro* **16,** 239.

Praeger, F. C., and Gilchrest, B. A. (1986). *Proc. Soc. Exp. Biol. Med.* **182,** 315–321.

Rheinwald, J. G., and Green, H. (1975). *Cell* **6,** 331–334.

Rheinwald, J. B., and Green, H. (1977). *Nature (London)* **265,** 421–424.

Rice, R. H., and Green, H. (1978). *J. Cell Biol.* **76,** 705–711.

Sandblum, P. H., Peterson, P., and Muren, A. (1953). *Acta Chir. Scand.* **105,** 252–257.

Serrero, G. R., McClure, D. B., and Sato, G. H. (1979). *In* "Hormones and Cell Cultures" (G. H. Sato and R. Ross, eds.), pp. 523–530. Cold Spring Harbor Lab., Cold Spring Harbor, New York.

Simpson, K. L., and Chichester, C. O. (1981). *Annu. Rev. Nutr.* **1,** 351–74.

Tindall, J. P., and Smith, J. G. (1963). *J. Am. Med. Assoc.* **186,** 1039–1042.

Viljanto, J. A. (1969). *Acta Chir. Scand.* **136,** 297–300.

Vitamin D Synthesis by the Aging Skin

Michael F. Holick

*USDA Human Nutrition Research Center on Aging at Tufts
and Departments of Physiology and Nutrition
Tufts University
Boston, Massachusetts*

I. INTRODUCTION: CONSEQUENCES OF BONE DISEASE IN THE AGED

It has been conservatively estimated that upward of 10 million elderly Americans suffer from marked reduction in bone mass that puts them at significant risk of fracturing their bones. It is well recognized that bone loss begins in women during the third and fourth decades and accelerates after menopause. In men, significant bone loss begins in the fifth and sixth decades. The magnitude of the public health prob-

45

lem posed by age-related bone loss (osteopenia) has recently gained wide public attention because of its association with fractures of the wrist, hip, and spine. It has been estimated that about 200,000 elderly Americans fractured their hips during this past year. The medical expenses associated with the acute care of these fracture patients are estimated to be 2 billion dollars annually (Cummings *et al.*, 1985). This staggering cost triples when all fractures related to age-dependent osteopenia are accounted for. Besides the enormous medical costs, about 10% of patients with hip fractures die within the first three months of the fracture. In the first year after fracture, the mortality rate in these patients is up to 20% higher than it is in persons of similar age and sex who have not suffered a fracture (Cummings *et al.*, 1985). Patients who survive hip fractures often suffer permanent disability, and many who were formerly independent need to enter a chronic-care facility. Osteopenia in the elderly is a silent epidemic that can cause physical and financial hardship to those who are afflicted. There are multiple causes for osteopenia. Many of these will be discussed in later chapters by Drs. DeLuca and Riggs. I will review the role of vitamin D nutrition on osteopenia in the aged.

II. HISTORICAL PERSPECTIVE

Although it is now common knowledge that vitamin D, the sunshine vitamin, is important for the development of a healthy skeleton, this association was not known when the industrial revolution took hold in northern Europe. People left the farms and migrated to the industrial centers for the promise of jobs and a better life. They lived in buildings several stories high that were in close proximity to each other. The children who played in the sunless alleyways were afflicted with a bone-deforming disease known as rickets. By 1650, this childhood malady was already recognized as a clinical syndrome that usually affected small children and was characterized by bowlegs, knucklelike projections along the rib cage (commonly known as the rachitic rosary), and deformities of the pelvis (Fig. 1). By the turn of the century, this disease was endemic in the industrial cities of northern Europe and in the northeastern United States. One study conducted in Leyden, the Netherlands, suggested that up to 90% of the children living in that industrial city were afflicted with this disease. Besides the permanent deformities of the legs and rib cage that resulted from this disease, young women who suffered from rickets during childhood often had deformities of the pelvis that were responsible for high maternal and infant mortality (Park, 1923).

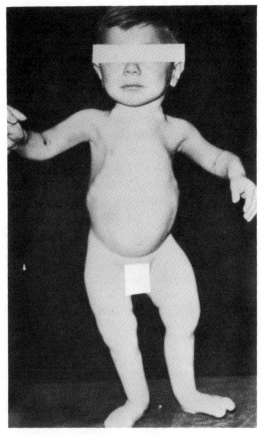

Fig. 1. Child with rickets showing rachitic rosary of the rib cage, bowed legs, deformity of the long bones, and muscle weakness. (Reproduced with permission, Fraser and Scriver, 1979. Grune & Stratton, New York.)

During the ensuing years, several theories were proposed as the cause for this childhood disease, including poor nutrition, infection, lack of activity, and inheritance. As early as 1822, J. Sniadecki had suggested that there was a strong association between the high incidence of rickets in the poor who lived in the overcrowded industrial cities of Poland and the lack of adequate exposure to sunlight (cited by Mozolowski, 1939). In 1890, Palm reported on his epidemiologic survey of the disease and concluded that exposure to sunlight was essential for the prevention and cure of rickets. He found that in the poor and starving populations in India and the Orient where malnutrition, tuberculosis, syphilis, and unsanitary living conditions prevailed, rickets was rarely seen, whereas in Great Britain, one of the wealthiest countries in the world, rickets was endemic among the working classes living in the crowded cities. By the process of exclusion he concluded that exposure to sunlight protected children in the Orient and India from rickets. He advocated the study of the therapeutic and beneficial effects of sunlight and encouraged the use of sunbaths to prevent and cure this crippling disease (Palm, 1890). However, at this time most physicians and scientists could not imagine that exposure to sunlight could have a therapeutic effect on bone, and therefore Palm's brilliant deductions were essentially disregarded.

At the turn of the century, several scientists investigated the use of different types of artificial lights as a treatment for rickets but without much success. In 1919, Huldschinsky reported that the exposure of four rachitic children to radiation from a quartz mercury-arc lamp resulted in the resolution of this bone-deforming disease. Two years later, Hess and Unger (1921) proved that exposure of the skin to sunlight did cure the rachitic lesions in eight children who were treated only with sunbaths outdoors.

These observations prompted Steenbock and Black (1924) and Hess (1925) to investigate whether exposure of food to radiation from a quartz mercury-arc lamp could prevent rickets in animals. They found that this process did indeed prevent rickets. These observations provided the impetus for the fortification of milk and other food stuffs with vitamin D that, in turn, led to the rapid eradication of rickets in the United States and in other countries that fortified foods with vitamin D.

III.   PRODUCTION OF VITAMIN D IN THE SKIN

When adult skin is exposed to sunlight, it is the high-energy ultraviolet photons that penetrate through the earth's atmosphere, with energies between 290 and 315 nm, that are ultimately responsible for producing vitamin D_3 in the skin (MacLaughlin et al., 1982). However, exposure to sunlight does not directly cause the skin to synthesize vitamin D_3. During exposure to sunlight, the high-energy photons enter the epidermis and are absorbed by 7-dehydrocholesterol, a precursor of cholesterol. Once the 5,7-diene of the 7-dehydrocholesterol (provitamin D_3) absorbs this radiant energy, the diene isomerizes, giving rise to a bond cleavage between carbons 9 and 10 to yield a 6,7-cis-secosteroid commonly known as previtamin D_3 (Holick et al., 1980). Once previtamin D_3 is formed in the epidermis, it immediately begins to convert to vitamin D_3 by a temperature-dependent isomerization (Fig. 2). At body temperature, about 50% of previtamin D_3 has been converted to vitamin

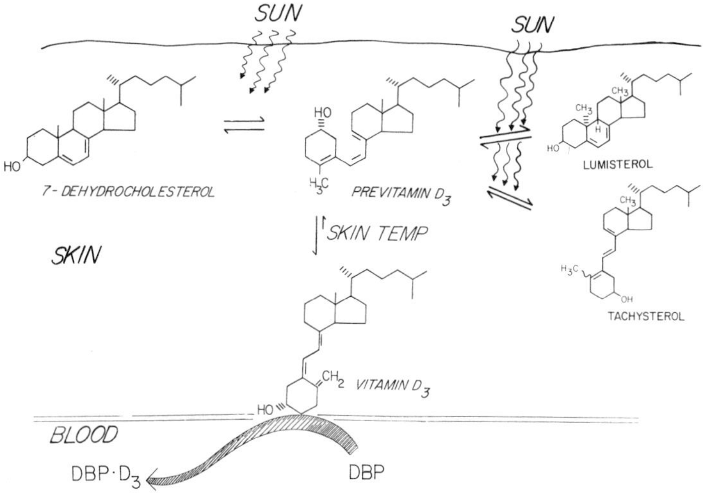

Fig. 2. Diagrammatic representation of the formation of previtamin D_3 in the skin during exposure to the sun and its subsequent thermal conversion to vitamin D_3, which, in turn, is bound to the vitamin D-binding protein (DBP) in plasma for transport into the circulation. Previtamin D_3 is photolabile and can undergo photoisomerization to lumisterol and tachysterol. (Reproduced with permission. Copyright 1981 by the American Association for the Advancement of Science, Holick *et al.*, 1981.)

D_3 within the first day, and, by three days, essentially all of the previtamin D_3 has converted to the vitamin (Holick *et al.*, 1980). Once formed, vitamin D_3 is translocated from the bloodless epidermis by plasma vitamin D binding protein into the dermal capillary bed (Fig. 2).

IV. METABOLISM OF VITAMIN D

On entering the circulation, vitamin D_3 is transported to the liver, where it is hydroxylated on carbon 25 to form 25-hydroxyvitamin D_3 (Fig. 3) (Holick and Potts, 1983). 25-Hydroxyvitamin D_3 (25-OH-D_3) is the major circulating form of vitamin D_3, and its concentration in the circulation is an excellent clinical indicator of the vitamin D nutritional status. The circulating normal range is between 8 and 55 ng/ml. Values below about 10 ng/ml are usually indicative of vitamin D deficiency. 25-OH-D_3 concentrations can fluctuate throughout the year owing to seasonal exposure to sunlight (Lester *et al.*, 1977; Omdahl *et al.*, 1982). The values are usually at the highest and lowest at the end of the summer and winter, respectively.

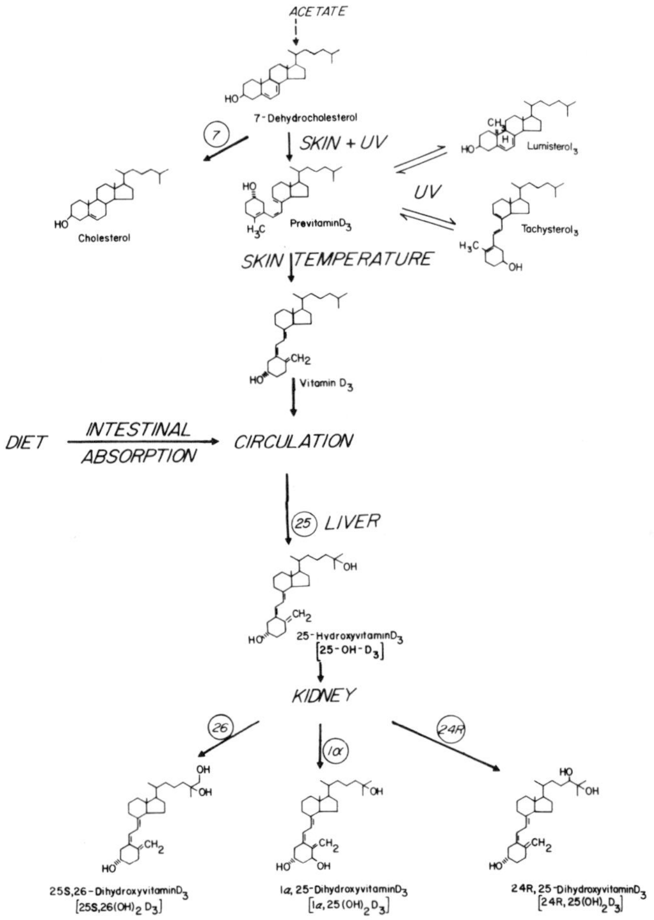

Fig. 3. Photobiogenesis and metabolic pathways for vitamin D production and metabolism. Circled letters and numbers denote specific enzymes: 7 = 7-dehydrocholesterol reductase; 25 = vitamin D-25-hydroxylase; 1α = 25-OH-D-1-hydroxylase; 24R = 25-OH-D-24R-hydroxylase; 26 = 25-OH-D-26-hydroxylase. (Reproduced with permission, Holick and Potts, 1983.)

However, 25-OH-D_3 is not the biologically active form of vitamin D_3. To become active, 25-OH-D_3 must journey to the kidney, where it is hydroxylated on carbon 1 to form 1,25-dihydroxyvitamin D_3 (1,25-$(OH)_2$-D_3). 1,25-$(OH)_2$-D_3 enters the circulation and enters the small intestine and bone, where it stimulates calcium absorption and bone calcium mobilization, respectively (Holick and Potts, 1983).

V. VITAMIN D NUTRITION IN THE AGED

Because of the recognition that vitamin D is essential for the development of healthy bones in growing children, vitamin D-deficiency rickets is a relatively rare occurrence in the United States. However, it is not well appreciated that vitamin D is also essential for adults for the maintenance of a healthy skeleton. In adults, because the bones no longer grow in length, the lack of vitamin D cannot cause rickets. Instead, vitamin D deficiency in adults results in a defect in bone mineralization called osteomalacia. In Great Britain, where dairy products are not routinely fortified with vitamin D as they are in the United States, adult vitamin D deficiency is a significant public health problem, especially as it relates to the incidence of hip fracture. It is well documented that upward of 30% of women and 40% of men who develop a hip fracture are found to be vitamin D deficient (Chalmers et al., 1967; Jenkins et al., 1973; Aaron et al., 1974).

In the United States, it has been generally accepted that vitamin D deficiency is not a health problem for either growing children or aging adults. Omdahl et al. (1982) investigated the vitamin D nutritional status of healthy free-living elderly persons in Albuquerque, New Mexico, and found that the circulating concentration of 25-OH-D in these subjects was about half that of the young adults. In about 15% of the elderly, the plasma concentrations of 25-OH-D were less than 8 ng/ml, which is considered borderline vitamin D deficiency. Nearly 80% of these people were not taking a vitamin D supplement. The greatest frequency (87%) of low plasma 25-OH-D concentrations occurred during the late winter and early spring.

In 1978, Sokoloff reported that low-grade osteomalacia was present in 8 of 31 midwestern patients who had a hip fracture and had normal serum calcium concentrations. Doppelt et al. (1983) found that an evaluation of 172 patients in a Boston hospital admitted with a hip fracture revealed that up to 40% had low or undetectable concentrations of 25-OH-D, and, of the bone biopsies obtained, 30% showed wide osteoid seams suggestive of osteomalacia.

There are various possible causes for vitamin D deficiency in the elderly, including (1) decreased activity outdoors, (2) impaired intestinal calcium absorption of vitamin D, (3) decline in the metabolism of vitamin D to 25-OH-D and 1,25-(OH)$_2$-D, (4) low dietary intake of vitamin D, and (5) decreased capacity of the skin to produce vitamin D$_3$. Omdahl et al. (1982) found that one of the primary causes of low vitamin D intake by the elderly in the United States is a decrease of, or complete abstinence from, the consumption of milk and milk products, often because of associated gastrointestinal discomfort caused by the lack of the enzyme lactase, which is responsible for digesting the lactose in milk.

VI. EFFECT OF AGING ON THE CAPACITY OF THE SKIN TO PRODUCE VITAMIN D_3

In the United Kingdom, where vitamin D supplementation is not widely practiced, and in the United States, where dairy products that are fortified with vitamin D are often avoided, the elderly are dependent on their skin to synthesize adequate quantities of vitamin D_3. It is well known, however, that aging causes various changes in the skin. After about the age of 20 years, skin thickness decreases linearly with time (Tan *et al.*, 1982). The age-related changes principally occur in the dermis, where the elastic fiber structure sinks and sags (Montagna and Carlisle, 1979).

Lester *et al.* (1977) were among the first to provide evidence that aging might decrease the efficiency of the skin to produce vitamin D_3. They found that during the summer months the circulating concentrations of 25-OH-D were lower in the nonhousebound elderly than they were in the healthy young British subjects. To determine whether aging influences the capacity of the skin to produce vitamin D_3, MacLaughlin and Holick (1985) determined the concentrations of the vitamin D precursor in the whole epidermis and dermis in a defined area, inasmuch as the cutaneous production of vitamin D_3 ultimately depends on the amount of skin surface that is exposed to sunlight. Our laboratory reported that the epidermal concentrations of 7-dehydrocholesterol decreased with increasing age (Fig. 4). This reduction was not accounted for by any significant decrease in the total mass of the epidermis (Table I). It was found that the dermal concentrations of the vitamin D precursor were not influenced by age, although the total mass of the dermis (weight of whole skin minus the weight of the epidermis) was reduced (Table I).

To ascertain that aging affected the capacity of the skin to produce vitamin D_3, representative skin samples from young and old subjects were exposed to simulated sunlight. As shown in Table II, the epidermis in the young and older subjects was the major site for the photosynthesis of previtamin D_3, accounting for greater than 80% of the total previtamin D_3 formed in the skin. A comparison of the amount of previtamin D_3 produced in the skin of the younger subjects with the amount produced in older subjects revealed that aging can decrease by greater than twofold the capacity of the skin to produce previtamin D_3. Hence, aging decreases the capacity of the skin to produce vitamin D_3.

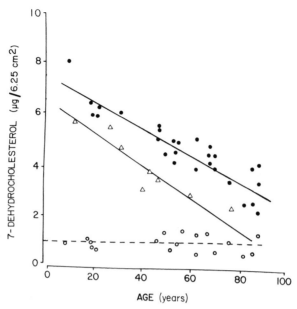

Fig. 4. Effect of aging on 7-dehydrocholesterol concentrations in human epidermis and dermis. Concentrations of 7-dehydrocholesterol (provitamin D_3) per unit area of human epidermis (●), stratum basale (△), and dermis (○) obtained from surgical specimens from donors of various ages. A linear regression analysis revealed slopes of -0.05, -0.06, and -0.0005 for the epidermis ($r = -0.89$), stratum basale ($r = -0.92$), and dermis ($r = -0.04$), respectively. The slopes of the epidermis and stratum basale are significantly different from the slope of the dermis ($p < .001$). (Reproduced with permission, MacLaughlin and Holick, 1985.)

TABLE I

The Effect of Aging on the Weight of the Whole Skin and Epidermis and on the Concentration of 7-Dehydrocholesterol (7-DHC) in the Epidermis.[a]

Age (years)	Wet weight of whole skin (g/cm²)	Wet weight of epidermis (g/cm²)	7-DHC (ng/cm²)	7-DHC (μg/g)
21	0.77	0.15	1747	11.65
29	0.64	0.14	1614	11.53
47	0.66	0.15	1350	9.00
58	0.72	0.16	1409	8.81
77	0.58	0.14	338	2.41
88	0.58	0.12	838	6.98

[a] Surgically obtained human skin was weighed and separated, and the 7-DHC concentrations were quantitated as previously described (MacLaughlin and Holick, 1985).

TABLE II

7-Dehydrocholesterol (7-DHC) Content before Exposure to Ultraviolet Radiation and Previtamin D_3 (PreD$_3$) Content after Exposure to Ultraviolet Radiation in 1 cm^2 of Human Epidermis and Dermis and the Percentage of PreD$_3$ Formed in the Epidermis and Dermis Relative to That in the 8-Year-Old Subject

| | Epidermis | | Dermis | | Epidermis and Dermis | |
| | | | | | PreD$_3$ (ng/cm^2) | Percent formation PreD$_3$ compared to 8-year-old |
Age	7-DHC (ng/cm^2)	PreD$_3$ (ng/cm^2)	7-DHC (ng/cm^2)	PreD$_3$ (ng/cm^2)		
8	1308	406	1800	36	442	100
18	1056	346	1125	22	368	80
77	605	144	1630	24	168	37
77	490	141	—	—	—	—
82	659	163	1040	20	183	40

VII. RECOMMENDATIONS FOR MAINTAINING VITAMIN D NUTRITION FOR THE ELDERLY

If an elderly adult does not consume milk or other dairy products or take vitamin D supplements it then becomes absolutely essential for that person to sunbathe in order to generate enough vitamin D to maintain a healthy skeleton. There is no question, however, that excessive sunbathing can cause skin cancer and other dermatologic changes such as wrinkles and dry skin. These facts have become a concern for the elderly. The dilemma is that, to prevent sun-induced dermatologic changes, the elderly are often advised to cover their skin with clothing or a sunscreen before going outdoors, and, by doing so, they prevent not only the damaging effects of solar irradiation on the skin but also the beneficial effect, i.e., the cutaneous photosynthesis of vitamin D_3. It is often asked how much exposure to sunlight is enough to provide adequate vitamin D nutrition. Unfortunately, there can be no one recommendation because there are multiple factors that influence the cutaneous production of vitamin D_3. The amount of previtamin D_3 that will be synthesized in a person will depend on (1) how much surface area is exposed to sunlight; (2) the amount of melanin skin pigmentation, inasmuch as melanin absorbs solar ultraviolet radiation and therefore limits the number of UV photons that can reach the epidermal stores of 7-dehydrocholesterol; (3) whether a sunscreen was applied before going outdoors (sunscreens absorb the solar radiation that is responsible for the sunburn and the production of vitamin D_3 and therefore inhibit both from occurring in the skin); (4) the time of day, because at the noon hours (11 A.M.–2 P.M.) the solar UV radiation is strongest; (5) the season, because in summer a greater amount of solar UV radiation penetrates to the earth's surface; and (6) the latitude, because the closer to the equator, the greater amount of solar UV radiation.

In addition to these factors, sunlight itself regulates the amount of previtamin D_3 that is produced in the skin. It had been assumed, for example, that if one is on the beach in the summertime, more time of body exposure to the sun would result in an increased production of vitamin D_3. In fact, this is not necessarily a correct assumption. Holick *et al.* (1981) reported that when a light-skinned Caucasian was outdoors on a bright sunny day in the summertime, the initial 10 to 15 minutes of exposure would effect a gradual increase in the photosynthesis of previtamin D_3 from 7-dehydrocholesterol that amounted to about 20% of the original 7-dehydrocholesterol stores. Thereafter, further exposure to the sun did not significantly increase the concentrations of previtamin D_3 in the skin (Fig. 5) because previtamin D_3 is sensitive to ultraviolet irradiation and is isomerized to two biologically inert photoproducts, lumisterol and tachysterol.

Therefore, for those persons who rely on sunlight for part or most of their vitamin D nutrition, it is important to recognize that only short exposures to sunlight are necessary to maintain normal calcium and bone metabolism. We have estimated in our laboratory that if young adults exposed their bodies to sunlight for a period that would cause a mild erythema of the skin, they would produce approximately 10,000 IU or 250 μg of vitamin D_3. On the basis of these data, we recommend that elderly Caucasians in Boston in the summertime expose hands, arms, and face to suberythemal doses (on a clear day usually 10 to 15 minutes, depending on the person's skin pigmentation) two to three times a week. If the person wants to remain outdoors after this initial exposure and is concerned about the harmful effects of sunlight, we encourage the use of a topical sunscreen.

VIII. CONCLUSIONS

It has generally been an accepted fact that aging causes a gradual and relentless reduction in bone mass that can result in fracture of the hip, wrists, and spine. The new revelations about the role of vitamin D metabolites in immunoregulation and in recruiting bone-marrow stem

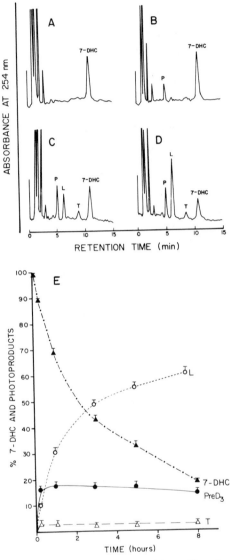

Fig. 5. High-performance liquid chromatographic profiles of a lipid extract from the basal cells of surgically obtained hypopigmented skin that was previously shielded from (A) or exposed to (B to D) equatorial simulated solar ultraviolet radiation for 10 minutes (B), 1 hour (C), or 3 hours (D). (E) An analysis of the photolysis of 7-dehydrocholesterol (7-DHC) in the basal cells and the appearance of the photoproducts previtamin D_3, lumisterol (L), and tachysterol (T) with increasing time of exposure to equatorial simulated sunlight. (Reproduced with permission. Copyright 1981 by the American Association for the Advancement of Science, Holick *et al.*, 1981.)

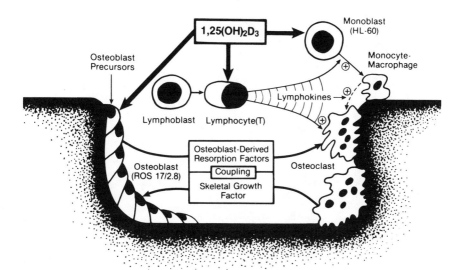

Fig. 6. Proposed function of 1,25-(OH)$_2$-D$_3$ and its receptor in bone remodeling and immunomodulation. (Reproduced with permission, Haussler *et al.*, 1985.)

cells to form new bone cells (Fig. 6) may open up new avenues for treating osteoporosis (Haussler *et al.*, 1985). Equally important is the new awareness that sufficient calcium and vitamin D intake throughout life is important for optimum skeletal mineralization. It is absolutely essential for the elderly to obtain adequate vitamin D nutrition. If they are unable to obtain this nutrition from their diet or a supplement, they then should take advantage of the natural source of vitamin D that is provided to them by exposing their skin to sunlight.

REFERENCES

Aaron, J. E., Gallagher, J. C., Anderson, L., Stasiak, E. B., Longton, B. E., Nordin, C., and Nicholson, M. (1974). *Lancet* **1**, 229–231.

Chalmers, J., Conacher, D. H., Gardner, D. L., and Scott, P. J. (1967). *J. Bone Jt. Surg., Br. Vol.* **49B**, 403–423.

Cummings, S. R., Kelsey, J. L., Nevitt, M. C., and O'Dowd, K. J. (1985). *Epidemiol. Rev.* **7**, 178–208.

Doppelt, S. H., Neer, R. M., Daly, M., Bourret, L., Schiller, A., and Holick, M. F., and Mankin, H. (1983). *Orthop. Trans.* **7**, 512–513.

Fraser, D., and Scriver, C. R. (1979). *In* "Endocrinology" (L. DeGroot *et al.*, eds.), Vol. 2, pp. 653–668. Grune & Stratton, New York.

Haussler, M. R., Donaldson, C. A., Kelly, M. A., Mangelsdorf, D. J., Marion, S. L., and Pike, J. W. (1985). *Proc. Workshop Vitamin D, 6th, 1985*, pp. 83–92.

Hess, A. F. (1925). *JAMA, J. Am. Med. Assoc.* **84,** 1910–1913.

Hess, A. F., and Unger, L. J. (1921). *JAMA, J. Am. Med. Assoc.* **77,** 39.

Holick, M. F., and Potts, J. T., Jr. (1983). *In* "Harrison's Principles of Internal Medicine" (K. J. Isselbacher, E. Braunwald, R. G. Petersdorf, and J. D. Wilson, eds.), 10th ed., pp. 1944–1949. McGraw-Hill, New York.

Holick, M. F., MacLaughlin, J. A., Clark, M. B., Holick, S. A., Potts, J. T., Jr., Anderson, R. R., Blank, I. H., Parrish, J. A., and Elias, P. (1980). *Science* **210,** 203–205.

Holick, M. F., MacLaughlin, J. A., and Doppelt, S. H. (1981). *Science* **211,** 590–593.

Huldschinsky, K. (1919). *Dtsch. Med. Wochenschr.* **45,** 712–713.

Jenkins, D. H., Roberts, J. G., Webster, D., and Williams, E. O. (1973). *J. Bone Jt. Surg., Br. Vol.* **55B,** 575–580.

Lester, E., Skinner, R. K., and Mills, M. R. (1977). *Lancet* **1,** 979–980.

MacLaughlin, J. A., and Holick, M. F. (1985). *J. Clin. Invest.* **76,** 1536–1538.

MacLaughlin, J. A., Anderson, R. R., and Holick, M. F. (1982). *Science* **216,** 1001–1003.

Montagna, W., and Carlisle, K. (1979). *J. Invest. Dermatol.* **73,** 47–53.

Mozolowski, W. (1939). *Nature (London)* **143,** 21.

Omdahl, J. L., Garry, P. J., Hunsaker, A., Hunt, W. C., and Goodwin, J. S. (1982). *Am. J. Clin. Nutr.* **36,** 1225–1233.

Palm, T. A. (1890). *Practitioner* **45,** 270–279, 321–342.

Park, E. A. (1923). *Physiol. Rev.* **3,** 106–159.

Sokoloff, L. (1978). *Am. J. Surg. Pathol.* **2,** 21–30.

Steenbock, H., and Black, A. (1924). *J. Biol. Chem.* **62,** 408–422.

Tan, C. Y., Statham, B., Marks, R., and Payne, P. A. (1982). *Br. J. Dermatol.* **106,** 657–667.

Implications of Gastric Atrophy for Vitamin and Mineral Nutriture

Robert M. Russell

USDA Human Nutrition Research Center on Aging at Tufts
Boston, Massachusetts

I. INTRODUCTION

The prevalence of atrophic gastritis and gastric atrophy is known to increase with advancing age, and 30% of those over the age of 60 have one or the other condition (Vanzant *et al.*, 1932; Siurala *et al.*, 1968; Villako *et al.*, 1976). In atrophic gastritis, hypochlorhydria is caused by a decrease in the number of gastric glands, whereas achlorhydria is a result of total gastric atrophy. Atrophic gastritis and gastric atrophy may be considered as part of a continuum, with gastric atrophy at the most severe end of the spectrum and the cause of pernicious anemia.

59

The diagnosis of atrophic gastritis and gastric atrophy may be based on endoscopic examination and/or histologic changes seen in biopsy specimens of the stomach. However, such techniques are not amenable to the routine testing of populations. Blood tests which have been used to test for atrophic gastritis and gastric atrophy include the presence of parietal cell antibodies, intrinsic factor antibodies and elevated serum gastrin levels (Bock et al., 1963; Adams et al., 1964; Coghill et al., 1965; Irvine et al., 1965; Fischer and Taylor, 1965; Ganguli et al., 1971; Korman et al., 1971; Stockbrugger et al., 1976; Varis et al., 1979). The former two serologic tests are specific for severe atrophic gastritis and gastric atrophy but are not sensitive tests for picking up less severe forms of the disorder.

Samloff and colleagues have recently described a radioimmunoassay for circulating pepsinogen I and pepsinogen II, and have related these levels to the histologic appearance of the gastric mucosa (Samloff et al., 1982). Most pepsinogen I and pepsinogen II originates from the chief and mucous cells of the *fundic gland mucosa*. However, pepsinogen II is also produced by the glands in the cardiac portion of the stomach, the gastric antral glands, and Brunner glands of the proximal duodenum (Samloff, 1982). Higher levels of pepsinogen I than pepsinogen II normally circulate in blood. Loss of fundic glands in atrophic gastritis therefore results in a fall in serum pepsinogen I levels with little fall in serum pepsinogen II levels, and indeed pepsinogen II levels may increase in atrophic gastritis due to pyloric gland metaplasia of the fundus (Samloff, 1982). It has been shown that with increasing severity of chronic atrophic gastritis, a progressive decrease in the ratio of serum pepsinogen I to pepsinogen II levels occurs. Because of the nonparallel changes in pepsinogen I to pepsinogen II levels, the ratio of pepsinogen I to pepsinogen II in combination with the absolute pepsinogen I level has been shown to be highly predictive of gastric mucosal histology (Samloff, 1982). The pepsinogen I to II ratio has been shown to decrease progressively with increasing severity of the histology associated with atrophic gastritis.

In a survey among free-living Boston elderly using the serum pepsinogen I to II ratio to diagnose atrophic gastritis it was found that prevalence of atrophic gastritis was approximately 30% over the age of 60 (Russell et al., 1984a). The criterion used for diagnosing atrophic gastritis was a serum pepsinogen I to II ratio of <2.9. In a few other population studies using different techniques the prevalence of atrophic gastritis has similarly been reported to be 20–28% with an increase in prevalence with advancing age (Siurala et al., 1968; Villako et al., 1976; Kreuning et al., 1978).

The relation of gastric atrophy to pernicious anemia is well known. However, other nutritional consequences of this lesion are now being studied. The purpose of this paper is to review what is presently known about the physiologic consequences of atrophic gastritis and the effect of atrophic gastritis on vitamin and mineral absorption and bioavailability in humans and in animal models.

II. PHYSIOLOGIC CONSEQUENCES OF ATROPHIC GASTRITIS

There are conflicting reports on the influence of age alone on gastric emptying. In one study, the rate of gastric emptying was significantly different in young versus elderly volunteers (50 versus 123 minutes, respectively) (Evans *et al.*, 1981). Further, in a study by Davies *et al.* (1971), gastric emptying time was found to be significantly increased in individuals with gastric atrophy versus control subjects. A changed gastric emptying could confound the interpretation of the absorption data if timed blood or urinary collections after a given dose of nutrient were employed to reflect absorption. With delayed gastric emptying, blood and urine collections might need to be extended for longer periods and the area under a tolerance curve (rather than peak height) might better reflect absorption.

A decreased secretion of intrinsic factor for vitamin B_{12} absorption is a second concomitant of atrophic gastritis, but only when the atrophic gastritis has progressed to its most severe form (gastric atrophy). The stomach with mild or moderate atrophic gastritis continues to secrete sufficient intrinsic factor to prevent vitamin B_{12} malabsorption, and pernicious anemia only occurs with complete atrophy of the gastric mucosa (Allen, 1982).

Small intestinal bacteria overgrowth is a third consequence of atrophic gastritis. Intestinal bacteria concentrations are elevated in 50–100% of subjects with achlorhydria, since bacteria which are swallowed or ingested in food are mostly destroyed by gastric acid (Draser *et al.*, 1969). Bacteria which grow in the upper small bowel in gastric atrophy do not usually result in bile salt deconjugation and fat malabsorption (Tabaqhali, 1970). However, these bacteria may bind or metabolize nutrients and reduce bioavailability.

Finally, the pH of the proximal small intestine may be raised in atrophic gastritis. If a nutrient's absorption process is pH-sensitive and if it is absorbed in the proximal small intestine, the absorption of that nutrient might be greatly influenced by hypo- or achlorhydria. Also a high intraluminal pH of the proximal small intestine could prevent the release of specific nutrients from food complexes due to lack of pH-dependent dissociation and acid pepsin digestion.

III. VITAMIN B_{12}

The prevalence of low serum vitamin B_{12} levels among the elderly ranges from 0 to 23% (Elwood et al., 1971; Bailey et al., 1980; Magnus et al., 1982; Garry et al., 1984; Hayes et al., 1985). Dietary vitamin B_{12} is attached to food protein. In the stomach, acid and pepsin digestion of dietary protein releases the vitamin B_{12}. At the acid pH of the stomach, vitamin B_{12} is bound to R-binders, which are nonintrinsic factor vitamin B_{12} binding proteins that are present in saliva, gastric juice, and other body secretions (Allen et al., 1978; Toskes, 1980). When vitamin B_{12} bound to R-binder reaches the higher pH of the proximal small intestine, dissociation of the R-binder protein and vitamin B_{12} occurs. Vitamin B_{12} is then free to join with intrinsic factor with which it travels to the terminal ileum for active absorption. The dissociation between R-binder and vitamin B_{12} occurs not only because of the higher intraluminal pH in the proximal small intestine but also because of pancreatic proteases which digest R-binder protein off. In the terminal ileum, specific receptors are present for the vitamin B_{12} intrinsic factor complex and binding to this receptor requires the presence of calcium and a pH greater than 5.6 (Hooper et al., 1973).

It has been shown that vitamin B_{12} malabsorption from the gut does not decline with age in normal elderly subjects (Glass et al., 1956; Chow, 1958; Hyams, 1964; Fleming and Barrows, 1982; McEvoy et al., 1982). However, in humans with atrophic gastritis vitamin B_{12} malabsorption may occur by several mechanisms. First of all, in gastric atrophy there is lack of secretion of intrinsic factor, which over time will result in pernicious anemia. However, the stomach usually secretes intrinsic factor in great excess, and therefore in milder degrees of atrophic gastritis lack of intrinsic factor secretion is not an issue (Allen, 1982).

A second mechanism whereby B_{12} absorption may occur in people with atrophic gastritis is via lack of acid pepsin digestion of dietary protein from the vitamin B_{12}. If this does not occur, vitamin B_{12} is not free to join with the B_{12} binding proteins (i.e., R-binders, intrinsic factor). King et al. (1979) have demonstrated a subset of patients with gastric atrophy who malabsorb protein (chicken serum) -bound vitamin B_{12} but not crystalline vitamin B_{12}. Similar results have been reported by Doscherholmen et al. (1978) using vitamin B_{12} bound to egg, ovalbumin, and chicken meat (Doscherholmen and Swain, 1973; Doscherholmen et *al.*, 1976). The exogenous administration of acid and pepsin to some of these individuals corrected the vitamin B_{12} malabsorption. Thus, in subjects with gastric atrophy the Schilling test using crystalline vitamin B_{12} may be normal, whereas if the Schilling test is carried out using protein-bound vitamin B_{12}, the test may be abnormal. This phenomenon has also been noted among individuals on long-term cimetidine therapy, which suppresses acid, pepsin, and intrinsic factor secretion by the stomach. Although it has been shown that the patients with gastric atrophy may malabsorb protein-bound vitamin B_{12}, it is not clear if patients with a milder form of atrophic gastritis (which make up a greater proportion of the elderly population) also malabsorb protein bound vitamin B_{12}.

A final reason why patients with atrophic gastritis could malabsorb vitamin B_{12} is bacterial overgrowth of the proximal small bowel. As mentioned previously, acid is an important factor in keeping the proximal small bowel relatively sterile. Bacteria could act on vitamin B_{12} in two ways: first, there could be binding of vitamin B_{12} (free or protein-bound) thus making it unavailable for absorption; second, the bacteria could synthesize analogues from the dietary vitamin B_{12} which are inactive in humans. It has been shown that bacteria in the small intestine can synthesize vitamin B_{12} analogues as well as modify ingested vitamin B_{12} even in the presence of intrinsic factor (Brandt *et al.*, 1977). Therefore, production of vitamin B_{12} analogues by bacteria in atrophic gastritis could significantly reduce the bioavailability of vitamin B_{12} and contribute to vitamin B_{12} deficiency in this elderly group.

IV. FOLIC ACID

The prevalence of low serum folate levels among elderly studied in the U.S. Health and Nutrition Examination Survey (Hanes I) was 6% (Lowenstein, 1982). Most dietary folates are in the form of folate polyglutamates. The polyglutamate side chain must be digested off of the folate molecule (pteryolmonoglutamic acid) prior to absorption by the intestinal epithelial cell. This digestion takes place by intestinal conjugates in the lumen of the small intestine or at the surface of the small intestinal epithelial cell. Conjugases are present both in the pancreas and in the small intestinal mucosa, although in the human, the small intestinal source of conjugase appears to be more important (Rosenberg, 1981). Pteryolmonoglutamic acid is transported across the intestine by a dual parallel mechanism: one is an energy-dependent saturable system occurring when physiologic concentrations of folate are presented to the small intestine epithelial cell, and the second is an energy-independent linear process of passive diffusion when higher unphysiologic concentrations of folate are presented. It has been found that the absorption of folic acid across the proximal small intestine is highly influenced by the pH of the intestinal milieu. The optimal pH for uptake of pteryolmonoglutamic acid by the small intestinal epithelial cell is 6.3 (Russell et al., 1979). Raising or lowering the pH of the intestinal lumen above or below 6.3 markedly diminishes the uptake of folic acid by the small intestine. This has been in both in vitro and in vivo studies using rats and humans (Russell et al., 1979). It was originally suggested that the pH effect on folic acid transport was mediated by changes in ionization of the molecule and diffusion of the neutral species; however, it is now known that the effect of pH is exerted on the energy-dependent uptake process of the intestinal cell (Russell et al., 1979).

There has been no demonstrable effect of age alone on folic acid absorption (Bhanthumnavin et al., 1974). Although Kesavan and Noronha (1983) demonstrated a decrease in the ability to absorb folate polyglutamates with age, this has not been born out by more recent studies. However, in preliminary studies in individuals with gastric atrophy, it has been reported that folic acid is malabsorbed and that this malabsorption is correctable by the administration of dilute hydrochloric acid (0.1 N) (Russell et al., 1984b). It is unclear if subjects with gastric atrophy have a higher prevalence of low serum folate levels. Bacterial synthesis of folate could make up for a relative defect in absorption of folate and thus prevent a deficiency state from occurring (due to the greater number of bacteria residing in the proximal small intestine in atrophic gastritis). High serum folate levels in patients with small intestinal bacterial overgrowth were first described in the 1960s (Hoffbrand et al., 1966). Thus, there could be a built-in mechanism for protection of atrophic gastritis individuals from folate depletion despite folate malabsorption.

V. IRON

Decreased iron absorption has been reported in old age, however, many early studies were not well controlled for iron status or the presence of gastrointestinal disease.

It has been clearly demonstrated that the absorption of ferric iron is diminished in achlorhydric subjects (Choudhury and Williams, 1959; Goldberg et al., 1963; Jacobs et al., 1964). Subsequently it has been shown that ferric iron absorption may be enhanced by the administration of hydrochloric acid alone (Biggs et al., 1962). Presumably, the beneficial effect of acid is to keep the ferric iron in solution until reaching the absorptive sites of the duodenal mucosa. Ferric iron is essentially insoluble above pH 5, whereas the ferrous iron and heme iron remain in solution at neutral or slightly alkaline pHs (Chaberek and Martell, 1959; Jacobs et al., 1964). Substances which form ligands with iron, such as ascorbic acid, amino acids, and sugars, increase the absorption of the ferric iron at a neutral or slightly alkaline pH range. However, the chelation with the ferric iron will only occur when the iron is in solution, that is, at acid pH (Conrad and Schade, 1968). Thus, acidity is needed for the chelation of the ferric ion to take place, which will then remain in solution at the higher pH of the proximal small intestine (Schade et al., 1968). In contrast, it has been shown that there is no diminished ability of atrophic gastritis individuals to absorb heme iron, and that the addition of hydrochloric acid will not enhance nonheme absorption further (Biggs et al., 1961; Jacobs et al., 1964; Bjorn-Rasmussen et al., 1974). A depressive effect of cimetidine on ferric iron absorption has been demonstrated, and antacids have been reported to cause a 52% decrease in ferric iron absorption.

Finally, it has also been shown that the absorption of ferric iron given to patients with achlorhydria can be increased by the administration of neutral gastric juice (Jacobs and Owen, 1969). This observation raises the question of whether gastric juice itself can promote absorption of ferric iron even when the effect of acid is eliminated. It is possible that gastric juice contains chelators that combine with iron at low pH. Thus, the increase of iron absorption produced by neutral gastric juice is greater when all iron is first incubated with gastric juice at an acid pH prior to neutralization than if incubated with already neutralized gastric juice (Jacobs and Owen, 1969).

It is not known how important atrophic gastritis is in reducing iron absorption in the elderly population. Population studies are now needed to relate iron status to atrophic gastritis.

VI. CALCIUM

Calcium must be dissociated from food complexes, and calcium salts must remain dissolved for calcium absorption to take place. Both of these processes depend on an acid pH and thus it is reasonable to presume that gastric acid secretion could play an important role in calcium absorption (Ivanovich et al., 1967; Nordin, 1968). It is thought that calcium carbonate reacts with hydrochloric acid to form soluble calcium chloride, which is subsequently absorbed in the proximal small intestine

(Clarkson *et al.*, 1966). The efficiency of absorption of calcium salts is becoming an important issue because of the use of calcium supplements in the prophylactic treatment of osteoporosis.

There have been two recent studies which have examined the role of hydrochloric acid in calcium absorption which gave conflicting results. In a study by Bo-Linn *et al.* (1984), large doses of cimetidine were given to 16 normal healthy subjects to reduce acid secretion. In addition, one female patient with pernicious anemia (age 57) was studied. The following meals were administered: a normal calcium meal (852 mg from milk) or a low-calcium meal which was supplemented with either calcium carbonate or calcium citrate. The method used to study calcium absorption included giving each individual subject a preparatory washout of the gastrointestinal tract. The subject was then given a meal containing calcium and a nonabsorbable marker. After 12 hours the intestine was once again cleansed by another washout. The rectal effluent was analyzed for calcium, and the completeness of the collection was evaluated by the recovery of the nonabsorbable marker. Net calcium absorption was then calculated. It was found that cimedtidine, which markedly reduced gastric acid secretion in the normal subjects, had no effect on calcium absorption. Also the achlorhydric patient with pernicious anemia was found to absorb calcium normally. This was true regardless of whether the source of dietary calcium was milk, insoluble calcium carbonate, or soluble calcium citrate. Finally, calcium absorption after calcium carbonate ingestion was the same whether the intragastric pH was maintained at 7.4 or 3.0, suggesting that dietary calcium absorption is not increased by increasing intragastric acidity.

Using a different method, Recker (1985) compared the absorption of calcium carbonate to calcium citrate in a group of 11 fasting subjects with achlorhydria and 7 normal fasting subjects. Fractional calcium absorption was measured using a double isotope procedure with 250 mg of calcium being used as the carrier. In the subjects with achlorhydria, calcium carbonate was markedly malabsorbed as opposed to normal subjects. However, the absorption of calcium citrate (pH adjusted to 5.8) in achlorhydric subjects was higher than in normal subjects.

The studies of Bo-Linn *et al.* and Recker differed in several respects. All Bo-Linn's patients with the exception of one were studied after cimetidine and their gastric pHs were in the range of 5.5 to 4.9, whereas in Recker's study the gastric pHs of the achlorhydric subjects were near 7.0. Also 7.2 liters of a balanced solution was used for lavage of each subject in Bo-Linn's study and this could have dissolved some of the calcium carbonate, permitting its absorption. Further investigations are needed, particularly in view of the high prevalence of calcium supplement taken by the elderly population at the present time.

VII. OTHER MICRONUTRIENTS

Gastric atrophy could theoretically affect the absorption of vitamins A and E. Hollander (1981) has shown that the absorption of these vitamins is decreased at an increased intraluminal pH. The possible role of bacteria in synthesizing folic acid has already been mentioned. Bacteria may also be active in synthesizing thiamin, vitamin B_6, biotin, and vitamin K. Atrophic gastritis might indirectly result in greater amounts of these vitamins being available to the host.

Thus, this rather common condition of the elderly known as atrophic gastritis should be studied in more detail with regard to its nutritional effects. Not only should the direct absorption of specific nutrients be studied, but also the bioavailability of nutrients when ingested with food. This condition could require altered dietary recommendations for certain micronutrients for a large subgroup of the elderly.

REFERENCES

Adams, J. F., Glen, A. I. M., Kennedy, E. H., McKenzie, I. L., Morrow, J. M., Anderson, J. R., Gray, K. G., and Middleton, D. G. (1964). *Lancet* **1**, 401–403.

Allen, R. H. (1982). *Gastroenterology* **14**(5), 17–20.

Allen, R. H., Seetharam, B., Podell, E., and Alpers, D. H. (1978). *J. Clin. Invest.* **61**, 47–54.

Bailey, L. N., Wagner, P. A., Christakis, G. J., Araujo, P. E., Appledorf, H., Davis, C. G., Doresey, E., and Dinning, J. S. (1980). *J. Am. Geriatr. Soc.* **28**, 276–278.

Bhanthumnavin, K., Wright, J. R., and Halsted, C. H. (1974). *Johns Hopkins Med. J.* **135**, 152–160.

Biggs, J. C., Bannerman, R. M., and Callender, S. T. (1962). *Proc. Congr. Eur. Soc. Haematol., 8th, 1961*, **1**, 236.

Bjorn-Rasmussen, E., Hallberg, L., Isaksson, B., and Arvidsson, B. (1974). *J. Clin. Invest.* **53**, 247–255.

Bock, O. A. A., Arapakis, G., Witts, L. J., and Richards, W. C. D. (1963). *Gut* **4**, 106–111.

Bo-Linn, G. W., Davis, G. R., Buddrus, D. J., Morawski, S. G., Santa Ana, C., and Fordtran, J. S. (1984). *J. Clin. Invest.* **73**, 640–647.

Brandt, L. J., Bernstein, L. H., and Wagle, A. (1977). *Ann. Intern. Med.* **87**, 546–551.

Chaberek, S., and Martell, A. E. (1959). "Organic Sequestering Agents", pp. 187–198. Wiley, New York.

Choudhury, M. R., and Williams, J. (1959). *Clin. Sci.* **18**, 527–532.

Chow, B. F. (1958). *Gerontologica* **5**, 651–658.

Clarkson, E. M., MacDonald, S. J., and De Wardner, H. E. (1966). *Clin. Res.* **30**, 425–438.

Coghill, N. F., Doniach, D., Roitt, I. M., Mollin, D. L., and Williams, A. W. (1965). *Gut* **6**, 48–56.

Conrad, M. E., and Schade, S. G. (1968). *Gastroenterology* **55**, 35–45.

Davies, W. T., Kirkpatrick, J. R., Owen, G. M., and Shields, R. (1971). *Scand. J. Gastroenterol.* **6**, 297–301.

Doscherholmen, A., and Swaim, W. R. (1973). *Gastroenterology* **64**, 913–919.

Doscherholmen, A., McMahon, J., and Ripley, D. (1976). *J. Haematol.* **33**, 261.

Doscherholmen, A., McMahon, J., and Ripley, D. (1978). *Am. J. Clin. Nutr.* **31**, 825–830.

Draser, B. S., Shiner, M., and McLeond, G. M. (1969). *Gastroenterology* **56**, 71–79.

Elwood, P. C., Shinton, N. K., Wilson, C. I. D., Sweetnam, P., and Frazer, A. C. (1971). *Br. J. Haematol.* **21**, 557–563.

Evans, M. A. Triggs, E. J., Cheung, M., Broe, G. A., and Creasey, H. (1981). *J. Am. Geriatr. Soc.* **29**, 501.

Fischer, J. M., and Taylor, K. B. (1965). *N. Engl. J. Med.* **272**, 499–503.

Fleming, B. B., and Barrows, C. H. (1982). *Exp. Gerontol.* **17**, 121–126.

Ganguli, P. C., Cullen, D. R., and Irvine, W. J. (1971). *Lancet* **1**, 155–158.

Garry, P. J., Goodwin, J. S., and Hunt, W. C. (1984). *J. Am. Geriatr. Soc.* **32**, 719–726.

Glass, G. B. J., Goldbloom, A. A., Boyd, L. J., Laughton, R., Rosen, S., and Rich, M. (1956). *Am. J. Clin. Nutr.* **4**, 124–133.

Goldberg, A., Lockhead, A. C., and Dagg, J. H. (1963). *Lancet* **1**, 848–850.

Hayes, A. N., Willams, D. J., and Skelton, D. (1985). *Clin. Biochem. (Ottawa)* **18**, 56–61.

Hoffbrand, A. V., Tabaqchali, M. B., and Mollin, D. L. (1966). *Lancet* **1**, 1339–1342.

Hollander, D. (1981). *J. Lab. Clin. Med.* **97**(4), 449–462.

Hooper, D. C., Alpers, D. H., Burger, R. I., Mehlman, C. S., and Allen, R. H. (1973). *J. Clin. Invest.* **52**, 3074–3083.

Hyams, D. E. (1964). *Gerontol. Clin.* **6**, 193–206.

Irvine, W. J., Davies, S. H., Teitelbaum, S., Delamore, F. W., and Williams, A. N. (1965). *Ann. N.Y. Acad. Sci.* **124**, 657–691.

Ivanovich, P., Fellows, H., and Rich, C. (1967). *Ann. Intern. Med.* **66**, 917–923.

Jacobs, A., and Owen, G. M. (1969). *Gut* **10**, 488–490.

Jacobs, P., Bothwell, T., and Charlton, R. W. (1964). *J. Appl. Phys.* **29**, 187–188.

Kesavan, V., and Noronha, J. M. (1983). *Am. J. Clin. Nutr.* **37**, 262–267.

King, C. E., Leibach, J., and Toskes, P. P. (1979). *Dig. Dis. Sci.* **24**, 397–402.

Korman, M. G., Strickland, R. G., and Hansky, J. (1971). *Br. Med. J.* **2**, 16–18.

Kreuning, J., Bosman, F. T., Kuiper, G., deWol, A. M., and Lindeman, J. (1978). *J. Clin. Pathol.* **31**, 69–77.

Lowenstein, F. W. (1982). *J. Am. Coll. Nutr.* **1**, 165–177.

McEvoy, A. W., Fenwick, J. D., Boddy, K., and James, O. F. W. (1982). *Age Ageing* **11**, 180–183.

Magnus, E. M., Bache-Wiig, J. E., Aanderson, T. R., and Melbostad, E. (1982). *Scand. J. Haematol.* **28**, 360–366.

Nordin, B. E. C. (1968). *Gastroenterology* **54**, 294–301.

Recker, R. R. (1985). *N. Engl. J. Med.* **313**, 70–73.

Rosenberg, I. H. (1981). *In* "Physiology of the Gastrointestinal Tract" (L. R. Johnson, ed.), pp. 1221–1230. Raven Press, New York.

Russell, R. M., Jeelani Dhar, G., Dutta, S. K., and Rosenberg, I. H. (1979). *J. Lab. Clin. Med.* **93**, 428–436.

Russell, R. M., Krasinski, S. D., Jacob, R. A., and Samloff, I. M. (1984a). *Gastroenterology* **86**, 1226.

Russell, R. M., Krasinski, S. D., and Samloff, I. M. (1984b). *Am. J. Clin. Nutr.* **39**, 656.

Samloff, I. M. (1982). *Gastroenterology* **82,** 26–33.

Samloff, I. M., Varis, K., Ihamaki, T., Siurala, M., and Rotter, J. I. (1982). *Gastroenterology* **83,** 204–209.

Schade, S. G., Cohen, R. J., and Conrad, M. E. (1968). *N. Engl. J. Med.* **13,** 672–674.

Siurala, M., Isokoski, M., Varis, K., and Kekki, M. (1968). *Scand. J. Gastroenterol.* **3,** 211–223.

Stockbrugger, R., Andervall, L., and Lundquist, G. (1976). *Scand. J. Gastroenterol.* **11,** 713–719.

Tabaqchali, S. (1970). *Scand. J. Gastroenterol.* **6,** 239–263.

Toskes, P. P. (1980). *J. Clin. Gastroenterol.* **2,** 287–297.

Vanzant, F. R., Alvarez, W. C., Eusternan, G. B., Dunn, H. C., and Berkson, J. (1932). *Arch. Intern. Med.* **49,** 345–359.

Varis, K., Samloff, I. M., Ihamaki, T., and Siurala, M. (1979). *Dig. Dis. Sci.* **24,** 187–191.

Villako, K., Tamm, A., Savisaar, E., and Ruttas, M. (1976). *Scand. J. Gastroenterol.* **11,** 817–827.

7

Trace Elements and the Needs of the Elderly

Walter Mertz

USDA Human Nutrition Research Center
Beltsville, Maryland

I. INTRODUCTION

It has been said that the aging process begins at conception; beyond this statement there is no general agreement as to the definition of the "elderly." This is not surprising, because age-related changes in the metabolism of nutrients become effective at widely different phases of the life cycle and, except for iron, are gradual and difficult to quantify. Iron is at

71

present the only known example for an acute, quantifiable change of metabolism and requirement with age, namely, the reduction of the requirement as a consequence of the cessation of blood loss in postmenopausal women. Age-related changes in bone metabolism affecting calcium from accretion to gradual depletion begin toward the end of the third decade, and the diminution of body pools for many trace elements as a function of the diminishing body mass shows great variation among individuals, possibly related to physical activity.

This uncertainty is reflected in the wide divergence of national and international recommendations for nutrient intake of the elderly (Committee 1/5 of the International Union of Nutrition Sciences, 1983). The recommendations of the Food and Agricultural Organization/World Health Organization do not address the needs of the elderly at all; their oldest age group is that of "adults." The Ninth Edition of the Recommended Dietary Allowances of the United States treats all those above the age of 51 in one category, an age beyond menopause in women and more than a decade before the time when most people change their lifestyle with retirement (National Academy of Sciences, 1980). At the other extreme are the nutrient recommendations for Bulgarians with a separate category for those 90 years and older (Committee 1/5 of the International Union of Nutrition Sciences, 1983). These few examples demonstrate that a valid, universal definition of the "elderly" cannot be made as yet. For the purpose of this discussion the aging process will be treated as a continuum with breaking points and rates differing not only among individuals but also among the mineral elements. From this definition follows the hypothesis that the nutritional status and, probably, the nutrient requirements of the elderly are much more determined by past history than by the current intake.

II.   DEFINITION OF REQUIREMENT AND RECOMMENDED INTAKE

There is general agreement that recommended intakes or allowances should meet the nutritional needs of nearly all healthy persons, they are therefore higher than the average need and provide a margin of safety for all but those with extreme requirements. This definition is clear when applied to young or middle-aged groups of people, but there is much discussion whether age-related functional impairment, for example, the decline of glomerular function, should be considered "normal" or pathological. That function is essential for the homeostasis of several elements. Regardless of the answer, the example suggests that what may be a margin of safety in younger people may well represent an added burden in the elderly. It is evident that recommended intakes for the elderly must not be derived from extrapolations of the needs of the young. Extrapolations are, however, the predominant method of today for lack of better methods.

If there is uncertainty with regard to recommendations for the elderly, there is controversy when it comes to the definition of requirements. Requirements can be defined in three ways, with the resulting definitions being basically and philosophically different and mutually exclusive. First, a requirement can be set as the amount in the daily diet that will prevent signs of deficiency. This interpretation assumes that no further benefit accrues from higher intakes. Although no recommendations suggest an intake at the requirement by that definition, the latter is an important argument in the deliberations of committees setting intake recommendations, modified only by the inclusion of a safety factor. Second, a requirement can also be determined on the basis of more liberal criteria, for example, saturation of a nutrient-dependent enzyme system, or the results of specific load tests, or simply the desire to maintain the existing nutritional status and the existing nutrient intake. The apparent scientific basis for the latter argument is the balance test for mineral elements which, in reality, measures that amount of an element that maintains the status quo (Levander and Morris, 1984). Finally, a requirement can be defined as that intake that provides maximal protection against the stresses of the environment, infectious, peroxidative, and chemical, resulting in acute and chronic infectious degenerative and neoplastic disease, and possibly affecting the aging process. What the three definitions of requirement mean for recommended intakes can be illustrated for the essential element selenium. Twenty micrograms per day prevent the only known deficiency in man, the Keshan Disease; a recommended intake of 30 μg would include an adequate safety factor (Yang, 1985). That amount maintains the existing nutritional status of New Zealanders, but not the saturation of the Se-specific enzyme, glutathione peroxidase, in individuals of that country (Levander and Morris, 1984). Balance studies have shown that Americans need approximately 70 μg/day to maintain their selenium status; this is the amount of the average intake in the United States. On the other hand, many animal studies have clearly demonstrated a protective effect of high doses of selenium against chemical and viral carcinogenesis and epidemiological correlations in man are consistent with these findings. Correspondingly, selenium intakes of 200–300 μg/day have been recommended by some, resulting in a 10-fold difference of estimated requirements (Schrauzer, 1978). The example of selenium is particularly pertinent to the elderly not only because neoplastic disease affects the elderly more than the young, but also because peroxidative processes, which selenium counteracts, may be intimately involved in the aging process.

As already stated, there is no consensus among those who set recommendations as to which of the criteria should be applied. At this time, expert bodies apply the first two criteria even within one document, whereas the third criterion is defended by a few scientists and many producers of nutrient supplements. The National Academy of Sciences, U.S.A., examined these criteria in two meetings held in 1985. Pending a consensus from these conferences, it will be necessary to qualify any statement pertaining to requirements by asking "requirements for what?"

III. THE PRESENT STATE OF KNOWLEDGE PERTAINING TO MINERAL REQUIREMENTS OF THE ELDERLY

Although several studies of the mineral intake of elderly population groups have been published, it is not known whether that intake is adequate, marginal, or inadequate. Whatever estimates of requirement have been made are based on extrapolations from results in the middle-aged or the young, with one exception: The sharply diminished iron requirement of postmenopausal women is easily calculated on the basis of the cessation of the monthly blood loss. Direct studies in the elderly are of the highest priority in view of the projected increase of their number in the population. Lacking the results of such studies, consideration of a few well-established facts that impinge on requirements might allow some general, but very preliminary estimates. The lean body mass diminishes with age (Munro, 1985). The rate of loss depends on factors such as physical activity, health status, and, possibly, nutrition; the end point is also a function of the maximal mass at the time when the decline began. Analytical measurements of mineral elements in autopsy material have shown that for most elements the concentrations change little from young adult age onward (Schroeder et al., 1966, 1967, 1970), except for some heavy metals, which tend to accumulate, and for chromium (Schroeder et al., 1962) and silicon (Loeper et al., 1978), which tend to decline with age. The decline in lead body mass in the presence of nearly constant concentrations leads to a diminution of the metabolic pools of most elements. As the obligatory loss of most mineral elements is a function of the pool size, one could conclude that the minimal requirement of the elderly, i.e., the amount to offset obligatory losses, decreases with the diminishing lean body mass. That interpretation presupposes that the decline is a "natural" phenomenon, as is, for example, the acceleration of bone loss in postmenopausal women, due to hormonal imbalances. Alternatively, one could consider the contraction of body mass (including bone mass) a pathological event that should be counteracted. Hormone therapy of osteoporosis is effective in many cases, but nutritional intervention by itself in the elderly with osteoporosis calls for very high calcium intakes that cannot be provided by even the best of balanced diets (Nilas et al., 1984). High *therapeutic* supplements can restore zero balance, but certainly not in all cases. For other elements, such as iron or copper, attempts to force zero or positive balance by supplements would run the risk of increasing tissue concentrations of these highly prooxidative elements, a potential insult to the elderly.

The consequences for health of the changing pool size with age, except for calcium, are not yet known. Until such knowledge is firmly established it appears prudent not to force increases by high amounts of individual supplements.

IV. EFFICIENCY OF INTESTINAL ABSORPTION

It is well known that the absorption efficiency of several mineral elements can be grossly impaired in the elderly. If this were a true "normal" aging phenomenon, it would call for an increase in the dietary recommendations in order to allow the absorption of amounts adequate to meet the absolute requirement for these elements. The impairment, however, is almost always caused by a pathological process, such as atrophy of the gastric mucosa or marginal vitamin D deficiency. The former affects the absorption of cobalt in the form of vitamin B_{12} through lack of intrinsic factor and of iron and possibly other elements, through achlorhydria. These conditions call for substitution of the missing agent; they are not indicative of a depressed absorptive function of mineral elements in the healthy elderly. Although the beneficial effects of substitution therapy with vitamin D, estrogens, intrinsic factor, or hydrochloric acid on the absorption of calcium, cobalt, and iron are well documented, very little is known of the consequences of achlorhydria for other trace elements.

Some animal experiments have shown a gradual decline of absorption efficiency for several trace elements with age. When such results are reinforced by analytical studies showing a decline in the concentration of an element in tissues with age, as is the case with chromium, they indicate a true impairment of absorption in that animal species and, by extrapolation, possibly in man. Only the demonstration of a consistent impairment of a physiological function, specific for that element as a consequence of the low tissue levels, is an indication of adverse health effects and an argument for higher intakes. Again, this is the case for chromium (Mertz, 1982).

In the absence of such confirmatory data, a diminshed absorption efficiency may only signal adequate body stores and a slightly decreased absolute requirement. This has been amply demonstrated for iron. These considerations suggest that the predominant concern with regard to the mineral absorption in the elderly should be with pathological conditions, gastric mucosal atrophy, and others that affect absorbability.

V. DETERMINATION OF REQUIREMENTS FOR MINERAL ELEMENTS IN THE ELDERLY

Because of the lack of direct, reliable measurements of requirements in the elderly, estimates have been made by extrapolation from data obtained in younger subjects, most often college students. Extrapolation is beset with many uncertainties and is inadequate for the determination of nutrient needs that are believed to affect the aging process itself in a rapidly expanding proportion of the population. The establishing of two USDA Human Nutrition Research Centers, one at Boston dedicated to research on nutritional needs of the elderly and the other at San Francisco concerned with methods of nutritional status diagnosis, promises much needed new approaches. This raises the question: What are the feasible approaches to determine in direct studies the mineral requirements of elderly subjects?

A. Daily Intake of Mineral Elements

Determination of the daily intake of mineral elements in an elderly, supposedly "healthy" population group rests on the assumption that the measured intake must be adequate to maintain health. Even if the assumption is accepted, there are two uncertainties, one practical, the other theoretical. Apart from the known difficulties of obtaining accurate food intake records even from younger people (Hallfrisch et al., 1982), the food composition tables are inadequate at this time with regard to important elements, such as magnesium, zinc, copper, chromium, and selenium (Beecher and Vanderslice, 1984). In addition, a quantitative calculation of the biologically available element is as yet impossible, except for iron, in view of the multitude of dietary interactions affecting biological availability (Monsen *et al.*, 1978). The theoretical uncertainty lies with the definition of health in the elderly. There is little agreement as to which of the processes of aging are physiological and which could be delayed or prevented by, among several measures, nutritional intervention. This approach almost inevitably arrives at lower estimates of requirement for the elderly than for younger age groups because of the former population's lower food intake, a conclusion that should not be accepted without additional proof.

B. Balance Studies

Balance studies have been widely used in younger individuals to determine apparent requirements for mineral elements. Their interpretation rests on the assumption that an intake of an element equal to or greater than the sum of fecal, urinary, dermal, and menstrual losses meets the requirement, and that a negative balance represents an inadequate intake. Balance studies are beset by very substantial technical problems which have not yet been overcome. One is the uncertainty in the use of fecal markers which determine the length of the collection period, and another is the inadequacy of the analytical methods available. The best of our methods under ideal circumstances have a coefficient of variation of ±5%, totally inadequate to deal with an element of an absorption efficiency of less than 5%, or with the small but important dermal losses. More important are problems in the interpretation of balance studies, even if the data are accepted as accurate. It is well known that the excretion kinetics for most trace elements follows a series of exponential equations which describe rates of loss from usually two or three compartments. These equations allow the calculation of losses; they can be simplified in the general statement that the daily losses are a constant fraction of the existing, metabolically interchangeable pools. This constant fraction translates into a high amount when the pools are large and into a low amount when the pools are small. Therefore, the amount of a dietary intake to offset the daily losses is a function of the existing pool size. It determines not the requirement in general, but *the requirement to maintain the existing pool size*. An intake greater than that resulting in balance will increase the pool until a new equilibrium is reached, and one smaller will reduce the pool, until again losses equal the absorbable intake. Thus, balance studies do not relieve the nutritionist of a most important judgment as to the most desirable pool size. They do not, by themselves, establish a requirement.

C. Biochemical Indices

Biochemical indices are reliable for only four elements, iron, iodine, cobalt, and selenium. Iron status is determined by measurement of a storage protein or the saturation of a transport protein, iodine and cobalt status by measurement of specific chemical species, and selenium status by measurement of a specific enzyme, glutathione peroxidase. Analysis of the concentration of the remaining trace elements in blood, hair, or urine yields results that can be interpreted only in cases of extreme deficiencies and are subject to many interacting influences (Mertz, 1985; Hambidge, 1982).

D. Experimental Induction of Deficiencies

Experimental induction of deficiencies has been used in the past for several vitamins and two trace elements, copper and zinc. It provides an accurate estimate of minimum requirements, but is beset with ethical problems which question its application in young, healthy individuals and rules out its use in the elderly.

E. The Epidemiological Approach

The epidemiological approach is, in the opinion of the author, the optimal method, and indicative of future development of nutrition research. Although it has to cope with all of the technical difficulties described above under Section A, its advantages are that it integrates the results of many experiments that Nature herself has performed. The correlation between the health status and dietary patterns of different populations integrates lifetime exposure to diet with the only really important criterion of public health, namely, disease risk and longevity. This approach is not yet universally accepted with its assumption that nutritional status affects disease risk, nor do correlations establish cause and effect relations. Yet, a committee of the National Research Council on Diet, Nutrition, and Cancer has used this approach and has stimulated many studies in experimental animals and man (Committee on Diet, Nutrition, and Cancer, 1982).

The acceptance of criteria of minimal risk for chronic degenerative and neoplastic disease in relation to nutrition as opposed to the criterion of absence of even the mildest form of deficiency is by no means universal and, as discussed previously, has led to substantial current controversies (Toufexis, 1985). Even so, the epidemiological approach has the distinct advantage that it deals with lifetime patterns of dietary intake which are much more meaningful than any ad hoc nutritional study to determine requirements could be. The demonstration of significantly better bone mass and bone health in a Yugoslav population group with a high-calcium dietary pattern as compared to a similar group with a low-calcium pattern is a convincing argument for recommending high intakes of calcium throughout the lifetime (Matkovic et al., 1979). Similarly, the strong negative correlation between serum selenium levels in individuals who also exhibit low levels of vitamins A and E and cancer risk suggests dietary selenium intakes that maintain "protective" concentrations of the element in serum (Willett et al., 1983).

The epidemiological approach is applicable at this time to only a small number of nutrients. In addition, any conclusions resulting from it need confirmation of a cause–effect relationship by properly designed experiments, at least in animals, and ideally also in man. As evidenced by the elements calcium and selenium, progress is rapid.

The epidemiological approach, with its reliance on long-term dietary patterns in relation to diseases of slow progression, emphasizes the importance of nutrient intake during younger ages for the health of the elderly. Dietary recommendations for the young should be influenced by the concern for health of these same persons when they grow older.

VI. THE CATEGORIES OF MINERAL ELEMENTS

Requirements and recommendations for mineral elements of concern in the elderly have been discussed in a previous publication (Mertz, 1986). They can be summarized in three categories of increasing priorities. In the following discussion those priorities are set strictly by nutritional, not medical, criteria; they do not take into account physiological (e.g., hormonal) or pathological changes (i.e., achlorhydria) that affect mineral metabolism and that must be treated according to their cause. Furthermore, the proposed categories are meant to apply to the population of the United States and not necessarily to populations of other regions where special environmental conditions may occur.

The first group of elements is of relatively small nutritional concern; it comprises manganese, molybdenum, iron, cobalt, and iodine. The supply of the first two elements from practically any diet is more than adequate, and deficiencies in man, other than experimental, are not known (National Academy of Sciences, 1980). In contrast to the substantial, worldwide problems of iron deficiency in premenopausal women, there is no evidence of deficiency in the elderly in the presence of normal gastric secretory function. Disturbances of that function affecting the utilization of iron and cobalt (as vitamin B_{12}) require medical treatment, not nutritional supplements. The intake of iodine in the United States is more than adequate to meet requirements; in addition, severe iodine deficiency affects primarily the developing fetus, not the elderly.

The second category, comprising magnesium, copper, zinc, and fluorine, is of potential concern in the elderly because each member element has been implicated as possibly protecting against diseases of old age and because of uncertainties concerning the adequacy of intake throughout the lifetime. Epidemiological and experimental data have postulated increased risk for cardiovascular diseases from marginal intake of magnesium (Seelig and Heggtveit, 1974) and copper (Klevay *et al.*, 1979), and the dietary allowances for these two elements are not readily supplied by even well-balanced diets. High environmental concentrations of fluorine have been correlated with bone health of the exposed populations (Bernstein *et al.*, 1966). Zinc is a problem element for the younger age groups, but recent evidence for the involvement of that element in immune functions points out the great potential importance of zinc for the health of the elderly (Chandra *et al.*, 1985). There is no agreement as to the zinc requirement, and the recommendations differ widely among countries. In the United States the habitual intake does not meet the Recommended Dietary Allowance.

Calcium, selenium, chromium, and silicon, representing the third category, can be considered as the true problem elements of geriatric nutrition. Calcium loss from the skeleton results in osteoporosis. Selenium protects against the damages from peroxidation products, which have been linked not only to cancer risk but also to the aging process itself. Chromium and silicon have in common the decline of tissue concentrations with increasing age. The decline of chromium concentrations in all tissues, except for the lungs, is associated with deterioration of glucose metabolism, as evidenced by the age-related increase of fasting serum glucose concentrations and the worsening of glucose tolerance. Silicon is one the "new trace elements" and practically nothing is known of requirements or intake by man (Carlisle, 1978). Yet the evidence is strong for a fundamental role of that element in bone metabolism. Experimental silicon deficiency in two animal species results in gross bone deformities, and the accretion of that element precedes calcification of bone (Carlisle, 1978).

The micronutrients of the third category have in common a *gradual* decline of the health functions in which they are involved, beginning years, perhaps decades, before clinical disease manifests itself. The treatment of diseases by nutritional intervention (i.e., by supplements or physiological amounts of nutrients) is extremely difficult if not useless. Chromium supplementation improves impaired glucose tolerance in many middle-aged subjects (Anderson *et al.*, 1983), but is of dubious value once the impairment has developed into clinical diabetes (Rabinowitz *et al.*, 1983). To restore calcium balance in postmenopausal women, calcium supplements severalfold in excess of what can be obtained from a balanced diet must be given (Nilas *et al.*, 1984). These facts emphasize the conclusion repeatedly made in this discussion that the nutritional status of the elderly is strongly determined by dietary practices during middle age.

VII. INTERACTIONS

Thousands of animal experiments in the past have examined the role of individual elements in various disease processes and have resulted in an almost automatic association in the minds of many between individual elements and a disease, for example, calcium and osteoporosis, selenium and cancer, or chromium and diabetes. This approach is justified as a scientific tool, but its conclusions can be applied to the situation in man only with great caution. Dietary calcium concentrations that are effective in animal experiments result in death from urolithiasis when accompanied by a slight reduction of protein quality and quantity (Roginski and Mertz, 1974), and selenium concentrations that reduce experimental carcinogenesis border on the toxic (Schrauzer, 1978). Hundreds of interactions among mineral elements and between those and other nutrients are known, but have not been quantified (Sandstead, 1980). The quantitative description of these interactions is probably the greatest challenge to future nutrition research.

The second type of interaction, the synergism of several micronutrients on a particular health function, is often neglected but holds great promise. Although the multifactorial nature of many of our public health problems is generally recognized, few studies have examined the influence of more than one or two factors simultaneously. For example, the function of five mineral elements in bone metabolism is firmly established. These are calcium, phosphorus, fluorine, copper, silicon. Epidemiological correlations point to a synergism of selenium, vitamin A, and vitamin E in relation to cancer risk. Calcium and potassium and polyunsaturated fatty acids must be considered with sodium in relation to hypertension, and glucose tolerance is regulated by several trace elements, among them chromium, manganese, copper, and zinc. The promise arising from these synergisms is in the postulate that control of several, if not all, of the interacting nutrients may obviate the need for intervention with excessive amounts of one.

VIII. CONCLUSIONS

1. Existing estimates of mineral requirements and recommendations for the elderly that are derived by extrapolations from younger age groups are unsatisfactory.

2. Nutrition-related health problems of the elderly are in part determined by nutritional practices of preceding decades; effective intervention should begin early in life.

3. The multifactorial approach to the prevention of age-related diseases of the elderly, taking into account synergistic (and antagonistic) interactions among nutrients, holds great promise.

REFERENCES

Anderson, R. A., Polansky, M. M., Bryden, N. A., Roginski, E. E., Mertz, W., and Glinsmann, W. H. (1983). *Metab., Clin. Exp.* **32**, 894–899.

Beecher, G. R., and Vanderslice, J. T. (1984). *In* "Modern Methods of Food Analysis" (K. K. Stewart and J. R. Whitaker, eds.), pp. 29–55. AI Publ. Co., Westport, Connecticut.

Bernstein, D. S., Sadowsky, N., Hegsted, D. M., Guri, C. D., and Stare, F. J. (1966). *JAMA, J. Am. Med. Assoc.* **198**, 499–504.

Carlisle, E. (1978). *In* "Biochemistry of Silicon and Related Problems" (G. Bendz and I. Lindqvist, eds.), pp. 231–252. Plenum, New York.

Chandra, S., Vyas, D., and Chandra, R. K. (1985). *Nutr. Res. Suppl.* **1**, 693–699.

Committee 1/5 of the International Union of Nutrition Sciences (1983). *Nutr. Abstr. Rev., Clin. Nutr., Ser. A* **53**, 939–1015.

Committee on Diet, Nutrition, and Cancer (1982). "Diet, Nutrition, and Cancer." Natl. Acad. Sci., Washington, D.C.

Hallfrisch, J., Steele, P., and Cohen, L. (1982). *Nutr. Res.* **2**, 263–273.

Hambidge, K. M. (1982). *Am. J. Clin. Nutr.* **36**, 943–949.

Klevay, L. M., Reck, S., and Barcome, D. F. (1979). *JAMA, J. Am. Med. Assoc.* **241**, 1916–1918.

Levander, O. L., and Morris, V. C. (1984). *Am. J. Clin. Nutr.* **39**, 809–815.

Loeper, J., Loeper, J., and Fragny, M. (1978) *In* "Biochemistry of Silicon and Related Problems" (G. Bendz and I. Lindqvist, eds.), pp. 281–296. Plenum, New York.

Matkovic, V., Kostial, K., Simonovic, E., Buzina, R., Brodarec, A., and Nordin, B. E. C. (1979). *Am. J. Clin. Nutr.* **32**, 540–549.

Mertz, W. (1982). *Chem. Scr.* **21**, 145–150.

Mertz, W. (1985). *Nutr. Res., Suppl. I*, pp. 169–174.

Mertz, W. (1986). *In:* "WHO Scientific Publication on Nutrition in the Elderly" (in press).

Monsen, E. R., Hallberg, L., Layrisse, M., Hegsted, D. M., Cook, J. D., Mertz, W., and Finch, C. A. (1978). *Am. J. Clin. Nutr.* **31,** 134–141.

Munro, H. N. (1985). *Drug-Nutr. Interact.* **4,** 55–74.

National Academy of Sciences (1980). "Recommended Dietary Allowances," 9th ed. NAS, Washington, D.C.

Nilas, L., Christiansen, G., and Rodbro, P. (1984). *Br. Med. J.* **289,** 1103–1106.

Rabinowitz, M. B., Gonick, H. C., Levine, S. R., and Davidson, M. B. (1983). *Biol. Trace Elem. Res.* **5,** 449–466.

Roginski, E. E., and Mertz, W. (1974). *J. Nutr.* **104,** 599–604.

Sandstead, H. H. (1980). *Ann. N.Y. Acad. Sci.* **355,** 282–284.

Schrauzer, G. N. (1978). *Adv. Exp. Med. Biol.* **91,** 323–344.

Schroeder, H. A., Balassa, J. J., and Tipton, I. H. (1962). *J. Chronic Dis.* **15,** 941–969.

Schroeder, H. A., Nasen, A. P., and Tipton, I. H. (1966). *J. Chronic Dis.* **19,** 1007–1034.

Schroeder, H. A., Nason, A. P., Tipton, I. H., and Balassa, J. J. (1967). *J. Chronic Dis.* **20,** 179–210.

Schroeder, H. A., Balassa, J. J., and Tipton, I. H. (1970). *J. Chronic Dis.* **23,** 451–499.

Seelig, M. S., and Heggtveit, H. A. (1974). *Am. J. Clin. Nutr.* **27,** 59–79.

Toufexis, A. (1985). *Time* **126,** 61.

Willett, W. C., Morris, J. S., Pressel, S., Taylor, J. O., Polk, B. F., Stampfer, M. J., Rosner, B., Schneider, K., and Hames, C. G. (1983). *Lancet* **1,** 130–134.

Yang, G. Q. (1985). *In* "Trace Elements in Nutrition of Children" (R. K. Chandra, ed), pp. 273–287. Raven Press, New York.

Role of Dietary Antioxidants in Aging

Jeffrey B. Blumberg and
Simin Nikbin Meydani

Nutritional Immunology and Toxicology Laboratory
USDA Human Nutrition Research Center on Aging at Tufts
Boston, Massachusetts

I. INTRODUCTION

How can people achieve long, healthy lives? The most common and best substantiated response to this question is by reducing risk factors such as smoking and excessive alcohol consumption. Is there a way to extend life expectancy or life span through a positive intervention other than reducing the impact of specific diseases? Our current, admittedly primitive, state of understanding of aging suggests there are probably multiple mechanisms underlying the aging process at molecular, cellular, and organ levels. Consequently, it would seem unlikely that a single "magic bullet" will reverse or

85

arrest all aging processes. However, interventions which affect one or just a few aging processes, i.e., "segmental" interventions, may be developed which could have a significant impact. The attempt to prevent or retard the decline in immune function that occurs with aging, for example, could increase the ability of older individuals to combat infectious disease and cancer with a subsequent increase in life expectancy.

II. FREE RADICAL THEORY OF AGING

Many of the theories proposed to explain aging have focused on one mechanism and encouraged the belief that a single global intervention will arrest the aging process. The free radical theory of aging proposed by Harman (1956) hypothesizes that the degenerative changes associated with aging might be produced by the accumulation of deleterious side reactions of the free radicals produced during cellular metabolism. Free radical damage could contribute to the aging process via several mechanisms. Free radical-induced DNA cross-links could lead to somatic mutations and loss of essential enzyme expression. Oxidation of sensitive sulfhydryl groups could cause cellular damage to mitotic and cytoplasmic microtubules. Membrane lipid peroxidation could destroy the integrity of subcellular organelles. Macromolecular cross-links of connective tissue could impede nutrient diffusion and impair tissue viability. Continuous oxidative stress on a cell could divert energy and reducing equivalents from biosynthetic processes to repair reactions that reduce oxidized cellular components. While it is accepted that free radical reactions and lipid peroxidation do occur in living cells, the degree to which these reactions contribute to the pathology of senescence remains to be determined (Pryor, 1976–1982).

III. ANTIOXIDANT DEFENSE SYSTEMS

Organisms have evolved enzymatic and nonenzymatic systems for scavenging free radicals and destroying potentially harmful products before further damage can occur. These antioxidant systems are compartmentalized and appear to be located near sites of generation of the peroxidative intermediates which they are best suited to nullify. Superoxide dismutases, metalloenzymes requiring copper and zinc or manganese, catalyze the dismutation of the superoxide radical in cytosol and mitochondrial intermembrane space (Fridovich, 1976). Catalase, containing an iron–protoporphyrin complex at its active site, is an important intracellular regulator of hydrogen peroxide located in peroxisomes and microperoxisomes (Chance et al., 1979). Glutathione peroxidase in cytoplasm and mitochondria catalyzes the reduction of hydroperoxides in a process dependent on the availability of dietary sulfur amino acids, glutathione, and selenium (Chance et al., 1979).

Nonenzymatic protection against free radical damage derives primarily from dietary micronutrients. Vitamin E is one of the most important biological free radical quenchers because of its long, hydrophobic isoprenoid side chain, which intercalates into endoplasmic reticulum and mitochondrial membranes, where unsaturated fatty acids are located (Green, 1972). Vitamin C is an effective scavenger of superoxide radicals and is found in high concentrations in the eye and extracellular fluid of the lung (Dubrick et al., 1982). Beta-carotene displays chain-breaking antioxidant behavior in membranes and organelles exposed to low partial pressures of oxygen; carotenoids and retinoids may complement the radical trapping action of vitamin E occurring at high oxygen concentrations (Burton and Ingold, 1984). Ceruloplasmin, a copper-containing protein, is an effective inhibitor of iron-dependent lipid peroxidation and DNA degradation (Gutteridge et al., 1980). Uric acid, present at high levels in blood and saliva, is a strong antioxidant whose concentration is influenced by dietary purines (Ames et al., 1981).

IV. AGE-RELATED ALTERATIONS IN ANTIOXIDANT PROTECTION

One approach taken to examine the free radical theory of aging has been to determine whether any age-related changes occur in cellular antioxidant protective mechanisms. The specific activity and concentration of superoxide dismutase has been found to be inversely correlated with age or longevity in some studies (Reiss and Gershon, 1976; Kellogg and Fridovich, 1976; Bartosz et al., 1978, 1979) but not in others (Ueda and Ogata, 1978; Joenje et al., 1978; Yamanaha and Deamer, 1974; Nohl et al., 1979). Levels of mitochondrial catalase and selenium-dependent glutathione peroxidase activity were found to be higher in old adult compared to young rats (Nohl et al., 1979). Glutathione tissue content has been found to be one-fifth to one-third lower in old mice than in adult animals (Hazelton and Lang, 1980.) Thomson et al. (1977) and Robinson et al. (1979) have described elderly populations with lower blood selenium levels and erythrocyte glutathione peroxidase activity than young adults although they did not establish whether these differences were due to diet or age-related changes. Serum mercaptan concentration decreases by 20% in 80-year-old men compared to 20- to 40-year-old men (Harman, 1960).

Garry et al. (1982) in assessing nutritional status of a healthy elderly population found 25% consumed less than 50% of the Recommended Dietary Allowance (RDA) for tocopherol. Several studies have demonstrated an age-related increase in total serum tocopherol through middle age (Chen et al., 1977; Wei Wo and Draper, 1975; Kelleher and Losowsky, 1978) followed by a decline after age 65 (Wei Wo and Draper, 1975; Barnes and Chen, 1981), which probably reflects similar changes in plasma lipid levels (Horwitt et al., 1972). Although Vatassery et al. (1983) found that platelet vitamin E concentrations decline with age, Underwood et al. (1970) found no age-related change in liver tocopherol concentrations of people who died accidentally. The vitamin E content of most rat tissues increases with age (Weglicki et al., 1969) although some brain regions show decreases with age (Meydani et al., 1985). Lower serum tocopherol levels have been found in aged mice than in young (Meydani et al., 1986a). Many elderly appear to have suboptimal intakes of vitamin C (Bowman and Rosenberg, 1982), i.e., below RDA levels, and several studies have reported an inverse correlation between age and levels of ascorbate in tissue and blood fractions (Schorah, 1979). Andrews et al. (1969) suggested that uptake of vitamin C by white blood cells may be less efficient in the elderly than in the young as they require greater doses to maintain the same ascorbate concentration. Grimble and Hughes (1968) found that old guinea pigs possess lower dehydroascorbic acid reductase activity than young animals.

V. LIFE SPAN MODIFICATION BY
DIETARY ANTIOXIDANTS

A more direct way to test whether free radical reactions contribute to or cause aging is to feed animals antioxidants and examine changes in life span or functional capacity of body systems where age-related changes have been demonstrated, such as the immune system. To date, unequivocal interpretation of existing data from survival studies is not possible. It is critical in longevity studies to separate effects due to prevention of disease from those due to modification of the basic aging process. Life span extension requires the longest-lived survivors to pass beyond the maximum limit reported for the species under optimal conditions. Extending the mean life span (MLS) of the population can be attributed to prevention or curing of disease rather than altering the basic aging rate.

Harman (1957) first attempted to prolong life span by supplementing the natural antioxidant protective mechanisms with chronic dietary administration of ascorbic acid, 2-mercaptoethanol, cysteine HCl, 2-mercaptoethylamine (2-MEA), or 2,2'-diaminodiethyl disulfide HCl. The latter three compounds extended the MLS of the short-lived (7.5-month MLS), lymphatic leukemia-prone AKR mouse strain while none of the antioxidants had an effect on the longer-lived (14.5-month MLS), mammary cancer-prone C3H strain. The antioxidants appeared to "square up" the mortality curve, possibly by delaying the development of leukemia in the AKR mice. Harman (1961) subsequently demonstrated that chronic administration of 2-MEA or hydroxylamine could extend the MLS of C3H mice but not Swiss mice (22-month MLS). Harman (1968) further reported that chronic 2-MEA or butylated hydroxytoluene (BHT) supplementation extended MLS in LAF_1 mice (20-month MLS), a strain with a low tumor incidence.

While Clapp *et al.* (1979) found that BHT increased MLS of the BALB/c mice, Kohn (1971) found no increase in MLS or maximum life span with 2-MEA or BHT treatment in C57 BL mice when care was taken to ensure that the control animals lived as long as possible. Similarly, Harman (1961) could not replicate the MLS extension with 2-MEA in AKR mice when control animals lived longer (9.6-month MLS). Comfort *et al.* (1971) have extended the MLS and maximum life span of C3H mice with ethoxyquin treatment. Injection of cysteine or thiazolidine carboxylic acid has been reported to increase the life spans of mice and guinea pigs but not rats (Oeriu and Vochitu, 1965).

Even the successful antioxidant feeding experiments described above do not show a dramatic effect on the life span of the animals tested. In trying to reconcile this data with the free radical theory of aging, it must be recognized that most of the synthetic antioxidants were developed for industrial uses such as stabilizing rubber or petroleum products. Vitamin E is distributed principally in membrane lipids of endoplasmic reticulum and mitochondria near sites of free radical generation. The synthetic antioxidants are found predominately in the cytosol and nonspecifically distributed in fat and are relatively quickly metabolized and eliminated (Witting, 1980). Tissue levels of the synthetic antioxidants were not measured in most experiments even though they are known to be poorly absorbed. Thus, the limited biologic effect demonstrated by antioxidant feeding experiments may be related to poor absorption, inadequate subcellular distribution, and/or rapid turnover. Moreover, many of the reports indicate moderate to significant weight loss in the treated animals. Caloric restriction is the most effective method of extending life span in laboratory animals (Masoro, 1985), thus the unintentional food restriction which occurred with antioxidant-supplemented diets confounds interpretation of the results. However, it has been proposed that food restriction itself might act to enhance coupling of oxidative phosphorylation to electron transport and thereby reduce free radical generation and lipid peroxidation (Weindruch *et al.*, 1980; Chipalkatti *et al.*, 1983). In studies conducted to date, it appears that antioxidant administration can extend the MLS of laboratory animals only when they have a genetic predisposition to life-shortening diseases or exposure to suboptimal environmental conditions which reduce survival.

Vitamin E, alone or in combination with other antioxidants, has been administered to mice (Tappel *et al.*, 1973; Ledvina and Hodanova, 1980; Blackett and Hall, 1980, 1981), rats (Berg, 1959; Porta *et al.*, 1980), fruit flies (Miguel *et al.*, 1973), rotifers (Enesco and Verdone-Smith, 1980), nematodes (Epstein and Gershon, 1970), human cell cultures (Packer and Smith, 1974, 1977; Sakagami and Yamada, 1977), and fungi (Munkves and Minssen, 1976) in an attempt to extend their longevity. Most of these studies report a reduction in lipofuscin accumulation with vitamin E supplementation. Intracellular lipofuscin, representing the accumulation of lipid peroxide breakdown products from lysosomes and mitochondria, is one of the strongest pieces of evidence that free radical processes occur *in vivo* (Logani and Davies, 1980). However, the majority of these experiments demonstrated only small increases in MLS or survival time and no increase in maximum life span (except with fruit flies and nematodes).

VI. ROLE OF DIETARY ANTIOXIDANTS IN DEGENERATIVE CONDITIONS

Ames (1983) has suggested that cancer and other age-associated degenerative diseases are due to damage to DNA and other macromolecules from oxygen radicals and lipid peroxidation. It has been postulated that many promoters of carcinogenesis, including fat and hydrogen peroxide, share a common ability to generate oxygen radicals and lipid peroxidation (Emerit *et al.*, 1983). Dietary fat also appears to be a major risk factor for heart disease as well as for colon and breast cancer (Correa *et al.*, 1982). Atherosclerotic-like lesions have been produced by injecting rabbits with lipid hydroperoxide or oxidized cholesterol (Yagi *et al.*, 1981). Furthermore, products of oxidative degradation of arachidonic acid, e.g., prostaglandins, have been implicated in the development and pathogenesis of amyloidosis, arthritis, atherosclerosis, and cancer.

Associations have been made between the selenium status of various populations and their incidence of cancer, although most studies lack the strength needed for unequivocal conclusions (Ip, 1985). Studies have also suggested that low selenium levels may be associated with an increased risk of cardiovascular death and myocardial infarction (Salonen *et al.*, 1982). Lipid peroxidation occurs readily in the brain with potential consequences including senile dementia or other brain abnormalities (Harman, 1981). Meydani *et al.* (1985) demonstrated an increased susceptibility of several brain regions of aged rats to lipid peroxidation following oxidant challenge, which was prevented by dietary vitamin E supplementation. Senile cataracts have been associated with light-induced oxidative damage and retinal degeneration occurs with vitamin E/selenium deficiency (Varma *et al.*, 1982; Katz *et al.*, 1982).

VII. ROLE OF DIETARY ANTIOXIDANTS IN IMMUNE FUNCTION

It has been suggested by Harman (1982) that vitamin E and other antioxidants may increase longevity by influencing the immune system and reducing age-related diseases. An immunological basis for many of the age-associated diseases discussed above has been proposed (Walford and Weindruch, 1981).

Age-related functional changes have been defined for both humoral and cell-mediated immune responses. In the cell-mediated response, the decline has been observed both *in vitro* and *in vivo*, primarily in the T-cell limb of the immune system. *In vivo* T-cell-dependent cell-mediated functions such as primary delayed hypersensitivity (Roberts-Thompson *et al.*, 1974; Goodwin *et al.*, 1982), graft versus host reaction (Kay, 1979), and resistance to challenge with syngeneic and allogeneic tumor cells and parasites (Makinodan, 1981) are depressed with age. *In vitro*, the proliferative response of human and rodent lymphocytes to the T-cell mitogens phytohemagglutinin (PHA) and concanavalin A (ConA) and allogeneic target cells is depressed with age (Kay, 1979; Hallgren, *et al.*, 1973; Pisciotta *et al.*, 1967; Inkeles *et al.*, 1977). Several reports indicate that humoral immune responses decrease in old mice (Makinodan *et al.*, 1971; Buckley *et al.*, 1974). In humans an age-dependent drop in serum immunoglobulin levels has been detected (Buckley *et al.*, 1974).

The decline in immune response of the aged has been attributed to intrinsic alterations within the cells (Price and Makinodan, 1972) and extrinsic factors in the milieu of the cells. Inkeles *et al.* (1977) demonstrated that the hyporesponsiveness of lymphocytes from elderly subjects is due both to a reduction in the number of mitogen

(PHA) -sensitive cells and to their less vigorous proliferative response compared to in young people.

Recent studies by Rosenberg *et al.* (1983) indicate that cell–cell interaction and cooperation via lymphokines and other regulatory molecules is impaired in aged mice. Prostaglandin E_2 (PGE_2), formed by oxygenation and subsequent peroxidation of arachidonic acid, is produced by human peripheral blood mononuclear cells and by mouse splenocytes in response to mitogen or antigen stimulation and inhibits subsequent T-cell proliferation (Goodwin and Webb, 1980). *In vitro*, PGE_2 inhibits T-cell proliferation (Goodwin *et al.* 1977), lymophokine production (Gordon *et al.* 1976), and the generation of cytoxic cells (Plant, 1979). Both cellular and humoral immune responses appear to be under negative control by PG. *In vivo* administration of PG synthetase inhibitors enhance delayed hypersensitivity skin test response (Muscoplat *et al.* 1978), secondary antibody response (Goodwin *et al.* 1978), and cytotoxicity (Brunda *et al.* 1980). Goodwin and Messner (1979) demonstrated that PHA-stimulated cultures of peripheral blood mononuclear cells from subjects over 70 years old are more sensitive to inhibition by PGE_2 than are control cultures from young subjects; this sensitivity to PGE_2 did not increase gradually with age but was only apparent in subjects over 70 years old. A positive correlation existed between PGE_2 sensitivity and a depressed response to PHA; the depressed PHA responsiveness was partially reversed by indomethacin, an inhibitor of PG synthesis.

Delfraissy *et al.* (1982) also found that aged lymphocytes display a high sensitivity to the suppressive effect of exogenous PGE_2 and that elimination of radiosensitive T-suppressor cells restores normal T-helper cell function. It has been reported that macrophages from elderly individuals secrete more of the E series PGs than do macrophages from young donors (Rosenstein and Strauser, 1980). Splenocytes from old mice have also been found to have significantly more *ex vivo* synthesis of PGE_2 than those from young mice (Meydani *et al.* 1986a).

The increase in prostanoid synthesis during aging is not limited to PGE_2 nor does it seem to be specific for splenocytes. In our laboratory, lung homogenates from 24-month-old C57BL/J6 mice were found to have significantly greater *ex vivo* syntheses of thromboxane and prostacycline than those from 3-month-old mice (unpublished data). Similarly, in F344 rats there was an age-related increase in PGE_2 synthesis in midbrain although other brain regions showed a decrease in their synthetic ability (Meydani *et al.* 1985). The reasons for this altered prostanoid synthesis are not clear, however, the age-associated increase in lipid peroxidation could be a significant contributing factor. Lands (1984) showed that PG synthetase is regulated by lipid hydroperoxides. Therefore, products of lipid peroxidation could affect the immune system directly or by virtue of their effect on arachidonic acid metabolism.

Tengerdy (1980) reported that chickens given vitamin E significantly increased the generation of anti-sheep red blood cell (SRBC) plaque-forming cells (PFC). Mice fed diets supplemented with vitamin E significantly increased their humoral immune response as measured by PFC and antibody responses to SRBC and tetanus toxoid. Vitamin E deficiency decreased the PFC response to SRBC in mice, an effect restored to normal by vitamin E but not by the antioxidant N-N-diphenyl-P-phenylene diamine. Corwin and Shloss (1980a,b) found that vitamin E supplementation in mice enhanced the proliferative response of lymphocytes to suboptimal doses of ConA and suggested that vitamin E and 2-mercaptoethanolamine are both mitogenic. Pigs supplemented with vitamin E show enhanced proliferation of peripheral blood lymphocytes to PHA (Larsen and Tollersrud, 1981), whereas vitamin E deficiency in dogs decreases the blastogenic response of lymphocytes to ConA (Langweiler et al. 1981). Bendich et al. (1983) reported that low splenic vitamin E levels in spontaneously hypertensive rats (SHR) were correlated with depressed splenic mitogen responses; tocopherol supplementation enhanced immune responsiveness in SHR and normotensive rats. The immunostimulatory effect of vitamin E has been attributed to its inhibition of PG synthesis. Vitamin E has been shown to affect the lipoxygenase and cyclooxygenase pathways of arachidonic acid metabolism (Karpen et al. 1981; Goetzel, 1980).

An increase in average life span of short-lived autoimmune-prone NZB/NZW mice was reported by Harman (1980). Furthermore, vitamin E supplementation of aged C57BL/J6 mice enhanced in vitro mitogenic response of splenocytes to ConA and B-cell mitogen bacterial-derived lipopolysaccharide and improved the delayed hypersensitivity skin test to 2,4-dinitro-1-fluorobenzene (Meydani et al. 1986a). This immunostimulatory effect of vitamin E was associated with a significant decrease in ex vivo synthesis of PGE_2 by splenocytes and an absence of histological signs of kidney amyloidosis. Vitamin E and other antioxidants as well as dietary fish oil decreased production of the 2 series PGs and the severity of experimentally induced amyloidosis (Meydani et al. 1986b; Cathcart et al. 1984).

The effect of other dietary antioxidant micronutrients on age-related immune system decline has not been studied. Nonetheless, vitamin C has been noted to increase the mobility of white blood cells, inhibit their autoxidation, and increase serum levels of immunoglobulins and antibody formation (Prinz et al. 1977; Banic, 1982). Mononuclear leukocytes normally contain the highest levels of ascorbate among the various cellular components of blood regardless of variations in the plasma ascorbate content (Evans *et al.* 1982). Mice receiving selenium supplementation have been found to have greater antibody titer and enhanced primary immune responses to SRBC (Spallholz *et al.* 1975). Selenium deficiency has been associated with decreased function and glutathione peroxidase activity in peritoneal exudate polymorphonuclear neutrophils and pulmonary alveolar and peritoneal exudate macrophages (Serfass and Ganther, 1975, 1976).

VIII. CONCLUSIONS

The age-related accumulation of deleterious free radical reactions and increased rate of lipid peroxidation may contribute to some of the chronic degenerative conditions associated with aging. These peroxidative changes influence arachidonic acid metabolism and autocoid formation, which may in turn contribute to the alterations in immune responsiveness observed in the elderly. Intervention in the aging process through increased intake of dietary antioxidants might be beneficial but further research is necessary to substantiate this hypothesis. Furthermore, peroxidative damage resulting from exposure to environmental pollutants and the increased vulnerability of the elderly to such external insults also suggest that dietary antioxidant allowances for the aged need to be reassessed.

REFERENCES

Ames, B. N. (1983). *Science* **221**, 1256–1265.
Ames, B. N., Cathcart, E., Schwiers, E., and Hockstein, P. (1981). *Proc. Natl. Acad. Sci. U.S.A.* **78**, 6858.
Andrews, J., Letcher, M., and Brook, M. (1969). *Br. Med. J.* **2**, 416–418.
Banic, S. (1982). *Int. J. Vitam. Nutr. Res.* **23**, 49.
Barnes, K. J., and Chen, L. H. (1981). *J. Nutr. Elderly* **1**, 41–49.
Bartosz, G., Tannert, C., Fried, R., and Leyko, W. (1978). *Experientia* **34**, 11–13.
Bartosz, G., Leyko, W., and Fried, R. (1979). *Experientia* **35**, 1193–1194.
Bendich, A., Gabriel, E., and Machlin, L. J. (1983). *J. Nutr.* **113**, 1920–1926.
Berg, B. N. (1959). *J. Gerontol.* **14**, 174–180.
Blackett, A. D., and Hall, D. A. (1980). *Mech. Ageing Dev.* **14**, 305–316.
Blackett, A. D., and Hall, D. A. (1981). *Age Ageing* **10**, 191–195.
Bowman, B. B., and Rosenberg, I. H. (1982). *Am. J. Clin. Nutr.* **35**, 1142–1151.
Brunda, M., Herberman, R. B., and Holden, H. T. (1980). *J. Immunol.* **124**, 2682–2688.
Buckley, C. G., Buckley, E. G., and Dorsey, F. C. (1974). *Fed. Proc., Fed. Am. Soc. Exp. Biol.* **33**, 2034.

Burton, G. W., and Ingold, K. V. (1984). *Science* **224**, 569–573.

Cathcart, E. S., Leslie A., Meydani, S., and Hayes, K. C. (1984). *Am. J. Clin. Nutr.* **39**, 685.

Chance, B., Sies, H., and Boveris, A. (1979). *Physiol. Rev.* **59**, 527–550.

Chen, C. H., Hsu, S. J., Huang, P. C., and Chen, J. S. (1977). *Am. J. Clin. Nutr.* **30**, 728–735.

Chipalkatti, S., De, A. K., and Aiyar, A. S. (1983). *J. Nutr.* **113**, 944–950.

Clapp, N. K., Satterfield, L. C., and Bowles, N. S. (1979). *J. Gerontol.* **34**, 497–501.

Comfort, A., Youhotsky-Gore, I., and Pathmanathan, K. (1971). *Nature (London)* **229**, 254–255.

Correa, P., Strong, J. P., Johnson, W. D., Pizzolato, P., and Haenszel, W. (1982). *J. Chronic Dis.* **35**, 313–316.

Corwin, L. M., and Shloss, J. (1980a). *J. Nutr.* **110**, 916–923.

Corwin, L. M., and Shloss, J. (1980b). *J. Nutr.* **110**, 2497–2505.

Delfraissy, J. F., Galanaud, P., Wallon, C., Balavoine, J. F., Vazgrez, A., and Dormont, J. (1982). *Immunobiology* **163**, 372–373.

Dubrick, M. A., Heng, H. S., and Rucker, R. B. (1982). *Fed. Proc., Fed. Am. Soc. Exp. Biol.* **41**, 943.

Emerit, I., Levy, A., and Cerutti, P. (1983). *Mutat. Res.* **220**, 327–332.

Enesco, H. E., and Verdone-Smith, C., (1980). *Exp. Gerontol.* **15**, 335–338.

Epstein, J., and Gershon, D. (1970). *Mech. Ageing Dev.* **6**, 257–265.

Evans, R. M., Currie, L., and Campbell, A. (1982). *Br. J. Nutr.* **47**, 473–475.

Fridovich, I. (1976) *In* "Free Radicals in Biology" (W. A. Pryor, ed.), Vol. 1, p. 239. Academic Press, New York.

Garry, P. J., Goodwin, J. S., Hunt, W. C., Hooper, E. M., and Leonrd, A. G. (1982). *Am. J. Clin. Nutr.* **36**, 319–331.

Goetzel, E. J. (1980). *Nature (London)* **288**, 183–185.

Goodwin, J. S., and Messner, R. P. (1979). *J. Clin. Invest.* **64**, 434–439.

Goodwin, J. S., and Webb, D. R. (1980). *Clin. Immunol. Immunopathol.* **15**, 106–122.

Goodwin, J. S., Bankhurst, A. D., and Messner, R. P. (1977). *J. Exp. Med.* **146**, 1719–1734.

Goodwin, J. S., Selinger, D. S., Messner, R. P., and Reed, W. P. (1978). *Infect. Immun.* **19**, 430–433.

Goodwin, J. S., Searles, R. P., and Tung, K. S. K. (1982). *Clin. Exp. Immunol.* **48**, 403–410.

Gordon, D., Bray, M. A., and Morley, J. (1976). *Nature (London)* **262**, 401–402.

Green, J. (1972). *Ann. N.Y. Acad. Sci.* **203**, 29–36.

Grimble, R. F., and Hughes, R. E. (1968). *Life Sci.* **7**, 383–386.

Gutteridge, J., Richmond, R., and Halliwell, B., (1980). *FEBS Lett.* **112**, 269–271.

Hallgren, H. M., Buckley, C. E., Gilbertstein, V. A., and Yunis, E. J. (1973). *J. Immunol.* **4**, 1101–1111.

Harman, D. (1956). *J. Gerontol.* **11**, 298–300.

Harman, D. (1957). *J. Gerontol.* **12**, 257–263.

Harman, D. (1960). *J. Gerontol.* **15**, 38–45.

Harman, D. (1961). *J. Gerontol.* **16**, 247–254.

Harman, D. (1968). *J. Gerontol.* **23**, 476–482.

Harman, D. (1980). *Age* **3**, 64–73.

Harman, D. (1981). *Proc. Natl. Acad. Sci. U.S.A.* **78**, 7124–7128.

Harman, D. (1982). *In* "Free Radicals in Biology" (W. A. Pryor, ed.), Vol. 5, pp. 255–273. Academic Press, New York.

Hazelton, G., and Lang, C. (1980). *Biochem. J.* **188**, 25–31.

Horwitt, M. K., Harvey, C. C., Dahm, C. J., and Searey, M. T. (1972). *Ann. N. Y. Acad. Sci.* **203**, 223–236.

Inkeles, B., Innes, J. B., Juntz, M., Kadish, A., and Weksler, M. E. (1977). *J. Exp. Med.* **145,** 1176–1187.

Ip, C. (1985). *Fed. Proc., Fed. Am. Soc. Exp. Biol.* **44,** 2573–2578.

Karpen, C. W., Merola, A., Trewyn, R. W., Cornwell, D. G., and Pangamala, R. V. (1981). *Prostaglandins* **22,** 651–662.

Katz, M. L., Parker, K. R., Handelman, G. J., Bramel, T. L., and Dratz, E. A. (1982). *Exp. Eye Res.* **34,** 339–343.

Kay, M. M. B. (1979). *Mech. Ageing Dev.* **9,** 35–39.

Kelleher, J., and Losowsky, M. S. (1978). In "Tocopherol, Oxygen and Biomembranes" (C. de Duve and O. Hayaishi, eds.), pp. 311–327. Elsevier/North-Holland Biomedical Press, Amsterdam.

Kellogg, E. W., and Fridovich, I. (1976). *J. Gerontol.* **31,** 405–409.

Kohn, R. R. (1971). *J. Gerontol.* **26,** 378–380.

Lands, W. E. M. (1984). In "Icosanoids and Cancer" (H. Thaler-Dao, A. Crastes de Paulet, and R. Paoletti, eds.), pp. 41–48. Raven Press, New York.

Langweiler, M., Schultz, D., and Sheffy, B. E. (1981). *Am. J. Vet. Res.* **42,** 1681–1685.

Larsen, H. J., and Tollersrud, S. (1981). *Res. Vet. Sci.* **31,** 301–305.

Ledvina, M., and Hodanova, M. (1980). *Exp. Gerontol* **15,** 67–71.

Logani, M. K., and Davis, R. E. (1980). *Lipids* **15,** 485–491.

Makinodan, T. (1981). In "Biological Mechanisms in Aging" (R. T. Shimke, ed.), pp. 488–500. U.S. Dep. Agric., Natl. Inst. Health, Washington, D.C.

Makinodan, T., Perkins, E. H., and Chen, M. G. (1971). *Adv. Gerontol. Res.* **3,** 171–198.

Masoro, E. J. (1985). *J. Nutr.* **115,** 842–848.

Meydani, M., Meydani, S. N., Macauley, J. B., and Blumberg, J. B. (1985). *Prostaglandins Leuk. Med.* **18,** 337–346.

Meydani, S. N., Meydani, M., Verdon, C. P., Blumberg, J. B., and Hayes, K. C. (1986a). *Mech. Ageing Dev.* **34,** 191–201.

Meydani, S. N., Cathcart, E. S., Hopkins, R. E., Meydani, M., Hayes, K. C., Blumberg, J. B. (1986b). In "Amyloidosis" (G. G. Glenner, E. P. Osserman, E. Benditt, E. Cokins, A. S. Cohen, and D. Zucker-Franklin, eds.) pp. 683–692. Plenum, New York.

Miguel, J., Binnard, R., and Howard, W. H. (1973). *Gerontologist* **3,** 37.

Munkves, K. D., and Minssen, M. (1976). *Mech. Ageing Dev.* **5,** 79–85.

Muscoplat, C. C., Rakich, P. M., Theon, C. O., and Johnson, P. W. (1978). *Infect. Immun.* **20,** 625–631.

Nohl, H., Hegner, D., and Summer, K. (1979). *Mech. Ageing Dev.* **11,** 145–150.

Oeriu, S., and Vochitu, E. (1965). *J. Gerontol.* **20,** 417–419.

Packer, L., and Smith, J. R. (1974). *Proc. Natl. Acad. Sci. U.S.A.* **71,** 4762–4767.

Packer, L., and Smith, J. R. (1977). *Proc. Natl. Acad. Sci. U.S.A.* **74,** 1640–1641.

Pisciotta, A. V., Westring, D. W., DePrey, C., and Walsh, B. (1967). *Nature (London)* **215,** 193–194.

Plant, M. (1979). *J. Immunol.* **123,** 692–701.

Porta, E. A., Joun, N. S., and Nitta, R. T. (1980). *Mech. Ageing Dev.* **13,** 1–39.

Price, G. B., and Makinodan, T. (1972). *J. Immunol.* **108,** 403–417.

Prinz, W., Bortz, R., Bregin, B., and Hersch, M. (1977). *Int. J. Nutr. Res.* **47,** 248–256.

Pryor, W. A., ed. (1976–1982). "Free Radicals in Biology," Vols. 1-5. Academic Press, New York.

Reiss, V., and Gershon, D. (1976). *Eur. J. Biochem.* **63,** 617–621.

Roberts-Thompson, I. C., Yvonschairjud, V., and Whittingham, S. (1974). *Lancet* **2,** 368–370.

Robinson, M. F., Godfrey, P. J., Thompson, C. D., Rea, H. M., and van Rij, A. M. (1979). *Am. J. Clin. Nutr.* **32,** 1477–1485.

Rosenberg, J. S., Glimn, S. C., and Feldman, J. D. (1983). *J. Immunol.* **130,** 1754–1758.
Rosenstein, M. M., and Strauser, H. R. (1980). *J. Reticuloendothel. Soc.* **27,** 159–166.
Sakagami, H., and Yamada, M. (1977). *Cell Struct. Funct.* **2,** 219–227.
Salonen, J. T., Alfthan, G., Huttunen, J. K., Pikkarainen, J., and Puska, P. (1982). *Lancet* **2,** 175.
Schorah, C. J. (1979). *Int. J. Vitam. Nutr. Res.* **19,** 167–177.
Serfass, R. E., and Ganther, H. E. (1975). *Nature (London)* **255,** 640–641.
Serfass, R. E., and Ganther, H. E. (1976). *Life Sci.* **19,** 1139–1144.
Spallholz, J. E., Martin, J. L., Gerlach, M. L., and Heinzerling, R. H. (1975). *Proc. Soc. Exp. Biol. Med.* **184,** 37–40.
Tappel, A. L., Fletcher, B., and Deamer, D. (1973). *J. Gerontol.* **28,** 415–424.
Tengerdy, R. P. (1980) *In* "Vitamin E: A Comprehensive Treatise" (L. J. Machlin, ed.), pp. 429–445. Dekker, New York.
Thomson, C. D., Rea, H. M., Chapman, O. W., and Robinson, M. F. (1977). *Proc. Univ. Otago Med. Sch.* **55,** 18–19.
Ueda, K., and Ogata, M. (1978). *Acta Med. Okayama* **32,** 393–396.
Underwood, B. A., Seigel, H., Dolinski, M., and Weisell, R. C. (1970). *Am. J. Clin. Nutr.* **23,** 1314–1321.
Varma, S. D., Beachy, N. A., and Richards, R. D. (1982). *Photochem. Photobiol.* **36,** 623–627.
Vattassery, G. T., Johnson, G. J., and Krezowski, A. M. (1983). *J. Am. Coll. Nutr.* **4,** 369–375.
Walford, R. L., Weindruch, R. H. (1981). *Annu. Rev. Gerontol. Geriatr.* **2,** 3–49.
Weglicki, W. B., Luna, Z., and Padmanabhan, P. N. (1969). *Nature (London)* **221,** 185–186.
Weindruch, R. J. H., Cheung, M. K., Verity, M. A., and Walford, R. L. (1980). *Mech. Ageing Dev.* **12,** 375–392.
Wei Wo, C. K., and Draper, H. H. (1975). *Am. J. Clin. Nutr.* **28,** 808–813.
Witting, L. A. (1980). *In* "Free Radicals in Biology" (W. A. Pryor, ed.), Vol. 4, p. 295. Academic Press, New York.
Yagi, K., Ohkawa H., Ohishi, N., Yamashita, M., and Nakashima, T. (1981). *J. Appl. Biochem.* **3,** 58–62.
Yamanaha, N., and Deamer, D. (1974). *Physiol. Chem. Phys.* **6,** 95–98.

Aging Animal Models for the Study of Drug–Nutrient Interactions

Paul M. Newberne

Department of Pathology
Boston University School of Medicine
Boston, Massachusetts

I. INTRODUCTION

The adult human body contains about 10 trillion cells (10^{13}), some of which are incapable of undergoing cell division while others are actively dividing throughout our adult life. Still others retain the ability to divide but multiply rapidly only when tissues are undergoing regeneration usually as a result of having been damaged. There are precise systems that regulate cell division and during our adult life the gross and microscopic anatomy and the function of these systems are preserved in very well-defined and precise ways. As we grow

Nutrition and Aging

older we lose control of some of these regulatory processes and develop diseases associated with aging.

The average human in the United States today has a life span of about 74 years. This has increased dramatically over the past few decades and promises to continue to increase in the coming years. We have largely conquered diseases caused by infectious agents, for the most part a result of the remarkable increase in knowledge about the basic biology of disease and by developing antibiotics, vaccines, and other drugs and chemicals which permit us to prevent or control infections. We are now faced with the degenerative diseases, all of which are associated in one way or another with aging. It has been pointed out that the death rate from all combined causes increases logarithmically with advancing age and the probability of death doubles every eight years after a person reaches physical maturity (Kent, 1976). Despite the fact that there is an enormous range in longevity among various animal species including man, the mortality pattern is essentially the same in all respects.

The various species are born at different stages of maturity and the time at which they reach half-maturity differs. In the human species the mortality curve describes a high death rate during the perinatal period that steadily declines during infancy and youth. Following that there is a progressive increase after maturity. In medically advanced countries where mortality in the perinatal period has been sharply reduced, a high percentage of the people die from diseases associated with middle or old age (Shank, 1975).

The human infant develops very slowly. No other mammal species is helpless for such a long period of time; even rhesus infant monkeys are capable of locomotion after 1 week of age, yet it requires many months for the human infant to develop this ability. In apes, learning to walk takes a few months, a relatively long period, but still much less than the 9-month period in which a human infant is incapable of locomotion. While the infant is incapable of locomotion it has to be transported and there is a limit to the active exploration of its environment. This makes the human infant vulnerable to social deprivation, a well-known risk factor for developmental retardation and psychiatric deviations, and recent evidence suggests greater susceptibility to certain types of organic disease.

Alterations in the immune system are one of the more interesting aspects of aging that differ immensely in experimental animals. The increased incidence of antibodies directed against cell components (Aab) with aging is one of the most easily recognized phenomena in gerontology. An immunological aging theory was developed around Aab.

"Whereas development and maturation would be characterized by an increased ordering of the immunological repertoire, the age-related decline in biological function would start with a disorganization of the immune system resulting in autoaggressive Aab which hastens the aging process" (Walford, 1969). This concept has been further examined in *Mastomys* (*Praomys*) *natalensis*, a species that has been used for a number of years as a possible animal model for age-related Aab (Coolen *et al.*, 1981). The studies by Coolen *et al.* have suggested, in part, that the laboratory-bred *Mastomys* is probably exceptional in that its thymic maturation has an innate defect already at a young age and the T-cell repertoire is not balanced with the B-cell repertoire, a situation that is generally believed to be characteristic of the old immune system (Radl, 1979). This then suggests that the *Mastomys* may or may not be a good animal for the study of aging research particularly as it relates to the immune system. However, it does offer the possibility of testing a number of hypotheses which may lead to a better understanding of nonpathogenic autoantibody formation.

The National Institute of Aging (NIA) was created in May of 1974 with the passage of the Research on Aging Act (PL-93-296). This act designated the NIA as the principal federal agency responsible for studies related to the basic aging processes. The Research on Aging Act called for the development of a research plan on aging. A report entitled "Our Future Selves" outlined the state of aging research at that time and made recommendations for the new institute's research agenda. In 1980 the NIA undertook a comprehensive planning and evaluation project to assess more recent changes in the field and to chart a course for the 1980s. An important part of this evaluation was the animal models development program, and a report from this evaluation set forth a number of interesting developments in the field and is an important document for those engaged in aging research (NIA, 1982). Among other issues, this interesting report points out that one of the initial criteria for choosing animal models for research on aging is convenience. While this has served a purpose in the past it is no longer adequate to use as a criterion for selecting an animal model. Choices must now be made on the basis of other criteria not only for current ongoing work but for the future, that is, for the next ten or more years. Table I lists the two kinds of models which must be considered in approaches to investigation of aging.

This presentation addresses a part of the second category of models, that of drug–nutrient interactions and the relation of such interaction to the aging process.

TABLE I

Animal Models for Aging.

1. Models to study intrinsic aging processes
2. Models to study processes that give rise to diseases associated with aging

II. BASIC ASPECTS OF AGING

All species are affected by a physiological process categorized as aging. The process is associated with increased susceptibility to injury and a decreased capacity to resist or repair those injuries occasioned, to a large exent, by our life-styles (King, 1984). There is a range of life spans (Sachar, 1980) associated with the various species (Table II), with the human surviving longer than others that have been studied.

In all species, with aging there is a series of alterations in organs and tissues. The thymus atrophies, along with a decrease in its input into

TABLE II

Life Spans of Various Species, Estimated in Years

Common name	Recorded life span maximum	Common name	Recorded life span maximum
Human	>90	American Beaver	20
Finback whale	>80	European wild boar	19
Sperm whale	>65	New World Monkeys	<18
Asiatic elephant	70	Guinea pig	7
Orangutan	>50	Pack rat	7
Chimpanzee	>44	Black rat	4
Gray seal	41	House mouse	3
Lowland gorilla	>39	Commercial rat	<2
Giraffe	36	Commercial mouse	<3
Mongolia horse	34	Syrian hamster	<2
Polar bear	34	*Mastomys*	<2
Old World monkeys	33	Rabbits	<7
Gibbon	31		
Bengal tiger	26		
Red deer	26		
Jaguar	23		
Coyote	22		
Beagle dog	<15		
Cats	<15		

immunocompetence; reproductive organs lose functional capacity; also diminished in keenness of response are the endocrine system and central nervous system mechanisms of control which result in homeostasis. This is reflected in degenerative changes in the cardiovascular system, particularly in humans, in the kidney in all species, and in atrophy, compensatory hyperplasia, or hypertrophy in all organs and tissues. This results in structural disorganization of the extracellular components which produces a variety of lesions. There are significant alterations in the capacity of cells to repair DNA damage, to resist the age-related decline in protein synthesis, and, as noted above, to maintain the role of the endocrine and neuroendocrine systems in homeostasis at a high level of efficiency.

The changes associated with aging found in the CNS and endocrine and immune systems are to some extent under genetic control. However, one's life-style can override the genetic aspects related to defense mechanisms and hasten the aging process. Excesses in food, tobacco use, and alcohol consumption all can contribute to shortening of the life span, or to a decrease in the quality of life in the declining years. The use of animal models to probe these areas of concern offers considerable promise in limiting disease and in improving life for the elderly.

III. MAJOR ANIMAL GROUPS FOR RESEARCH ON AGING

Some features of aging are probably unique to humans but others seem to be expressed in a similar or identical fashion by both humans and experimental animals. A number of animal species have been characterized and their advantages and limitations presented with respect to their use as animal models in aging research [National Academy of Sciences/National Research Council (NAS/NRC), 1981]. Table III lists major animal groups and tissue culture systems available for aging research.

Since moral, ethical, and legal constraints prohibit most research on aging in humans, animals must be used as surrogates. Valid information developed through research in various animal species provides a basis for making scientific judgments regarding extrapolation of data from animals to humans.

Choosing an animal model in the past has been based largely on convenience. However, we must now approach the choice of an animal model by examining the relevance and appropriateness of the various species for use in aging research. Costs, complexity of raising and main-

TABLE III

Major Animal Groups and Culture Systems for Research on Aging

Rodents and Lagomorphs	
Mice	Hamsters
Rats	*Mastomys*
Gerbils	White-footed mice
Guinea pigs	Rabbits
Carnivores	
Dogs	
Cats	
Nonhuman Primates	
Apes	
Old World Monkeys	
New World Monkeys	
Prosimians	
Culture Systems	
Tissue explants—lung, bronchus, bladder, kidney <1 year	
Cell cultures—fibroblasts <50 of human, 8 of rodent	

taining old animals, limited availability, and the complex questions being asked by investigators in aging research must now be taken into account when selecting the model. Basic criteria for selecting animals include the following:

1. Comparability of parameter under study to human diseases
2. Life span of the animal
3. Frequency of phenomenon occurring
4. Genetic heterogeneity or homogeneity
5. Background data on animal
6. Unique features of animal (anatomical, physiological)
7. Techniques available for sophisticated research
8. Supply of animals
9. Cost factors
10. Convenience factors

An in-depth discussion on each of the criteria noted above, the advantages of which are readily obvious, can be found in the NAS/NRC monograph "Mammalian Models for Research on Aging" (1981). However, the individual investigator must focus more narrowly on animal models that will examine one or the other of two broad categories, namely, the biology of aging or the pathology of aging, which are clearly different with respect to experimental strategy, methodology, and perspectives on the relationship between aging and disease. While it is important to choose an appropriate species for an individual's research, it seems more significant to analyze, compare, or manipulate relationships across a variety of phylogenetic orders, genera, and species if one is to understand the mechanisms of aging in the broadest sense. For that reason, no recommendations as to model species are made here; instead, selected examples of research results with some of the species are provided and the selection of a model will ultimately depend on a number of factors which in concert satisfy the needs of the investigator as nearly as possible.

To turn now to the main thrust of this paper, the following section provides a brief discussion of human problems in drug–nutrient interactions.

IV. DRUG–NUTRIENT INTERACTIONS IN THE ELDERLY

As defined by Roe (1984), drug–nutrient interactions are "events and outcomes that ensue as a result of physical, chemical, physiological, or physiopathological relationships between drugs and nutrients." Centuries of observations and decades of research into the cause and effect of drug–nutrient interactions have permitted a better understanding of clinically important events which may adversely affect the elderly. Significant improvement in our prediction and understanding, however, await much additional research, much of which of necessity must be done using experimental animals.

A drug–nutrient interaction or its outcome is clinically important when it reduces the intended response to a therapeutic drug, when it causes an acute or chronic drug toxicity, and when it results in impaired nutritional status. Effects of drug–nutrient interactions can then be divided into those which are pharmacological and those which are nutritional. Pharmacological effects include slowed or diminished response to the drug as well as development of an acute incompatibility reaction or drug intoxication. Nutritional effects are secondary to mineral loss, malabsorption, antinutrient properties of the compound, or a change in food intake, any of which may be associated with drug therapy. Many of these phenomena can be addressed by using appropriate animal models. A few illustrations are provided here, related to animal models, to indicate the types of problems encountered in clinical medicine. Selected animal data will then be addressed.

It is well established that foods can influence drug bioavailability through the effects on physicochemical or chemical interactions between drug molecules, nutrients, and other food components. In addition, physiological events in the gastrointestinal compartment also influence the bioavailability of drugs (Melander, 1978; Toothaker and Welling, 1980). Table IV lists some drugs whose absorption may be delayed or reduced by food and those foods which promote absorption. Tetracycline, for example, complexes with calcium, magnesium, iron, and zinc in the gastrointestinal tract to reduce its bioavailability (Cohn, 1961; Mattilla et al., 1972; Dearborn et al., 1957; Neuroven, 1976). Antacids which contain magnesium or aluminum also reduce availability of tetracyclines.

The bioavailability of chlorothiazide is enhanced by food; this may result as a secondary event from a delay in gastric emptying time which delivers the drug at a more appropriate rate to an absorptive site in the small intestine. The same is true for propranolol, perhaps via changes in splanchnic blood flow (Walle et al., 1981). Further examples of effects of food on absorption can be found in Welling (1977) and Roe (1984).

Foods affect drug metabolism in both the gastrointestinal tract and in the liver. Part of this results from altered metabolism of the drug in the liver but much of it derives from first pass metabolism in the gut mu-

TABLE IV

Food and Drug Bioavailability[a]

Drug	Form	Food	Effect
A. Absorption Reduced or Delayed by Food			
Cefaclor	Capsules	Breakfast	Absorption delayed
Cimetidine		Breakfast	Absorption delayed
Digoxin	Tablets	Breakfast	Absorption delayed
Ibuprofen	Capsules	Breakfast	Absorption delayed
Isoniazid	Tablets	Breakfast	Absorption reduced
Levo dopa	Tablets	Protein meal	Absorption reduced
Penicillin G	Suspension	Milk	Absorption reduced
Tetracycline	Capsule	Milk	Absorption reduced
Phenytoin	Suspension	Enteral Formula	Absorption reduced
B. Absorption Promoted by Food			
Chlorothiazide	Tablets	Breakfast	
Dicoumarol	Tablets	Breakfast	
Erythromycin	Suspension	Milk	
Nitrofurantoin	Tablets	Low-fat meal	
Propranolol	—	High-protein meal	

[a] From Welling (1977).

cosa. The sulfation and glucuronidation of salicylamide occur at the level of the gut mucosa and other important conversions of therapeutic agents also occur there (Barr and Riegelman, 1970; George, 1981). Some drugs are modified by intestinal microflora; sulfasalazine undergoes bacterial cleavage of the azo linkage, forming 5-aminosalicylate, the metabolite responsible for the anti-inflammatory action of the drug (Das *et al.*, 1974).

Perhaps the most important dietary effect on drug metabolism in the elderly is the amount of protein consumed. High-protein diets increase the rate of drug metabolism and low-protein diets slow the process. This is likely mediated by the liver mixed function oxidases (Anderson *et al.*, 1982), in which, overall, there is decreased activity in the aged. In addition to protein intake, other factors that modify drug metabolism in the aged include the sulfur-containing amino acids, charcoal-broiled meats, dietary fiber, the types of vegetables that are consumed (brussel sprouts, cabbage), methylxanthine-containing beverages (coffee, tea, cocoa), and the pattern of eating in relation to drug intake.

Thus, there is convincing evidence that drug–nutrient interactions in the elderly are important considerations in managing effective drug therapy and in decreasing the probability of drug toxicity. In all such responses, the liver is central to the manner in which the aged individual can react (Bach *et al.*, 1981).

Other aspects of drug–nutrient interactions in aging need to be dealt with if the elderly are to be adequately nourished, protected from toxic episodes, and effectively treated for age-related diseases (Florini, 1975). There are well-known drug-induced deficiencies of fat-soluble and water-soluble vitamins (i.e., vitamin A and alcohol; vitamin D and anticonvulsants; folate and anticonvulsants; alcohol and antifolates; vitamin B_6, niacin, and isoniazid; riboflavin and chlorpromazine). In addition, there are multifactorial etiologies for mineral depletion in the aged.

V. AGING AND DRUG EFFECTS IN ANIMAL MODELS

The pharmacological effects in aging animals are modified by a number of factors (Table V). These factors result in differences in absorption, binding, metabolism, and excretion of drugs (Bender, 1964, 1967; Bender *et al.*, 1970; Goldberg and Roberts, 1979; Ritchey and Bender, 1977). Table VI lists selected changes associated with aging that can affect pharmacokinetic parameters of drug action, most of which have been collected from studies with rats. Tables VII to IX show the effects of age,

TABLE V

Factors Influencing Pharmacological Effects in
Aging Animals

1. Genetic Factors
2. Environment
3. Nutritional status
4. Age-specific biological characteristics
5. Age-specific pathological characteristics
6. Life expectancy
7. Mean survival time
8. Sex

TABLE VI

Aging Changes That May Affect Pharmacokinetic Parameters of Drug Action[a]

Property	Direction of change	Effect
Gastrointestinal Motility	Decreased	Delayed absorption
Lean/fat body weight	Decreased	Change in drug distribution
Organ weight/body weight	Variable	Change in sensitivity
Body water (extracellular)	Decreased	Change in drug distribution
Binding to plasma proteins	Reduced	Increased free drug
Metabolism by liver	Decreased	Prolonged half-life; less active metabolite
Induction microsomal enzymes	Variable	Rate of metabolism variable

[a] From National Academy of Sciences/National Research Council (NAS/NRC) (1981).

TABLE VII

Age and Species Effects on Action of Atropine[a]

Species	Parameter/response	Effect of age
Dog	Anticholinergic	Sensitivity
Rabbit	Anticholinergic	Sensitivity
Rat	Anticholinergic	Sensitivity
Guinea pig	Anticholinergic	No effect
Human	Heart rate	Rate

[a] From Lasagna (1956), Farner and Verzar (1961), and Bender (1964).

TABLE VIII

Age, Species, and Strain Effects on Action of Barbiturates[a]

Species/strain	Parameter/response	Effect of age
Rat, Wistar	Enzyme induction	Decreased
Rat, CFN	Enzyme induction	No change
Rat, SD	Sleep time	Increased
Human	Sedative effect	Increased
Rat, Wistar	Hypnotic effect	Increased

[a] From Baird et al. (1975).

species, and strain on the action of several classes of drugs. Of possible relevance to these observations is the report of Bolla and Greenblatt (1982), who reported an age-related decline in liver cell protein and transferrin synthesis from 6 to 30 months of age in rats.

Since the liver is central to drug metabolism it is interesting that Nokubo (1985) has observed a sex-related difference in the microviscosity of liver cell plasma membranes, which are thought to be involved with hepatic uptake and release of various substances into plasma. Membrane microviscosity increased progressively with age after 2 months in male Fischer rats but the increase began only after 24 months in females of the same strain. This may explain in part the changes in drug metabolism with age and the sex differences in response to the biliary excretion of a number of endo- and xenobiotics and of bile formation. In addition, Hamm and Knisely (1985) have reported an age-related decline in an endogenous opioid system in rats from 5 to 24 months of age which confirms an effect of age on the neurochemical indexes of the opioid receptor system and the function of these receptors in producing analgesia in response to stimulation. Thus other systems, including the CNS

TABLE IX

Dose–Response Relationship in Rat Strains[a]

Drug	Species/strain	Response	Effect of age
Codeine	Rat, Wistar	Toxicity	No change
Morphine	Rat, Wistar	Toxicity	Decreased
Morphine	Rat, SD	Analgesic	Increased
Amphetamine	Rat, Wistar	Motor activity	Increased

[a] From Bender (1964), Braunlich (1966), and Ziem et al. (1970).

affected by age and by nutritional status, are also influenced by environmental stimuli.

VI. DRUG–NUTRIENT INTERACTIONS IN ANIMAL MODELS

Significant studies about interactions of drugs or chemicals and nutrients in aging animal species are few in number and generally do not address the complex of variables. Three examples of results from studies in our own laboratory are provided here to illustrate (1) an age and protein effect on response to an environmental toxin, (2) protein effects on liver microsomal characteristics, and (3) an interaction between vitamin A, a toxin, and age. Tables X to XII illustrate these interesting interactions and consequences in the rat.

Table X shows the reduction in incidence of tumors induced by aflatoxin B_1 (AFB$_1$) as the dietary protein level was reduced from 20 to 6%. In addition, fewer numbers of animals developed tumors under the same dosing schedule with a delay in dosing until the animals were 1 year old. Some of the year-old rats died during the dosing period and others were clinically ill but survived. This indicates that the older rats were more sensitive to the toxic effects but less so to the carcinogenic effect of AFB$_1$. Fewer in the older groups developed tumors at the end of the 24-month

TABLE X

Influence of Age and Dietary Protein on Response to Aflatoxin B_1

| | | Tumor incidence at 24 months | | | |
| | | AFB$_1$ at 6–9 weeks | | AFB$_1$ at 52–55 weeks | |
Group No.	Dietary treatment (% protein)	No.	%	No.	%
1	20	21/26	80.7	8/15	53.3
2	20[a]	17/28	60.7	6/16	37.5
3	15[a]	10/29	34.4	3/18	16.6
4	10[a]	4/30	13.3	2/16	12.5
5	6	2/27	7.4	2/18	11.1

[a] Pair-fed to 6% protein group. All rats were started on diet at weaning. AFB$_1$ was administered at 25 μg/day for 15 doses at times noted. Three, four, and one rat from groups 1, 3, and 4, respectively, were lost at dosing during 52–55 weeks.

TABLE XI

Influence of Dietary Protein and Age on Liver Microsomal Characteristics and AFB$_1$ Adduct Formation

Component parameter[a]	Age					
	12 months			24 months		
	Dietary protein					
	6	20 pr. fed	20 ad lib.	6	20[b] pr. fed	20 ad lib.
Microsomal protein, mg/g liver	6.8 (±0.49)	10.9 (±0.3)	12.2 (±0.10)	5.7 (±0.51)	8.2 (±0.81)	11.2 (±0.14)
CYT-P-450, nmol/mg protein	0.11 (±0.02)	0.43 (±0.08)	0.40 (±0.03)	0.07 (±0.02)	0.34 (±0.04)	0.35 (±0.06)
P-450 reductase, nmol P-450 reduced, mg/protein per hr	6.7 (±0.09)	16.8 (±0.09)	17.1 (±1.1)	4.7 (±0.07)	—[b]	14.6 (±1.3)
Covalent AFB$_1$ adducts, ng/mg DNA	6.7 (±0.09)	16.8 (±0.09)	17.1 (±1.1)	3.9 (±0.14)	—[b]	18.3 (±1.5)

[a] Six to ten rats per group, assayed in duplicate; for AFB$_1$ adduct studies, [^{3}H]AFB$_1$ and cold AFB$_1$ to S.A. 7 μCi/μmol at dose of 1 mg/kg, killed 6 hr later for assay.
[b] Some rats and some samples were lost and were not available for assay.

holding period. These observations may be criticized because the groups dosed at 12 months had only a further 12-month period to develp tumors after exposure to AFB$_1$, while the groups dosed during the early period had 24 months to respond. Nevertheless, there does appear to be an age–protein interaction that is of consequence in the response to exposure to AFB$_1$ and, perhaps, to other chemicals and drugs.

Table XI lists some interesting data which suggest an age–dietary protein interaction in liver microsomal characteristics and in the covalent binding of AFB$_1$ to DNA. It would appear that dietary protein is directly related to the components of the liver cell responsible for activation of the carcinogen and that advancing age as well as decreasing dietary protein diminished activation and binding of AFB$_1$ to DNA, which could, in part, explain the reduction in incidence of liver tumors.

Table XII lists data from studies with AFB$_1$ and vitamin A in two different age groups. In earlier studies (Newberne and Rogers, 1976) we observed that aflatoxin resulted not only in liver tumors in rats but that vitamin A deficiency was associated in a significant number with colon tumors. In those developing liver tumors only, however, there was a

TABLE XII

Vitamin A Deficiency and Response to AFB_1 in Two Different
Age Groups of Male Rats

Treatment or parameter	12 Weeks[a]	52 Weeks[a]
Liver vitamin A, $\mu g/g$		
Control	54.8 ± 4.8	47.2 ± 7.3
A-Deficient	6.9 ± 0.9	2.8 ± 0.2
LD_{50}, AFB_1 mg/kg[b]		
Control	7.1 (4.8–9.2)	15.3 (10.1–19.8)
A-Deficient	3.8 (3.0–6.1)	9.2 (6.9–13.1)
GSH, $\mu g/g$ liver		
Control	1541 ± 121	962 ± 83
A-Deficient	730 ± 60	448 ± 36
Microsomal protein, $\mu g/g$ liver		
Control	15.9 ± 0.91	13.6 ± 0.82
A-Deficient	14.8 ± 1.13	11.2 ± 0.94
AFB_1–GSH conjugate, nmol/g liver per hr[c]		
Control	0.08 (0.06–0.09)	0.12 (0.05–0.10)
A-Deficient	0.25 (0.06–0.10)	0.22 (0.06–0.09)

[a] Eight to twelve rats per group, on diet 7–8 weeks or 52 weeks prior to evaluation.
[b] LD_{50} with 95% confidence interval.
[c] [^{3}H]AFB_1: 150 μCi; S.A. 40 Ci/mmol, 24 hr prior to sacrifice.

significant reduction in the numbers of vitamin A-deficient rats of both sexes with liver tumors. This suggested a difference in the manner in which the deficient animals handled AFB_1, perhaps via metabolism, and may involve an additional target organ but also modify the susecptibility of the liver to the carcinogen.

Following up on these observations, we found that both liver and colon exhibit AFB_1 binding properties that are different in the vitamin A-deficient rat compared to supplemented controls and that this can be reversed by supplementing with retinol 48 hours prior to exposure to AFB_1 (Suphakarn et al., 1983). We have now extended those studies and, although still in progress, we have interesting data which clearly point to an age-related modification in properties of liver microsomal activities and in other parameters which could be responsible, in part, for variations in drug– or chemical–nutrient interactions. For example, the LD_{50} of AFB_1 increased from about 7 to 15 mg/kg between 12 weeks and 1 year of age, indicating less toxicity with age; vitamin A deficiency reduced the LD_{50} at both periods, suggesting less ability to deal with the toxic aspects of exposure and/or greater sensitivity of the liver to the toxin.

These data point to significant modifications in toxin–nutrient interactions, which changed with age, with apparent detriment to the host.

VII. CONCLUSION

The aging process results in modified capabilities for mammalian systems to deal with infectious and degenerative diseases. It is known that the endocrine and immune systems are markedly affected by aging but less is known about how the aging process affects interactions between drugs, other chemicals, and nutrients. There are a number of animal species which can serve as surrogates for humans and many of these are being used to explore the many facets of aging. One of the more important aspects of aging is that of the disposition of drugs in the aged individual and how this can influence the therapeutic efficiency or the toxicity of compounds needed to alleviate age-related diseases. It is clear that foods can either enhance or inhibit the absorption and the excretion of drugs. Moreover, the bioavailability of drugs, once consumed, can be modified by foods, presumably through effects on physicochemical or chemical interactions between drug molecules, nutrients, or other food components. In addition, physiological events in the gastrointestinal tract also influence bioavailability of drugs.

Foods and nutrients also influence drug metabolism in both the gastrointestinal tract and the liver. Microflora in the gastrointestinal tract influence drugs in a number of ways, by cleavage of the parent molecule to an active form or through other mechanisms. Dietary nutrients affect the metabolism of drugs. For example, as a general phenomenon, a high-protein diet enhances the metabolism of drugs whereas a low protein diet inhibits or slows the process. Much of this effect is mediated via the liver mixed function oxidase system, a system that generally decreases in activity with age.

There are numerous examples where drugs influence nutritive status in the elderly but little is known about mechanisms. This paper describes some examples and discusses selected aspects of a rapidly emerging, important field in the nutrition of the elderly, some of which can be examined in animals models.

ACKNOWLEDGMENTS

This work was supported in part by USDHHS-ES00597, EYO3126, CA32520, CA26731, AM32959, and grants from the Merrell–Dow and Hoffmann–LaRoche Pharmaceutical Companies.

REFERENCES

Anderson, K. E., Conney, A. H., and Kappas, A. (1982). *Nutr. Rev.* **40**, 161–170.

Bach, B., Hausen, J. M., Kampmann, J. P., Rasmussen, S. N., and Skovsted, L. (1981). *Clin. Pharmacokinet.* **6**, 389–396.

Baird, M. B., Nicolosi, R. J., Massie, H. R., and Samis, H. V. (1975). *Exp. Gerontol.* **10**, 89–99.

Barr, W. H., and Riegelman, S. (1970). *J. Pharm. Sci.* **59**, 164–168.

Bender, A. D. (1964). *J. Am. Geriatr. Soc.* **12**, 114–134.

Bender, A. D. (1967). *J. Am. Geriatr. Soc.* **15**, 68–74.

Bender, A. D., Kormendy, C. G., and Powell, P. (1970). *Exp. Gerontol.* **5**, 97–129.

Bolla, R. I., and Greenblatt, C. (1982). *Age* **5**, 72–79.

Braunlich, H. (1966). *Acta Biol. Med. Ger.* **16**, 178–186.

Cohn, K. W. (1961). *Nature (London)* **191**, 1156–1158.

Coolen, J., Solleveld, H. A., van Rossum, A. L., and Zurcher, C. (1981). *Clin. Immunopathol.* **19**, 238–244.

Das, K. M., Eastwood, M. A., McManus, J. P. A., and Sircus, W. (1974). *Scand. J. Gastroenterol.* **9**, 137–141.

Dearborn, E., Litchfield, J. T., Eisner, H. J. *et al.* (1957). *Antibiot. Med.* **4**, 627–641.

Farner, D., and Verzar, F. (1961). *Experientia* **17**, 421–422.

Florini, J. R. (1975). *Exp. Aging Res.* **1**, 137–144.

George, C. F. (1981). *Clin. Pharmacokinet.* **6**, 259–274.

Goldberg, P. B., and Roberts, G. (1979). *Proc. Int. Congr. Gerontol., 11th, 1978* Abstr., p. 88.

Hamm, R. J., and Knisely, J. S. (1985). *J. Gerontol.* **40**, 268–274.

Kent, J. (1976). *J. Geriatr.* **31**, 128–134.

King, D. W. (1984). *In* "Modern Aging Research, Comparative Pathobiology of Major Age-Related Diseases" (D. G. Scarpelli and G. Migaki, eds.), Vol. 4, pp. 3–18. Liss, New York.

Lasagna, L. (1956). *J. Chronic Dis.* **3**, 567–574.

Mattila, M. J., Neuroven, P. J., Golhoni, G., and Hackman, C. R. (1972). *Int. Congr. Ser—Excerpta Med.* **254**, 128–133.

Melander, A. (1978). *Clin. Pharmacokinet.* **3**, 337–351.

National Academy of Sciences/National Research Council (NAS/NRC) (1981). "Mammalian Models for Research on Aging." Inst. Lab. Anim. Resour., Assembly Life Sci., Natl. Acad. Press, Washington, D. C.

National Institute on Aging (NIA) (1982). "Animal Models Development Program," Report of the Panel Evaluation of the National Institute on Aging. U.S. Dep. Health Hum. Serv., Natl. Inst. Health/Natl. Inst. Aging, Bethesda, Maryland.

Neuroven, P. J. (1976). *Drugs* **11**, 45–54.

Newberne, P. M., and Rogers, A. E. (1976). *In* "Fundamentals in Cancer Prevention" (P.N. Magee, S. Takayama, T. Sugimura, and T. Matsushima, eds.), pp. 15–39. Univ. of Tokyo Press, Tokyo.

Nokubo, M. (1985). *J. Gerontol.* **40**, 409–414.

Radl, J. (1979). *Clin. Immunol. Immunopathol.* **14**, 251–256.

Ritchey, D. P., and Bender, A. D. (1977). *Annu. Rev. Pharmacol. Toxicol.* **17**, 49–65.

Roe, D. A. (1984). *In* "Toxicology: Determinants of Susceptibility and Predictability" (M. W. Anders and R. G. Carlson, eds.), pp. 109s–122s. Williams & Wilkins, Baltimore, Maryland.

Sachar, G. A. (1980). *Adv. Pathobiol.* **7**, 21–28.

Shank, R. E. (1975). *In* "Epidemiology of Aging" (A. M. Arstfeld and D. C. Gibson, eds.), DHEW Publ. No. 75-711, pp. 199–213. U.S. Department of Health, Education and Welfare, Washington, D.C.

Suphakarn, V., Newberne, P. M., and Goldman, M. (1983). *Nutr. Cancer* **5**, 41–50.

Toothaker, R. D., and Welling, P. G. (1980). *Annu. Rev. Pharmacol. Toxicol.* **20**, 173–179.

Walford, R. L. (1969). "The Immunologic Theory of Aging." Munksgaard, Copenhagen.

Walle, T., Fagan, T. C., Walle, U. K., Olxmann, M. J., Conradi, E. C., and Gaffney, T. E. (1981). *Clin. Pharmacol. Ther.* **30**, 790–795.

Welling, P. G. (1977). *J. Pharmacokinet. Biopharm.* **5**, 291–334.

Ziem, M., Caper, H., Broermann, G., and Strauss, S. (1970). *Naunyn-Schmiedebergs Arch. Pharmakol.* **267**, 208–223.

10

Biochemical Assessment of Vitamin Status in the Elderly: Effects of Dietary and Supplemental Intakes

Philip J. Garry and William C. Hunt

Department of Pathology
Clinical Nutrition Laboratory
University of New Mexico School of Medicine
Albuquerque, New Mexico

I. INTRODUCTION

There is currently no consensus on the vitamin requirements of the elderly. While overt vitamin deficiencies are rare, it has been suggested that "subclinical" deficiency states

117

Nutrition and Aging

may contribute to health problems such as dementia and chronic diseases of the aged. Some research has led to the suggestion that correction of hypovitaminosis can improve mental health status (Fleming, 1982; Goodwin *et al.*, 1983; Broatlehurst *et al.*, 1968), but such evidence is sparse.

The primary reason for interest in subclinical vitamin deficiency conditions in the elderly is the general decline in food intake, and intake of essential nutrients, with advancing age. Decline in physical activity and a lowered metabolic rate with advancing age may account for this observed decline in food intake (Durnin and Passmore, 1967). Economic conditions, educational level, and changes in life-style can influence the amount and type of foods eaten (O'Hanlon *et al.*, 1983). Chronic illness and age-related changes in digestion of food and in absorption, metabolism, utilization, and excretion can also affect vitamin status in the elderly (Balacki and Dobbins, 1974).

Both dietary analysis and biochemical measures have been used to assess the nutritional status of populations. Assessment of dietary intake has been a primary source of nutritional information on elderly populations. Difficulty in obtaining accurate estimates of intake and inability of intake data to account for variations in absorption of nutrients limit the usefulness of dietary information. Biochemical measures can corroborate the information obtained through dietary assessment as well as taking into account potential problems in absorption. However, biochemical assessment is generally limited to the analysis of specific micronutrients, such as vitamins. In this paper, we give a brief background on both dietary and biochemical measures of nutrition and present data of both types from an elderly population in New Mexico.

II. DIETARY INTAKE MEASUREMENTS

Dietary intakes of older persons have been estimated by a number of different methodologies which are designed to determine usual or habitual dietary intakes of individuals. These include dietary histories, food records, and 24-hour dietary recalls. Dietary history methods are primarily designed to estimate the habitual food intake over a long period of time ranging from one week to several months and in some instances up to one year. As pointed out by Mahalko *et al.* (1985), the subjectivity involved in describing a usual eating pattern makes the dietary history method vulnerable to memory lapses and psychological tendencies to exaggerate or minimize self-described behavior. Food record methodology requires an individual to record all foods eaten over a specified period of time, generally from a few days to one week. Unlike dietary history methodology, which requires a trained interviewer, the burden is placed on the subject to provide accurate intake information. This requires that the individual be highly motivated, especially if required to keep records for several days. There may also be a tendency to alter eating behavior during the record-keeping period in order to make the task easier (Garry *et al.*, 1985). Thus the dietary data may not accurately reflect usual intakes. The 24-hour dietary recall methodology also requires a trained interviewer and has been used successfully in large population surveys such as the first and second National Health and Nutrition Examination Surveys (NHANES). The major advantage of this methodology is the minimum amount of interviewer and subject time required to complete the intake recall. A major disadvantage of this technique, especially when used with elderly individuals, is the subjects' ability to accurately remember the food items and amounts eaten the previous day.

When estimating the usual or typical diet from the dietary intakes of a sample of daily observations, either by food record or recall, the error is from two sources. The first source of error is inaccuracy in the measurement of the dietary intake for a particular day. This can result from error in estimating quantities or the omission (or inclusion) of entire food items. The magnitude of this error is increased by incomplete or inaccurate knowledge of the nutrient content of the foods actually consumed. The second source of error is the use of a small sample of days to estimate the usual intake. In theory this error can be minimized or eliminated by use of a large enough sample. However, practical considerations make this impossible and error from this source can be considerable.

The effects of errors in estimating dietary intake are several. If the error is biased, that is, not centered about zero, the distributions of nutrient intake will be shifted and suggest intakes that are either too large or too small. It may be reasonable to assume that the error is unbiased from some sources, such as estimating quantities, but for other sources there is almost certainly bias. For example, incomplete information on the nutrient composition of foods biases the estimates of intake toward quantities less than those actually consumed. If the sample of days from which the usual intake is estimated is not random, the error from this source may also be biased. For example, intakes on weekends can be higher than on weekdays and the failure to include weekend days can lead to underestimating usual intake. Finally, the magnitude and bias of the error can differ for different nutrients.

Any amount of error, even if there is no bias, will increase the observed variance of nutrient intake in the population above the true variance. This will lead to overestimates of the proportions of the population in the extremes of the distribution, quite frequently the population segments of primary interest. Second, measurement error will cause observed statistical associations of nutrient intake with other factors to be lower than the true associations, with a subsequent loss in power for statistical tests (Liu *et al.*, 1978).

Despite these problems, dietary information can be reasonably accurate for some macronutrients. For example, the approximate energy content of foods is generally known and underestimation of daily energy intake is not a problem as long as reasonably accurate food records or recalls can be obtained. The error of measurement of energy intake (protein, fat, carbohydrate) has a variance that is about equal in magnitude to the true population variance in usual energy intake (Hunt *et al.*, 1983). This means that the observed population variance in energy intake, based on a one-day diet record, is twice the true variance. Similarly, it is only $1\frac{1}{3}$ times the true variance for a three-day record, and in this case the standard deviation is inflated by about 15%. This leads to only modest overestimations of the numbers of individuals in the tails of the distribution. Similarly, correlations of energy intake with other factors are only slightly diminished. For some macronutrients, however, the variance of the error can be three or four times the actual variance of the nutrient intake in the population and the consequences of estimating usual intake from a three-day record can be much worse. Dietary cholesterol and vitamin B_{12} intake are examples of nutrients where the error of measurement appears to be large.

In summary, it is probably necessary to view most estimates of the proportion of the population with intakes below (or above) a critical value in the tail of the distribution as being somewhat exaggerated, especially when based on only a few days of diet records or recall. Similarly, observed correlations of dietary intake with biochemical measures are probably smaller than the true correlations.

III. VITAMIN MEASUREMENTS

The use of analytical biochemical techniques to assess vitamin status of individuals and populations has undergone dramatic changes in the past 20 years. Most of these changes are related to improved instrumentation such as high-performance liquid chromatography (HPLC), which has been employed to measure plasma retinol, α-tocopherol, and β-carotene. Another area of improvement has been the development of functional enzyme assays of vitamin status. An example of a functional enzyme assay is the glutathione reductase assay (NADPH: oxidized glutathione oxidoreductase; EC 1.6.4.2) for assessment of riboflavin status. Glutathione reductase is one of two erythrocyte enzymes that requires flavin adenine dinucleotide (FAD) as a coenzyme. The ratio of enzyme activity (with FAD/without FAD) is termed the activity coefficient (AC) and the erythrocyte glutathione reductase activity coefficient (EGR-AC) has been used successfully in a number of recent studies.

For most biochemical determinations, there are usually a number of procedures to choose from including the type of instrumentation. It is not always apparent whether a published procedure for a particular vitamin will provide accurate and useful data unless one has complete familiarity with all aspects of the assay.

An example of faulty analytical methodology can be demonstrated by the choice of methods used to measure serum vitamin A levels. With the introduction of inexpensive fluorometers in the early 1960s there was a movement away from the colorimetric methods used to measure serum vitamin A concentrations, primarily because of the toxic chromogens used in the assay (Garry, 1981). The major problem with one of the more popular fluorometric assays to appear in the literature (Hansen and Warwick, 1968) was that it was not specific for vitamin A. This procedure required only that the serum be extracted with an organic solvent and the extract excited at a specific wavelength and the fluormetric emission measured at a longer wavelength. The upper range of normal by this fluorometric procedure was approximately 200 μg/dl as compared to 70 μg/dl by the standard Carr–Price colorimetric assay. These differences in normal ranges led to a considerable amount of confusion when investigators tried to compare results between studies and the interpretation of results within a single study (Garry, 1975). Thompson *et al.* (1971) later found that serum contained variable amounts of phytofluene, which has fluorescence characteristics very similar to those of retinol. Phytofluene, a conjugated, long-chain hydrocarbon ($C_{40}H_{62}$), is widely found in vegetables, especially in tomatoes. Thus, even very slight contamination of serum by phytofluene will give biased results for serum vitamin A levels when measured with the fluorometric assay of Hansen and Warwick.

A related problem is the lack of standardized methodology, especially for the functional enzyme assays. For example, the erythrocyte glutathione reductase (EGR) assay requires for substrates oxidized glutathione and NADPH as well as the coenzyme flavin adenine dinucleotide in the reaction mixture. The activity of this enzyme is dependent not only on the sequence of substrate and coenzyme addition to the erythrocyte hemolysate (Beutler, 1969) but on the concentration of FAD required to activate the apoenzyme (Garry and Owen, 1976). In published manual procedures, concentrations of FAD used to stimulate EGR range from 1.0 to 10 μmol/liter (Beutler, 1969; Nichoalds et al., 1974; Vo-Khactu et al., 1976). However, final concentrations of FAD in the EGR reaction greater than 5.0 μmol/liter have been shown to inhibit the reaction if very little apoenzyme is present. As a consequence, EGR-ACs less than 1.0 are often found in studies in which riboflavin nutriture is adequate. In other words, a concentration of 10.0 μmol/liter FAD may be needed to maximally activate unsaturated enzymes in vitro, but this concentration of FAD inhibits enzyme which is already saturated by FAD resulting in an AC less than 1.0. This inhibitory effect of FAD is negated in the automated procedure (Garry and Owen, 1976) by preincubating the erythrocyte hemolysates with high concentrations of FAD followed by the subsequent reduction of FAD concentration to approximately 1.0 μmol/liter during the assay.

Because of the lack of a standardized methodology it is not surprising that there has been some disagreement regarding normal values for EGR-ACs. Tillotson and Baker (1972) suggested that a normal AC range should extend from 0.90 to 1.30, while Glatzle et al. (1970) and Vo-Khactu et al. (1976) suggested that the normal range for human adults was between 0.90 and 1.20. In the automated procedure mentioned above, the normal range was determined to be between 1.00 and 1.35. Frequently readers, and sometimes investigators themselves, are not aware of the existence of such variation in procedure. This can result in improper comparison of data from different studies examining vitamin status in populations. For example, a recent study (Mahalko et al., 1985) examining riboflavin status in a group of healthy elderly individuals used an AC of 1.2 as the upper range of normal and made reference that, in a similar study of riboflavin status in healthy elderly, Garry et al. (1982a) found a substantial number of elderly subjects with AC values over 1.20. This comparison is not valid and is misleading because of differences in normal ranges between the manual and automated methods used in these two separate studies.

Sample preparation is also important in assuring accurate determination of vitamin levels. For example, if serum ascorbic acid is to be measured by the dichlorophenolindophenol method (Garry et al., 1974), the sample must be treated soon after collection. Ascorbic acid is very labile and is easily oxidized to dehydroascorbic acid when plasma is separated from whole blood. If the plasma is not treated within 10 minutes with meta-phosphoric acid, the results obtained will be biased on the low side. It is also imperative that individuals be in a fasting state (12 hours or longer) for serum ascorbic acid levels to be free of influence from recent intakes of vitamin C. After a meal containing ascorbic acid, blood levels of ascorbic acid peak at around 3 hours and can remain elevated for up to 12 hours before returning to a steady-state level. If this fact is not realized, the values can be spuriously high and therefore misleading.

Given the correct methodology, accurate estimates of vitamin concentrations in the blood are possible to obtain, and one can further reduce any error of measurement by replicate determinations. This is an advantage over assessment of nutritional status by dietary measures.

IV. VITAMIN ASSESSMENT IN A HEALTHY ELDERLY POPULATION

A. Study Description

The data presented in this section were obtained from healthy elderly residents from the Albuquerque, New Mexico, area who were recruited in 1979 for a study entitled "A prospective study of nutrition in the elderly." Entrance to the study was limited to persons over the age of 60 years with no known medical illnesses and no prescription medication (other than occasional hypnotic, laxative, or analgesic). Subjects' ages ranged from 60 to 93 years and the median age in 1980 for both males and females was 72 years. Entrance was not limited to any ethnic group but all volunteers were Caucasian; only 3% were of Hispanic origin. More than 40% had college degrees. For a more complete description of the population the reader is referred to a previous publication (Garry *et al.*, 1982b).

Since 1980, volunteers were seen once each year as outpatients in the Clinical Research Center at the University of New Mexico Hospital. After an overnight fast, the volunteers came to the clinic for a complete physical examination. Approximately 50 ml of heparinized blood was obtained for various biochemical measurements. Dietary intakes were assessed from 3-day food records collected during 3 successive weekdays immediately following the annual examinations. The dietary and biochemical data as well as supplemental information in this report were collected in 1980 for folate and B_{12} and in 1981 for vitamins A, B_2, C, and E. In 1980 there were 124 men and 145 women; in 1981 there were 113 men and 141 women.

B. Dietary Intakes

Table I gives the mean and standard deviation (STD) as well as the median, 25th (Q_1) and 75th (Q_3) percentile values for dietary intakes of vitamins C, B_2, B_{12}, folic acid, A, and E. The mean and median intakes for these vitamins, with the exception of folic acid and vitmain E, are above the recommended dietary allowances (RDA) for these vitamins.

The low intake of folate raises a question about the adequacy of folate nutriture in this population. The data become less alarming considering the current state of knowledge about the folic acid content of food. Folate values were available for less than 40% of the 2400 food items on our computerized nutrient data base. Data were relatively complete for some food groups, such as beef and pork. For other groups—poultry, fruit, vegetables and legumes, breads and cereals—a substantial amount of information was missing. Therefore our estimates of folate intake are lower than the true intakes. It has been suggested that the RDA for folic acid (400 μg/day) may be higher than is necessary for healthy elderly persons (Rosenberg et al., 1982). In support of this suggestion, Milne et al. (1983) found that 200 $\pm$ 68 μg/day appeared to be adequate for the maintenance of folate stores in adult males.

Even though it appears that dietary vitamin E intakes in this population are on the low side, the current state of knowledge about vitamin E

TABLE I

Dietary Intakes of Vitamins in Albuquerque Elderly

Vitamin	Mean	STD	Q_1	Median	Q_3	RDA
			Men			
C (mg)	133	67.9	89	122	162	60 mg
B_2 (mg)	1.9	0.9	1.4	1.8	2.3	1.4 mg
B_{12} (μg)	4.5	4.9	2.3	3.2	4.8	3.0 μg
Folic acid (μg)	260	130	160	230	330	400 μg
A (IU)	8,853	7,390	4,515	7,061	10,819	5000 IU
E (mg)	7.5	5.6	3.4	6.4	10.5	10 mg
			Women			
C (mg)	123	62.9	78.5	113	157	60 mg
B_2 (mg)	1.5	0.6	1.0	1.3	1.7	1.2 mg
B_{12} (μg)	4.9	7.8	2.0	2.5	4.1	3.0 μg
Folic acid (μg)	230	120	160	210	270	400 μg
A (IU)	7,742	6,649	3,702	5,932	8,604	4000 IU
E (mg)	7.4	5.0	3.2	6.6	10.1	8 mg

content of foods is limited and therefore the intakes are biased on the low side.

In general, the median dietary intake of all vitamins noted in Table I shows that men had larger dietary intakes of vitamins than women. This finding reflects the differences between men and women in total caloric intake.

C. Supplemental Intakes

Table II gives the percentage of elderly taking various vitamin supplements along with the mean, STD, median, and the 25th (Q_1) and 75th (Q_3) percentile intake values.

Supplementary vitamin C was taken by the greatest proportion of the elderly even though more than 90% of them received at least 100% of the RDA from diet alone. Median supplemental intake ranged from a high of more than 50 times the RDA for vitamin E (women) to an amount equal to the RDA in the case of folic acid. Analysis showed little statistical difference in dietary intake for those individuals taking a vitamin supplement when compared to those who did not take supplements.

In summary, we found that 31% were ingesting a daily multivitamin

TABLE II

Supplemental Intakes of Vitamins in Albuquerque Elderly

Vitamin	Mean	STD	Q_1	Median	Q_3	Percentage taking supplements
			Men			
C (mg)	608	530	200	500	937	60.1
B_2 (mg)	14.5	17.1	2.6	10	17.5	46.9
B_{12} (μg)	20.9	31.6	5.0	6.0	16.5	42.7
Folic acid (μg)	320	190	100	400	400	31.9
A (IU)	9,743	7,181	5,000	10,000	10,000	46.0
E (mg)	278	307	25	200	415	55.8
			Women			
C (mg)	810	1241	200	500	993	59.6
B_2 (mg)	18.8	22.2	2.0	10	26	50.4
B_{12} (μg)	27.9	43.2	5.0	6.0	35.5	45.5
Folic acid (μg)	340	220	100	400	400	32.6
A (IU)	11,874	10,206	5,000	10,000	15,000	45.4
E (mg)	384	454	30	400	430	49.7

preparation, and approximately 95% of these individuals were also taking one or more additional vitamin and/or mineral supplements.

D. Biochemical Measurements

Blood samples were obtained from these elderly volunteers following an overnight fast. It should be stressed that the dietary food records were collected during the 3 days after blood samples. This juxtaposition of diet and biochemical measurements is of some importance when viewing the relationship of diet and biochemical assessment of vitamin status.

Plasma ascorbic acid measurements were performed by an automated 2,6-dichlorophenolindophenol procedure (Garry *et al.*, 1974). The biochemical measure of riboflavin status was determined by the *in vitro* response of erythrocyte enzyme glutathione reductase (NADPH$_2$: glutathione oxidoreductase; EC 1.6.4.2) to the addition of flavin adenine dinucleotide. The ratio of glutathione reductase activity with added coenzyme (FAD) to that without is defined as the erythrocyte glutathione reductase activity coefficient. The greater the EGR-AC, the greater the deficiency. Samples were assayed by the automated method of Garry and Owen (1976) and the normal range of EGR-ACs by this procedure is 1.00 to 1.35.

Plasma and erythrocyte folate and vitamin B$_{12}$ levels were determined by a simultaneous radioassay kit purchased from Becton-Dickinson Immunodiagnostics, Orangeburg, N. Y. A more complete description of these assays can be found in a previous publication (Garry *et al.*, 1984). Plasma vitamin A (retinol) and vitamin E (α-tocopherol) levels were determined by high-performance liquid chromatography according to the procedure published by Biere *et al.* (1979). This procedure allows for simultaneous determination of retinol and α-tocopherol from a single hexane extraction of plasma and utilized retinyl acetate as an internal standard.

Tables III and IV show the results for all biochemical measures of vitamin status. These are given separately for those men (Table III) and women (Table IV) taking and not taking a supplement for the particular vitamin. The percentage of men and women taking vitamin supplements is noted in Table II. With the exception of plasma retinol levels, all biochemical measures of vitamin status in both men and women were significantly increased in those taking supplements in comparison with those not taking supplements. It should be remembered that there is an inverse relationship between riboflavin intake and EGR-ACs. Women who were not taking supplements tended to have biochemical measures

TABLE III

Biochemical Measures of Vitamin Status in Men According to Use of Supplements

Vitamin	Mean	STD	Q_1	Median	Q_3
	No Supplement				
C^a (mg/dl)	0.95	0.37	0.77	1.14	1.19
B_2 (EGR-AC)	1.14	0.07	1.09	1.14	1.19
$B_{12}{}^b$ (pg/ml)	476	177	331	460	600
Folate^c (ng/ml)	5.38	2.08	3.75	5.20	6.60
Folate^d (ng/ml)	277	117	192	260	319
A^e (μg/dl)	59.9	12.9	50.5	56.0	70.0
E^f (mg/dl)	1.08	3.28	8.66	1.04	1.28
	Supplement				
C^a (mg/dl)	1.33	0.36	1.13	1.30	1.44
B_2 (EGR-AC)	1.07	0.06	1.03	1.06	1.09
$B_{12}{}^b$ (pg/ml)	659	325	490	578	807
Folate^c (ng/ml)	7.46	2.50	5.22	6.95	9.17
Folate^d (ng/ml)	423	168	323	393	508
A^e (μg/dl)	65.6	13.3	54.5	64.0	75.5
E^f (mg/dl)	1.80	6.85	1.34	1.63	2.12

^{a} Plasma ascorbic acid.
^{b} Plasma true cobalamin.
^{c} Plasma folate.
^{d} Erythrocyte folate.
^{e} Plasma retinol.
^{f} Plasma α-tocopherol.

of vitamin status that were equal to or greater than those seen in men. This unexplained finding is interesting considering that men had higher dietary intakes of vitamins.

E. Relationships between Total Intake and Biochemical Measures of Vitamin Levels

Table V shows the correlations between total intake (diet plus supplement) and biochemical measures for each of the vitamins examined. In most cases the relation between intake and blood level is not linear; therefore, we applied transformations to diet or biochemical measures or both to linearize the relationship before we computed the correlations.

The relationship of total daily intake of ascorbic acid and plasma concentration is shown in the scatter plot of Fig. 1. Two things are evident

TABLE IV

Biochemical Measures of Vitamin Status in Women According to Use of Supplements

Vitamin	Mean	STD	Q_1	Median	Q_3
	No Supplement				
C^a (mg/dl)	1.17	0.36	1.00	1.24	1.31
B_2 (EGR-AC)	1.15	0.09	1.10	1.14	1.18
$B_{12}{}^b$ (pg/ml)	551	229	405	515	660
Folate^c (ng/ml)	5.58	2.61	4.00	5.00	6.60
Folate^d (ng/ml)	298	132	210	271	350
A^e (μg/dl)	57.9	11.6	48.7	56.0	65.2
E^f (mg/dl)	1.20	2.42	1.06	1.22	1.37
	Supplement				
C^a (mg/dl)	1.53	0.39	1.28	1.46	1.68
B_2 (EGR-AC)	1.07	0.05	1.03	1.05	1.08
$B_{12}{}^b$ (pg/ml)	749	398	460	600	1050
Folate^c (ng/ml)	8.60	2.91	6.82	8.20	10.15
Folate^d (ng/ml)	435	196	296	401	565
A^e (μg/dl)	62.0	12.2	53.5	58.0	72.0
E^f (mg/dl)	1.92	5,51	1.44	1.82	2.28

[a] Plasma ascorbic acid.
[b] Plasma true cobalamin.
[c] Plasma folate.
[d] Erythrocyte folate.
[e] Plasma retinol.
[f] Plasma α-tocopherol.

TABLE V

Correlations of Biochemical Measures with Total Intake (Diet Plus Supplements, $N = 254$)

Biochemical measure	r
Plasma ascorbic acid	0.59
EGR-AC	−0.55
Plasma true cobalamin	0.45
Plasma folate	0.50
Erythrocyte folate	0.49
Plasma retinol	0.13
Plasma α-tocopherol	0.64

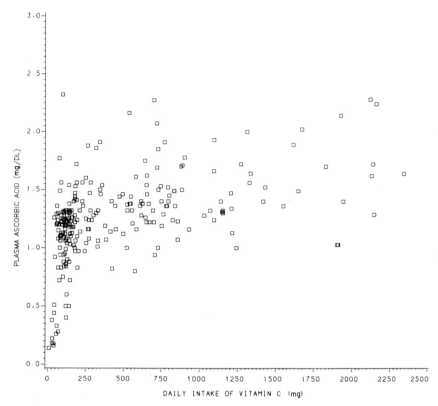

Fig. 1. Plasma ascorbic acid versus estimated total daily intake of vitamin C (diet plus supplement) (N=254).

from this plot. First, all eleven individuals who had low plasma ascorbic acid levels (<0.4 mg/dl) also had intakes of vitamin C below 92 mg. Of these eleven individuals all but three were males. As noted in Section IV,D, men had significantly lower plasma ascorbic acid levels than women. This finding held true regardless of the level of total vitamin C intake and suggests, as previously reported (Garry *et al.*, 1982c), that elderly men may have a higher requirement for vitamin C than elderly women. Second, there is a sharp rise in plasma ascorbic acid levels with intakes up to 150 mg/day followed by a plateauing or a very gradual rise to higher plasma levels with increasing intakes.

The relationship between EGR-AC and total daily riboflavin intake (diet plus supplement) is presented in Fig. 2. Total intake ranged from approximately 0.5 to 100 mg/day and is shown on a logarithmic scale in this plot. This plot shows that the EGR-ACs decreased with increasing

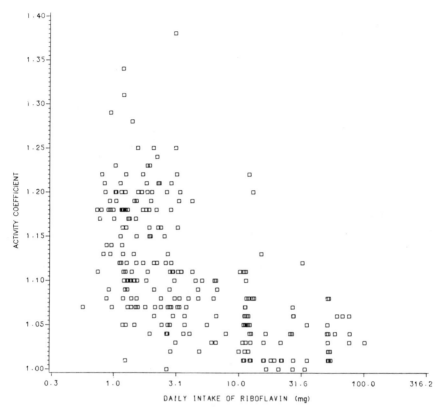

Fig. 2. Erythrocyte glutathione reductase activity coefficients versus estimated total daily intake of riboflavin (diet plus supplement) (N=254).

intakes up to approximately 4.0 mg/day. Variability in EGR-AC is clearly greater at lower levels of intake and reflects, in part, the greater error in measurement of dietary intake as compared to supplemental intake. The reduction in variability seen at riboflavin intakes above 4 mg/day also reflects the fact that a minimum level of 1.0 exists for the EGR-AC by the automated procedure used in this study. To quantify the relationship of EGR-AC and total riboflavin intake, a correlation between the reciprocal of the EGR–AC and the reciprocal of total intake was computed and resulted in a statistically significant correlation coefficient of −0.55 ($p <$ .0001). Several recent studies failed to find a significant correlation between riboflavin intake and EGR-ACs in the elderly (Vir and Love, 1977; Rutishauser et al., 1979; Mahalko et al., 1985). Two factors might explain the difference between our finding and others. The first is the large number of subjects and the second is a wider range of intakes in the present study compared to the studies noted above.

As pointed out in Section III, there is some confusion as to the exact EGR-AC to use as a cutoff level for evidence of inadequate riboflavin nutriture. The EGR-AC cutoff value we used to indicate a marginal or deficient riboflavin status was 1.35. We found only one individual with an EGR-AC greater than 1.35 in 1981 and only three individuals above this value in 1980 (Garry et al., 1982a). Thus, we feel that riboflavin intakes in this population are quite adequate based on EGR-AC data and are further supported by dietary intake data (See Table I).

As stated in Section IV,B, there is some question about the accuracy of the dietary folate values; therefore, the biochemical data versus intake probably give an inaccurate picture of the real relationship. Even considering the questionable nature of the dietary folate intake, correlations of total intake with plasma and erythrocyte folates were 0.50 and 0.49, respectively. The relationships are plotted in Fig. 3 and 4. Although there is some scatter, the relationships appear to be approximately lin-

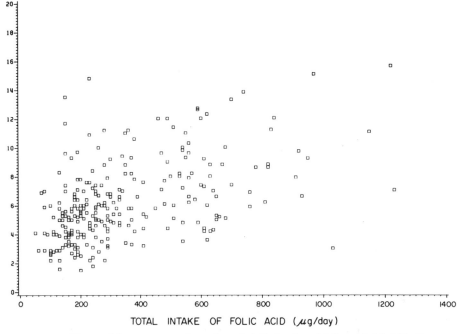

Fig. 3.   Plasma folate versus estimated total daily intake of folic acid ($N=269$). Reprinted with permission from the American Geriatrics Society, "Folate and Vitamin B_{12} Status in a Healthy Elderly Population", by Garry et al. (1984). J. Am. Geriatr. Soc. **32,** 719–726.

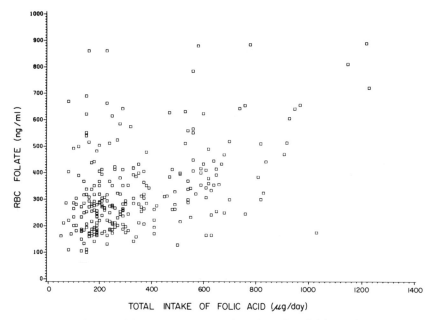

Fig. 4. Erythrocyte folate versus estimated total intake of folic acid ($N=269$). Reprinted with permission from the American Geriatrics Society, "Folate and Vitamin B_{12} Status in a Healthy Elderly Population", by Garry *et al.* (1984). J. Am. Geriatr. Soc. **32,** 719–726.

ear. We also found a significant relationship between plasma and erythrocyte folate ($r=0.50$).

The relationship between total daily vitamin B_{12} intake and plasma true cobalamin concentrations is shown in Fig. 5. There was a large range of vitamin B_{12} intakes, reflecting consumption of organ meats by some individuals. For this reason the plot of vitamin B_{12} intake with plasma true cobalamin is shown on a logarithmic scale. On this scale, the relationship is approximately linear, with a correlation of 0.45.

There have been suggestions that excessive intakes of ascorbic acid can destroy vitamin B_{12} resulting in lowering plasma values (Herbert *et al.*, 1978). As can be seen in Fig. 1, many individuals in this population had large supplemental intakes of ascorbic acid. We examined the association between ascorbic acid intake and plasma true cobalamin levels for those not taking a vitamin B_{12} supplement. There was a significant positive association between ascorbic acid intake and plasma true cobalamin even after adjusting for vitamin B_{12} intake (partial $r=0.2$, $p<.05$). Thus, our data would not support this hypothesis.

Only nine individuals (3.2%) were found to have low plasma true cobalamin levels (<220 pg/ml) and none of these had macrocytosis.

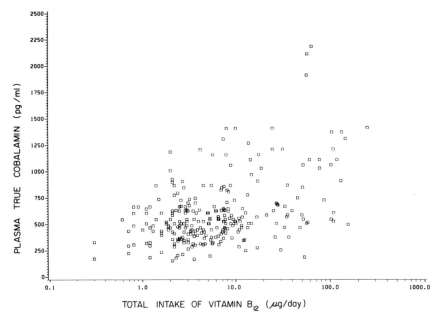

Fig. 5. Plasma true cobalamin versus estimated total intake of vitamin B$_{12}$ ($N=269$). Reprinted with permission from the American Geriatrics Society, "Folate and Vitamin B$_{12}$ Status in a Healthy Elderly Population", by Garry *et al.* (1984). J. Am. Geriatr. Soc. **32**, 719–726.

Thus, the combined dietary intake and biochemical data suggest that vitamin B$_{12}$ nutriture is adequate in this population.

Figure 6 shows the scatter plot of daily intake of vitamin E with corresponding plasma α-tocopherol values as determined by HPLC. There are several important things to point out in these data. First, usual dietary intakes of vitamin E are difficult to measure for two reasons. One is that the concentrations have not been determined in many foods and, second, if they have they are usually a mixture of tocopherols. Because α-tocopherol is the most biologically potent form of the vitamin, this is the form of most interest, and it is the predominant form found in plasma. Since it is almost impossible to get accurate data on α-tocopherol content in major food items containing vitamin E, one has to settle for total vitamin E intake. In fact most surveys do not even bother to calculate dietary intakes of vitamin E for reasons stated above. The use of supplements, in which the primary form is α-tocopherol, is largely responsible for the good association between intake and plasma α-tocopherol levels.

Plasma α-tocopherol levels have also been shown to increase as the total plasma lipid levels increase (Horwitt *et al.*, 1972). While we did not

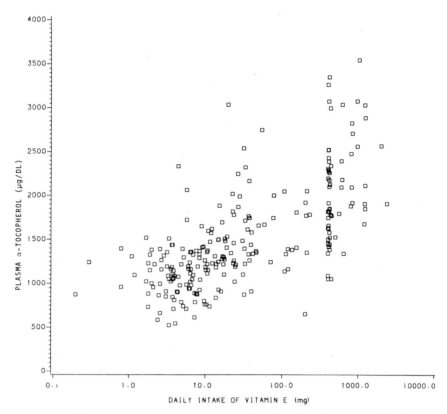

Fig. 6. Plasma α-tocopherol versus estimated total intake of vitamin E ($N=254$).

measure total plasma lipid concentrations we have determined plasma cholesterol and triglyceride concentrations in the same fasting samples which were used for the α-tocopherol measurements. When we calculated a multiple regression with cholesterol and triglycerides, the R^2 value increased from 0.42 to 0.62. In other words, we can explain 62% of the variability in plasma α-tocopherol values by knowing vitamin E intakes along with plasma cholesterol and triglyceride values. An R^2 value of 0.62 is quite remarkable considering the fact that actual dietary intakes of vitamin E are difficult to assess.

Figure 7 shows the scatter plot of total vitamin A intake and plasma retinol values. In contrast to the vitamin E scatter plot, there is little relationship between vitamin A intake and plasma levels. This finding was not unexpected as others have shown that large intakes of vitamin A have very little effect on plasma values (Willett *et al.*, 1983).

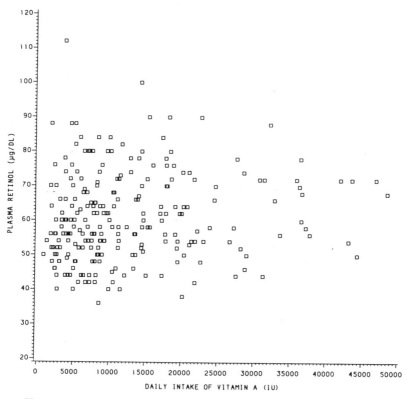

Fig. 7. Plasma retinol versus estimated total intake of vitamin A (N=254).

TABLE VI

Percentage of Subjects Taking Supplement by Quartile of Plasma Level

Quartile range	Percentage taking vitamin supplement
Vitamin E—Plasma α-tocopherol (mg/dl)	
0.53–1.10	12.7
1.11–1.36	32.3
1.37–1.80	61.5
1.81–4.43	96.8
Vitamin A—Plasma retinol (μg/dl)	
36–51	45.8
52–59	55.1
60–70	64.8
71–112	78.9

Another way to examine the effects of supplementation of vitamins E and A on plasma levels is to divide the plasma levels into quartiles and then examine the percentage taking supplements in each quartile. As we can see in Table VI, there is a good relation between quartile ranges and the proportion of individuals taking a vitamin E supplement. The plasma retinol values show a similar though much less strong relation with level and supplementation. Unlike plasma α-tocopherol levels, which respond quite promptly to supplemental intakes, we feel that it may take several years of supplementation to raise plasma retinol levels and then the increase is probably very gradual.

V. CONCLUSION

We have presented dietary and biochemical measures of vitamin status in a group of healthy elderly from Albuquerque, New Mexico, and have tried to evaluate these data in the light of some factors that are often ignored. Our data indicate that biochemical measures, especially of the water-soluble vitamins, correlate well with estimates of intake. These relations are stronger than some other investigators have found. We credit the use of supplements and the resultant increase in the range of intakes for these good associations. Given the difficulty of accurately measuring dietary intake, we conclude that biochemical measures of vitamin status are to be preferred in most cases.

ACKNOWLEDGMENTS

Supported by grants from the United States Public Health Service (AG02049 and RR-00997-05,06) and Grant-in-Aid from Hoffmann–LaRoche, Inc.

Collaborators in this study were Ms. J. Bandrofchak, Ms. J. Fleig, Ms. S. Frye, Ms. B. Gilbert, Ms. M. Marcial, and Ms. A. Safier.

REFERENCES

Balacki, J. A., and Dobbins, W. O. (1974). *Geriatrics* **29**, 157–166.

Beutler, E. (1969). *J. Clin. Invest.* **48**, 1957–1966.

Biere, J. G., Tolliver, T. J., and Catignani, G. L. (1979). *Am. J. Clin. Nutr.* **32**, 143–149.

Broatlehurst, J. C., Griffiths, C. C., Taylor, F., Marks, J., Scott, D. L., and Blackley, J. (1968). *Gerontol. Clin.* **10**, 309–317.

Durnin, J. V. G. A., and Passmore, R. (1967). "Energy, Work and Leisure." Heinemann, London.

Fleming, B. B. (1982). *In* "Nutritional Approaches to Aging Research" (G Moment, ed.), pp. 83–117. CRC Press, Boca Raton, Florida.

Garry, P. J. (1975). *Pediatrics* **55**, 899–900.

Garry, P. J. (1981). *In* "Clinics in Laboratory Medicine" (R. Labbe, ed.), pp. 699–711. Saunders, Philadelphia, Pennsylvania.

Garry, P. J., and Owen, G. M. (1976). *Am. J. Clin. Nutr.* **29**, 663–674.

Garry, P. J., Owen, G. M., Lashley, D. W., and Ford, P. C. (1974). *Clin. Biochem. (Owatta)* **7**, 131–145.

Garry, P. J., Goodwin, J. S., and Hunt, W. C. (1982a). *Am. J. Clin. Nutr.* **32**, 902–909.

Garry, P. J., Goodwin, J. S., Hunt, W. C., Hooper, E. M., and Leonard, A. G. (1982b). *Am. J. Clin. Nutr.* **36**, 319–331.

Garry, P. J., Goodwin, J. S., Hunt, W. C., and Gilbert, B. A. (1982c). *Am. J. Clin. Nutr.* **36**, 332–339.

Garry, P. J., Goodwin, J. S., and Hunt, W. C. (1984). *J. Am. Geriatr. Soc.* **32**, 719–726.

Garry, P. J., Hunt, W. C., and Goodwin, J. S. (1985). *Proc. Int. Nutr. Congr. 13th, 1984* (in press).

Glatzle, D., Korner, W. F., Christeller, S., and Wiss, O. (1970). *Int. J. Vitam. Res.* **40**, 166–83.

Goodwin, J. S., Goodwin, J. M., and Garry, P. J. (1983). JAMA, *J. Am. Med. Assoc.,* **249**, 2917–2921.

Hansen, L. G., and Warwick, W. J. (1968). *Am. J. Clin. Pathol.* **50**, 525–529.

Herbert, V., Jacob, E., Wong, K. T. J., Scott, J., and Pfeffer, R. D. (1978). *Am. J. Clin. Nutr.* **31**, 253–259.

Horwitt, M. K., Harvey, C. C., Dahm, C. H., and Searcy, M. T. (1972). *Ann. N. Y. Acad. Sci.* **203**, 223–236.

Hunt, W. C., Leonard, A. G., Garry, P. J., and Goodwin, J. S. (1983). *Nutr. Res.* **3**, 433–444.

Liu, K., Stamler, J., Dyer, A., McKeever, J., and McKeever, P. (1978). *J. Chronic Dis.* **31**, 399–418.

Mahalko, J. R., Johnson, L. K., Gallagher, S. K., and Milne, D. B. (1985). *Am. J. Clin. Nutr.* **42**, 542–553.

Milne, D. B., Johnson, L. K., Mahalko, J. R., and Sandstead, H. H. (1983). *Am. J. Clin. Nutr.* **37**, 768–773.

Nichoalds, G. E., Lawrence, J. D., and Sauberlich, H. E. (1974). *Clin. Chem. (Winston-Salem, N.C.)* **20**, 624–628.

O'Hanlon, P., Kohrs, M. B., Hilderbrand, E., and Nordstrom, J. (1983). *J. Am. Diet. Assoc.* **82**, 646–653.

Rosenberg, I. H., Bowman, B. B., Cooper, B. A., Halsted, C. H., and Lindenbaum, J. (1982). *Am. J. Clin. Nutr.* **36**, 1060–1066.

Rutishauer, I. H. E., Bates, C. J., Paul, A. A., Black, A. E., Mandel, A. R., and Patnaik, B. K. (1979). *Br. J. Nutr.* **42**, 33–42.

Thompson, J. N., Erdody, P., Brien, R., and Murray, T. K. (1971). *Biochem. Med.* **5**, 67–77.

Tillotson, J. A., and Baker, E. M. (1972). *Am. J. Clin. Nutr.* **25**, 425–431.

Vir, S. C., and Love, A. H. G. (1977). *Int. J. Vitam. Nutr. Res.* **47**, 336–344.

Vo-Khactu, K. P., Sims, R. L., Clayburgh, R. H., and Sandstead, H. H. (1976). *J. Lab. Clin. Med.* **87**, 741–748.

Willett, W. C., Stampfer, M. J., Underwood, B. A., Taylor, J. O., and Hennekens, C. H. (1983). *Am. J. Clin. Nutr.* **38**, 559–566.

11

Effectiveness of Nutrition Intervention Programs for the Elderly

Mary Bess Kohrs

Department of Community Health Sciences
University of Illinois at Chicago
Chicago, Illinois

I. INTRODUCTION

A. Factors Influencing Food Intake

Multiple factors influence food intake and nutritional status in the elderly, including physical, psychological, and sociological factors. Many of the physical factors are referred to in this book (Table I). Among those not already mentioned in-

139

Nutrition and Aging

TABLE I

Physical Factors Influencing Nutritional Status of the Elderly

Dental problems
Excretion problems (constipation, incontinence)
Physical weakness (e.g., generalized arteriosclerosis or arthritis
    with joint stiffness, making eating painful)
Lack of physical activity
Loss of sensation (smell, taste)
Chronic disease
Lactose intolerance
Drug interference
Reduced digestive capacity

clude the change in taste and smell perception (Kohrs, 1985). Contradictory evidence exists in the literature regarding changes in taste acuity with age. In part, confusion exists because of the multiple confounding factors that influence taste acuity such as drugs, nutrition, and disease. However, there is general agreement that the sensitivity to salt and sweet tastes declines with age. The ability of older persons to identify blended foods while blindfolded is decreased and may be attributed to a decreased ability to smell.

Psychological factors which predispose to decreased food intake include emotional depression, anorexia, personal taste preferences, lifetime eating habits, lack of socialization with meals, and recent changes in life-style (O'Hanlon et al., 1983). Among 445 elderly persons in Missouri, housing and work experience were associated with inadequacy of food intake. Significantly fewer persons who lived alone in federally funded high-rise apartments consumed adequate calories, iron, thiamine, and riboflavin than those who lived alone or with someone in privately owned housing (Fig. 1). Work experience, another parameter associated with change in life-style, was significantly associated with intake of two food groups—protein-rich foods and fruits and vegetables. A smaller percentage of individuals consumed <67% of the recommended servings of protein-rich foods and fruits and vegetables who worked at least part-time for the full year compared to those who only worked part of the year.

Social factors certainly influence food intake and nutritional status of the elderly (O'Hanlon et al., 1983; Kohrs et al., 1984). Among the 445 elderly individuals referred to above, sex and education were related to dietary intake of nutrients. Significantly more women consumed inadequate amounts of calcium, iron, thiamine, and riboflavin than men (Fig.

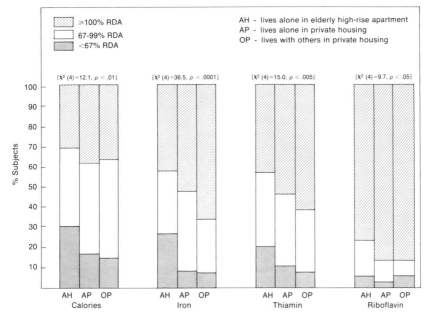

Fig. 1. Percentage of elderly subjects consuming ≤100%, 67 to 99%, and <67% of recommended dietary allowances (RDAs) according to housing (O'Hanlon *et al.*, 1983).

2). Education was significantly related to the consumption of calories, iron, thiamine, and niacin (Fig. 3). Financial restrictions, inconvenience of food preparation for one person, inability to adapt to unfamiliar surroundings, and erroneous dietary beliefs are other social factors which contribute to poor nutritional status of the elderly. The susceptibility of the elderly to "fad nutritional claims" is certainly substantiated by the high percentage of elderly persons consuming one or more vitamin and/or mineral supplements (Table II).

B. Food Programs

Food and nutrition programs have been developed in the United States as a result of national surveys conducted during the late sixties and early seventies. Table III lists the food programs which affect the elderly directly. The Title III Nutrition Program for Older Americans reaches almost two million persons over 59 years old and is designed to ameliorate some of the psychological and social factors which interfere with adequate food intake (U.S. Congress, Office of Technological Assessment, 1985).

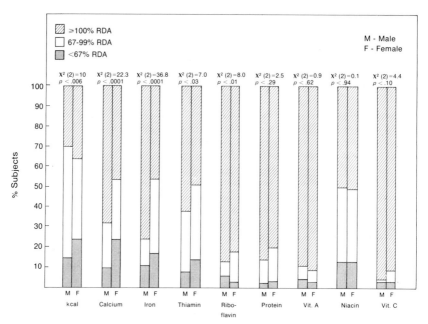

Fig. 2. Percentage of men and women consuming ≤100%, 67 to 99%, and <67% of the recommended dietary allowances (RDAs) (O'Hanlon *et al.*, 1983).

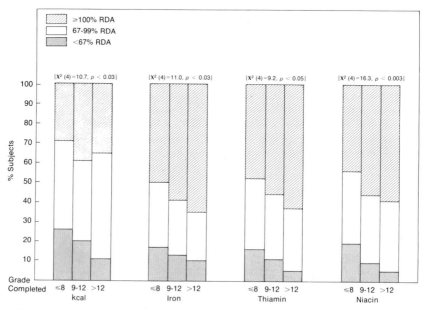

Fig. 3. Percentage of subjects consuming ≤100%, 67 to 90%, and <67% recommended dietary allowances (RDAs) according to education (O'Hanlon *et al.*, 1983).

TABLE II

Percentage of Elderly Subjects Who Consumed Vitamin and Mineral Supplements According to Sex and Frequency of Participation in the Program[a]

| | Participation (times/week) | | | | | |
| | Males | | | Females | | |
Supplement	0	<2	2–5	0	<2	2–5
Iron tablets	6	3	2	5	3	1
Calcium tablets	3	0	0	5	2	2
Multiple vitamins[b]	29	10	15	32	16	21
Vitamin C tablets[c]	19	1	9	11	4	7
Multiple vitamin and mineral	16	10	13	11	8	12
Geritol	3	0	4	0	1	2
Gelatin tablets	0	0	2	1	1	0
Other supplements	19	12	11	17	13	13
One or more of the above	58	34	39	56	38	47
Two or more of the above	29	3	6	19	6	9

[a] From Kohrs et al. (1980).

[b] Significant association between consumption by females and frequency of participation in the program ($X^2 = 7.23$, $p < .01$).

[c] Significant association between consumption by males and frequency of participation in the program ($X^2 = 9.83$, $p < .01$).

II. TITLE III NUTRITION PROGRAM FOR OLDER AMERICANS

The Older Americans Act was authorized in 1972 as the Nutrition Program for Older Americans under Title VII (Cross and Kohrs, 1986). This enacted a congregate meal program for persons 60 years and over who were unable to buy nutritious food, were unable to prepare nutri-

TABLE III

Federal Food Assistance Programs for the Elderly

Department of Agriculture
  Food Stamps
  Food Distribution
Department of Health and Human Services
  Nutrition Program for the Elderly
  Supplemental Security Income
Community Services Administration
  Community Food and Nutrition Program

tiously adequate meals, or who lacked incentive to prepare a meal. The program was designed to meet both nutritional and social needs of the elderly persons. The meal site was to be strategically located so that it could provide other supportive services such as outreach, escort and transportation, health services, information and referral, health and welfare counseling, nutrition education, and consumer education.

In 1978, the Older American Act was amended so that the Title VII Nutrition Program and Title V, Multipurpose Senior Centers, were consolidated under Title III, which then provided social services (Cross and Kohrs, 1986). At this time separate authorizations were established for congregate and home-delivered meals. As before, projects were to provide meals in a congregate setting. They would also be able to provide home-delivered meals depending on the need demonstrated by the recipient of the grant. State offices on aging distribute funds to area agencies within a state. Local sites contract with the area agencies that provide nutrition services. The federal guidelines suggest that each area agency have a board of directors consisting of local volunteers and senior citizens.

A. Perceptions of Benefits to Participants

The National Evaluation and an evaluation in Boston reported perceptions of the participants' health and benefits of the program to them (Opinion Research Corporation, 1983a,b; Posner, 1979). The National Evaluation reported that once a person enrolls in the program, program participation may keep them mobile. Those who have remained active in the program since Wave I have remained more mobile than respondents who either left the program or were never enrolled. The National Evaluation also reported that when age, minority status, sex, and self-reported health were controlled, program benefits were not apparent in terms of longevity. Although program participation did not benefit the longevity of the individuals participating in the program, the report stated that participation itself may help sustain the quality of life by enhancing social activity and maintenance of positive self-perceptions of the individual's health status. This is an area of investigation which needs further study—the hypothesis that participation in the program prolongs life.

The evaluation in Boston attempted to determine the perceptions of the participants in terms of the goals and the value to them personally (Posner, 1979). The primary determinants of program value to participants included the congregate meal, recreational and social activities, and indirect financial assistance. The majority of the participants (81%)

indicated that the program was achieving the following goals: provision of the meal, increased opportunities for socialization, and better health through improved nutrition. The evaluation found that the greatest impact of the program was through financial, social, and recreational areas. Even though the participants felt that the program was meeting the goal of improved health through nutrition, less than 5% felt the program impacted on improved diet or health. It was concluded that this group of participants, i.e., those with more frequent patterns of participation and those with greater need for financial dietary management assistance, realized significantly more impact on monetary savings, food preparation practices, food consumption, and food purchasing behavior. The author also felt it had an impact on the participants' socialization, recreation, and life satisfaction (Posner, 1979).

B. Adequacy of Meal Programs in Meeting Nutritional Goals

The adequacy of nutrition programs in meeting the nutritional needs of the elderly has been evaluated in one major national survey (Opinion Research Corporation, 1983a,b), one major area survey (Kohrs *et al.*, 1978, 1979; Kohrs, 1979), and six local evaluations (Caliendo, 1980; Caliendo and Smith, 1981; Grandjean *et al.*, 1981; Harrill *et al.*, 1981; LeClerc and Thornburg, 1983; Kim *et al.*, 1984). Among these only the major area evaluation and two of the local programs have attempted to utilize objective measures of health status such as biochemical measurements of nutrients in blood and anthropometric measurements (Kohrs, 1979; Kohrs *et al.*, 1980; Harrill *et al.*, 1981; Grandjean *et al.*, 1981) for determining weight status, including underweight indicative of undernutrition and overweight indicative of obesity. Nonetheless, the subjective measures of dietary intake using 24-hour recall, food records, and dietary histories do provide information on the effect of the congregate meal program on nutrient intake, the proportion of recommended dietary allowances as determined by the Food and Nutrition Board of the National Research Council contributed by the meal program, and the proportion of the total day's intake provided by the meal program.

Tables IV and V summarize the evaluations of the meal programs and give procedures, sample sizes, race, income, and advantages and limitations of each survey. Limitations of the surveys can be lumped into several categories, including sample selection procedures, dietary methodology, analytical procedures, and the generalizations which can be made from them. Only four of the studies appeared to select samples which were representative of the meal program participants (Caliendo,

TABLE IV

Description of Surveys for Evaluating Title III Congregate Meal Programs Funded by the Older Americans Act[a]

Survey	Sample selection	Sample size	N	Parameters measured	Limitations of survey
National (Opinion Research Corporation, 1983a,b)	Participants: Purposive	Participants: Ate a meal	800	Dietary intake: 24-hour recall	1. Use of 24-hour recall
		Did not eat a meal	920		2. No biochemical measures
	Nonparticipants: Purposive	Nonparticipants: Neighbors	1039		3. No health status measures
					4. No anthropometric measures
Missouri (Kohrs et al., 1980; Kohrs, 1982b)	Participants: Random sample from list of participants	Participants: Ate a meal	154	Dietary intake: Food record (1 day)	1. Area sample
		Did not eat a meal	213	Dietary histories	2. Only Caucasian participants
	Nonparticipants: Subjects most likely to participate in fact did participate one year later	Nonparticipants	99	Biochemical: Hct, Hb serum, iron, vitamins B_2, A, and C, albumin, cholesterol	
				Clinical: Height, weight, triceps, skin-fold thickness, blood pressure	

Location (Study)	Sample selection	Groups	N	Measures	Limitations
Nebraska (Grandjean et al., 1981)	Participants: Volunteers	Participants: Volunteers	30	Dietary intake: 24-hour recall Biochemical: Hct, Hb, vitamins B_6, B_{12}, A, and C, serum albumin Anthropometric: Height, weight, triceps, skin-fold thickness, arm girth, waist	1. Use of 24-hour recall 2. Small sample size 3. No comparison group
Colorado (Harrill et al., 1981)	Participants: Not stated Nonparticipants: Not stated	Participants Nonparticipants	59 32	Dietary intake: Food record (1 day) Biochemical: Hct, Hb, serum protein and albumin, serum vitamins A and C, serum iron, total iron binding capacity	1. Local site only 2. No anthropometric measures 3. Sample selection 4. Cross-sectional survey
New York (Caliendo, 1980)	Participants: Random selection from list of participants	Participants	73	Dietary intake: Food record (1 day)	1. Local site only 2. No biochemical measures 3. No anthropometric measures 4. No comparison group

(Continued)

TABLE IV (*Continued*)

Survey	Sample selection	Sample size	N	Parameters measured	Limitations of survey
Maryland (Caliendo and Smith, 1981)	Participants: Random selection from 11 site lists	Participants	169	Dietary intake: Food record (3 days)	1. County sample 2. No biochemical measures 3. No anthropometric measures 4. No comparison group
Illinois (Kim *et al.*, 1984)	Participants: Volunteers Nonparticipants: Volunteers	Participants Nonparticipants	8 32	Dietary intake: 24-hour recall	1. Local sample 2. Sample size and selection 3. Limited number of nutrients reported 4. No biochemical measures 5. No anthropometric measures
Maine (LeClerc and Thornburg, 1983)	Participants: Not stated Nonparticipants: Not stated	Participants Nonparticipants	27 26	Dietary intake: Food record (3 days)	1. Sample size 2. No biochemical measures 3. No anthropometric measures

[a] Adopted from United States Congress, *Technology and Aging in America*, 1985.

TABLE V

Description of Subjects and Advantages of Each Evaluation Survey[a]

Survey	Race	Income	Advantage
National (Opinion Research Corporation, 1983a,b)	Participants: 19% minority Nonparticipants: 19% minority	<6000 (1981) Participants—52% Nonparticipants—36%	1. National sample and sample size 2. Minorities represented 3. Longitudinal
Missouri (Kohrs et al., 1978, 1979, 1980; Kohrs, 1979)	97% White	NA (state guidelines did not permit)	1. Representative sample of area participants 2. Longitudinal 3. Dietary methodology 4. Biochemical evaluation 5. Clinical evaluation 6. Analysis of dietary data provided in meaningful ways 7. Sample size
Nebraska (Grandjean et al., 1981)	NS[b]	NS	1. Biochemical measures reported 2. Anthropometric measurements
Colorado (Harrill et al., 1981)	NS	NS	1. Dietary methodology 2. Biochemical measures
New York (Caliendo, 1980)	White	NS	1. Analysis of dietary data provided in meaningful ways
Maryland (Caliendo and Smith, 1981)	67% White 30% Black 3% Other	NS	1. Minorities represented 2. Sample size 3. Dietary methodology
Illinois (Kim et al., 1984)	Korean	NS	1. Minority evaluation
Maine (LeClerc and Thronburg, 1983)	NS	NS	1. Three-day food record

[a] Adapted from United States Congress, *Technology and Aging in America*, 1985.
[b] Not stated.

1980; Kohrs *et al.*, 1980; Opinion Research Corporation, 1983a; LeClerc and Thornburg, 1983). Although generalizations cannot be made based only on the findings from the other evaluations, they are valuable in that they provide supportive data for the surveys which are based on a representative sample. Second, methods for dietary intake may yield varying results. Generally, the use of the 24-hour recall may not be appropriate for use with the elderly, particularly the frail elderly, because they may have problems with memory (O'Hanlon and Kohrs, 1978). However, they are advantageous in view of the amount of time and effort necessary to obtain the data. Food records are particularly useful if they are obtained and reviewed by persons trained in foods and nutrition, i.e., dieticians. Dietary histories quantify nutrient intake based on the frequency and usual serving sizes. They are advantageous because they give an estimate of intake for a longer period of time. Larger sample sizes are required when only one day's intake is measured to get an estimate for a group. The most objective measures of nutritional status and/or improvement in nutritional status are biochemical assessment of vitamins and minerals and anthropometric measurements. The other difficulty encountered in comparing the data from the various evaluations was that not all evaluations used the same procedures for analyzing the data, i.e., the dietary intake data. The National Evaluation gave figures for porportions of persons meeting certain minimum dietary intake criteria, while others gave means for nutrient intakes. For the purpose of this paper, comparable results were found by the National Evaluation and the surveys.

The three studies which looked at the nutrient intake of participants compared to that of nonparticipants reported that the nutrient intake of vitamins and minerals was significantly increased by participation in the Title III Nutrition Program (Kohrs *et al.*, 1978; Harrill *et al.*, 1981; Opinion Research Corporation, 1983a). The National Survey used a 24-hour recall procedure while the other two evaluations used food records. The National Evaluation, the surveys in Missouri and Colorado, and an evaluation of elderly Korean Americans (Kohrs *et al.*, 1978; Harrill *et al.*, 1981; Opinion Research Corporation, 1983a; Kim *et al.*, 1984) indicated that the program significantly increased calcium intake, one of the major nutrients commonly lacking in diets of older women and implicated in prevention of osteoporosis and hypertension, two common diseases of the elderly. In Missouri the intakes of energy (Kilocalories) and protein were also greater for the participants who ate at the meal program than for the participants that did not eat at the meal program on the day of the food record and for nonparticipants (Kohrs *et al.*, 1978) (Fig. 4). Likewise, the energy and protein intakes were also greater for the participants that did

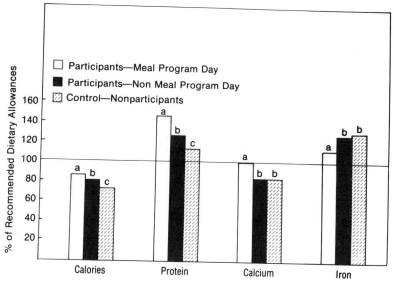

Fig. 4.   Influence of meal program on percentage of recommended dietary allowance (RDA) consumed (Kohrs *et al.*, 1978). Bars with different letters (a,b,c) are significantly different (*p* < .05).

not eat at the meal program than for nonparticipants. In Colorado, several other nutrients were greater for participants than for nonparticipants: fat and the B vitamins—thiamine, riboflavin, and niacin (Harrill *et al.*, 1981).

The second National Evaluation of the Title III program reported that the overall dietary source (inclusive of energy and eight nutrients) was greater for those who ate a program meal compared to nonparticipants but also compared to former participants and program participants who did not eat a program meal (Opinion Research Corporation, 1983a). Based on these findings, the report suggested that dietary intake improvement is largely a function of consuming a program meal rather than simply being enrolled in either congregate dining or home-delivery services. Slightly different results were reported for the intake of participants who did not eat the program meal the day of the food record in Missouri. They were found to consume a higher intake of energy and protein than the nonparticipants even though the intake was less than that for the participants who ate a program meal (Kohrs *et al.*, 1978; Kohrs, 1979). Thus, findings from the Missouri evaluation suggest that some of the other services such as transportation, shopping assistance, and nutrition education may contribute to improved intakes. It is also possible that the money saved by eating at the program meal may be used for buying additional food.

The guidelines for the federal programs state that a minimum of one-third of the recommended dietary allowances (RDAs) should be provided in the meal that is served to the older person. The results from the National Evaluation for both the congregate and home-delivered programs indicated that program meals were most successful in improving intake of the following nutrients for participants: protein, B vitamins (riboflavin, niacin, and thiamine), and iron (Opinion Research Corporation, 1983a) (Table VI). The National Evaluation documented a consistent effect of the program meal on enhancing dietary intake from 1976 to 1981, the years of dietary evaluation. Program meals were less successful in improving consumption of calcium, vitamin A, vitamin C, and energy. One is not able to determine from this evaluation whether these results reflected the nutritional content of the meals which were served or whether they reflected the food preferences of the participants. In Missouri, the total day's dietary intake of nutrients reflected the nutritional content of the menus (Kohrs et al., 1978; Kohrs, 1979) (Fig. 5). Those nutrients which were provided in the largest amounts—protein

TABLE VI

Percentage of Total Day's Nutrient Intake Supplied by Title III Meal[a]

	Meal program					
	Missouri[b]		Colorado[c]		New York[d]	
					Both	
Nutrient	Men	Women	Men	Women	sexes	Range
Energy	46.4[a]	52.4[b]	41 ± 3	48 ± 2	45 ± 3	29–72
Protein	47.5[a]	55.1[b]	54 ± 3	49 ± 2	51 ± 2	22–86
Calcium	42.4	45.2	48 ± 4[a]	61 ± 3[b]	44 ± 3	12–91
Iron	41.6[a]	46.7[b]	46 ± 3	52 ± 2	48 ± 3	12–79
Vitamin A	50.5	52.6	49 ± 5	59 ± 3	57 ± 4	19–70
Thiamine	38.8	42.2	39 ± 3	42 ± 2	48 ± 3	18–90
Riboflavin	41.4	44.4	50 ± 3	56 ± 2	47 ± 2	12–94
Niacin	45.6[a]	53.0[b]	53 ± 4	54 ± 2	52 ± 2	2–94
Vitamin C	48.4	46.3	36 ± 5	44 ± 4	48 ± 4	10–95

[a] Different letters in columns represent significant differences between men and women for the survey ($p < .05$).
[b] Based on 54 men and 100 women (Kohrs et al., 1978; Kohrs, 1979).
[c] Mean ± SEM based on 14 men and 45 women (Harrill et al., 1981).
[d] Mean ± SEM based on 53 subjects of both sexes (Caliendo, 1980).

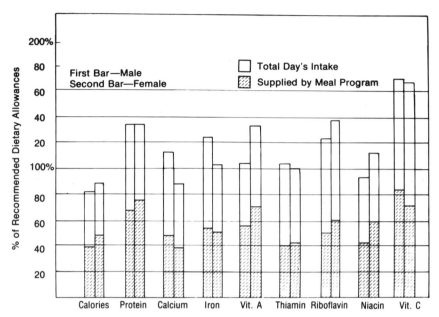

Fig. 5.   One-day intake of nutrients expressed as percentage of RDA by participants eating at the meal program (Kohrs *et al.*, 1978).

and vitamins A and C—were consumed in the greatest amount during the day. Nutrients which were provided by the menu in the smallest proportion of the RDA were also those for which the total day's consumption was less than 100% of the recommended amounts—energy and niacin for men and thiamine for both sexes.

The contribution to the total intake of nutrients for the day (percentage of total day's nutrient intake) was evaluated by the area evaluation and the two local evaluations (Table VI). All three evaluations indicated that a substantial proportion of the total day's intake was provided by the meal program (Kohrs *et al.*, 1978; Caliendo, 1980; Harrill *et al.*, 1981). All indicated that 40% or more of the total intake for most nutrients was provided by the meal. Figure 6 shows the results in Missouri, which were smaller to the findings from the other evaluations. In some cases, an average of 60% of the total day's nutrient intake was provided by the meal program (Table VI). In Missouri, the meal consumed at the meal program provided a larger mean proportion of energy, protein, iron, and thiamine to women than to men. As indicated by the range of values for percentage of total day's intake, the reuslts in the local evaluation in New York showed that for some people the meal provided more

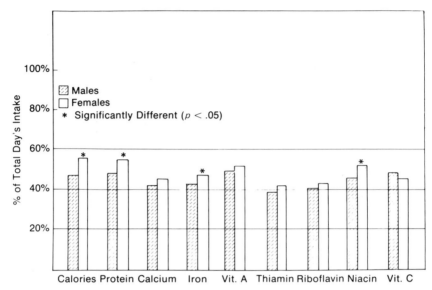

Fig. 6. Percentage of total day's intake of nutrients furnished by the meal program for males and females (Kohrs *et al.*, 1978).

than 75% of the protein, iron, calcium, riboflavin, niacin, vitamin C, and vitamin A for the day (Caliendo, 1980). The National Evaluation reported that the elderly who ate a program meal were more likely to meet one-third of the RDA for each nutrient between 11:00 A.M. and 4:00 P.M. (Opinion Research Corporation, 1983a) (Table VII).

The Administration on Aging commissioned an evaluation of the Food Service Delivery Systems used in the Title III program (Administration on Aging, 1981). One of the goals of the study was to determine the nutrient content of the meals provided by the program. An estimate of the nutrient content of the menus from a national sample was made, and Table VIII shows the results of this evaluation in comparison to two other evaluations on the percentage of RDA provided by the menus. Results from the National Evaluation indicated that for most of the nutrients analyzed the meals contributed over one-third of the recommended dietary allowances for those over 50 years old. The notable exception was the nutrient zinc, the menus providing less than one-third of the RDA for this nutrient. The report failed to note this exception. As the science of nutrition progresses and evaluations of the nutritional status of the elderly are reported, the significance of this nutrient to the health of the elderly is becoming more evident. Although the results are preliminary and need to be tested further, there is indication that zinc is an

TABLE VII

Percentage of Elderly Who Consumed One-third of the RDA during the 11 A.M.–4 P.M. Period[a]

	Ate a program meal		Did not eat a program meal			
Nutrient[b]	Congregate dining participants (N = 800)	Home-delivered meal recipients (N = 340)	Congregate dining participants (N = 920)	Home-delivered meal recipients (N = 63)	Non-participants (N = 1039)	Former participants (N = 249)
Calcium	51	50	26	30	25	25
Vitamin A	55	50	28	32	26	26
Vitamin C	59	52	36	44	34	36
Thiamine	70	67	54	49	52	54
Niacin	73	66	52	46	49	46
Iron	75	67	46	51	44	40
Riboflavin	78	75	57	54	56	55
Protein	87	83	64	63	60	58
Calories	53	48	35	30	32	31

[a] From Opinion Research Corporation (1983a).

[b] Elderly who ate a program meal were significantly more likely to meet one-third of the RDA for each nutrient (all X^2, 1 df, 90.0, all p's < .01).

important nutrient in maximum functioning of the immune system, which protects the body against invasion of foreign bodies, especially infections (Wagner et al., 1983). Another part of this report compared composition tables to chemical analyses of representative meals. Chemical analyses are particularly important for nutrients which are destroyed by overcooking, such as vitamin C, and for nutrients for which there are limited data available on amounts found in foods, such as folic acid and zinc (Bailey et al., 1979; Wagner et al., 1983) (Table IX). Thus, further evaluation by chemical analyses of the amounts of these nutrients available in meals is desirable.

The Nutrition Program for Older Americans is mandated to help meet the needs of the poor, ethnic minorities, socially isolated, those 75 years of age or older, and non-English speakers. The results from the National Evaluation and the Missouri Evaluation for dietary intake indicated that at least some of these groups benefited (Kohrs et al., 1979; Opinion Research Corporation, 1983a). The National Evaluation demonstrated that the energy intake for women less than 76 years of age who ate the program meal was greater for a larger proportion of persons than among the women of the same age who did not eat the program meal. The

Mary Bess Kohrs

TABLE VIII

Mean Percentages of Recommended Dietary Allowances Provided by Meal Served at
Congregate Meal Sites (Mean ± SEM)[a]

| | Area served by meals | | | | | |
| | National[b] | | Missouri[c] | | Colorado[d] | |
Nutrient	Men	Women	Men	Women	Men	Women
Protein	66 ± 1	84 ± 2	75 ± 3	91 ± 4	81 ± 12	99 ± 14
Calcium	61 ± 2	61 ± 2	65 ± 3	65 ± 3	60 ± 3	60 ± 3
Iron	51 ± 1	51 ± 1	53 ± 3	53 ± 3	62 ± 7	62 ± 7
Vitamin A	106 ± 10	133 ± 12	70 ± 12	87 ± 15	71 ± 28	90 ± 35
Thiamine	34 ± 1	48 ± 1	42 ± 4	49 ± 5	36 ± 1	43 ± 2
Riboflavin	64 ± 5	71 ± 3	63 ± 3	86 ± 3	61 ± 4	83 ± 4
Niacin	49 ± 1	57 ± 2	40 ± 3	54 ± 3	65 ± 10	86 ± 13
Vitamin C	73 ± 3	73 ± 3	83 ± 13	83 ± 13	52 ± 4	52 ± 4
Zinc	24 ± 1	24 ± 1	—	—	—	—

[a] Warning: Caution is needed in using these values because nutrients may have been
lost or destroyed during cooking process. These results are also based on the assumption
that there is adequate portion control.
[b] Based on 117 meals from selected sites representative of each region and the United
States (Opinion Research Corporation, 1983b).
[c] Based on 20 menus during survey days at five sites (Kohrs et al., 1978).
[d] Based on five meals served at site during survey (Harrill et al., 1981).

TABLE IX

Comparison of Analytical and Calculated Percentages of
Recommended Dietary Allowance Values in Meals Served to the
Elderly[a]

| | Analyzed | | Calculated | |
Nutrient	Men	Women	Men	Women
Protein	70 ± 2	90 ± 2	65 ± 2	83 ± 2
Calcium	53 ± 2	53 ± 2	59 ± 2	59 ± 2
Vitamin A	62 ± 6	78 ± 8	112 ± 20	140 ± 24
Thiamine	40 ± 4	56 ± 6	34 ± 1	48 ± 2
Riboflavin	51 ± 2	60 ± 6	64 ± 5	75 ± 6
Vitamin C	20 ± 2[b]	19 ± 2[b]	67 ± 6	67 ± 6
Zinc	29 ± 2[b]	29 ± 2[b]	24 ± 1[b]	24 ± 1[b]

[a] Administration on Aging (1981).
[b] Less than one-third of the RDA.

Missouri Evaluation demonstrated that program participants over 75 consumed a larger proportion of the total day's intake for energy and vitamin A than was the case for participants less than 75 years of age (Kohrs *et al.*, 1979).

Analysis of the data from the National Evaluation also revealed that income was significantly related to dietary intake in participant, home-delivered meal, and nonparticipant samples (Opinion Research Corporation, 1983a). A greater proportion of persons consuming a program meal consumed the minimum recommended amounts of calcium, vitamin A, and energy than was true for participants not eating a meal. Eating a program meal also significantly reduced income-related intake differences for calcium and energy. Although the evaluation in Missouri did not evaluate income, it reported that the meal program ameliorated the differences in nutrient intakes related to education and preretirement occupation (Kohrs *et al.*, 1979; Kohrs, 1979). None of the socioeconomic factors (education, preretirement occupation, and marital status) were related to the percentage intake of the RDA for nutrients for the group who ate at the meal program the day of the food record. However, socioeconomic factors were significantly related to intakes of energy and seven nutrients for the participants who did not eat at the program on the day of the food record and to energy and six nutrients for the nonparticipants (Figs. 7 and 8). Thus, using dietary intake as a measurement for meeting the nutritional goals of the Title III program, the oldest, those with the least income, and those of lower socioeconomic status benefited the most by eating a program meal.

The results in Central Missouri may not be reflective of the situation in other areas of the United States. However, state- and area-level administrative decisions appeared to influence the results of that evaluation (Kohrs *et al.*, 1980; Kohrs, 1982a). Registered dietitians at the state level reviewed the menus to make sure that each menu included a serving each of vitamin A- and C-rich fruits and vegetables. At the area level the University of Missouri Dietetics Department provided workshops for the local managers on preparation and serving of fruits and vegetables. Also the dietician at the area level purchased fruits and vegetables in bulk for the 15 sites in the Central Missouri area. The results from the food records for improvement in dietary intake of vitamins A and C were documented by results from the dietary histories and from analyses of blood samples for vitamins A and C (Kohrs *et al.*, 1980; Kohrs, 1982a). A greater intake of vitamin A- and C-rich fruits and vegetables was associated with regular participation in the meal program (two to five times per week). Fewer persons had low values (at risk for clinical symptoms of deficiency such as night blindness for vitamin A and

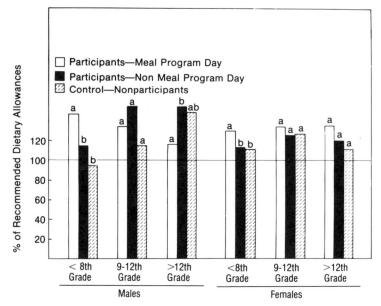

Fig. 7. Influence of group by sex and education on percentage RDA for protein (Kohrs *et al.*, 1979). Bars with different letters (a,b) are significantly different ($p < .05$) with each education group.

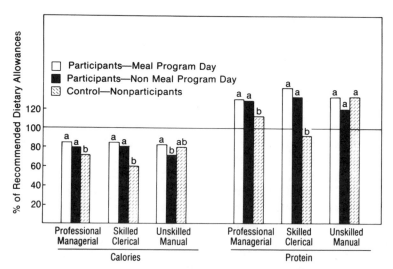

Fig. 8. Influence of group by occupation on percentage of RDA for calories and protein (Khors *et al.*, 1979). Bars with different letters (a,b) are significantly different ($p < .05$) within each occupation.

TABLE X

Percentage of Participants at One Site Who Had
Low Concentrations for Serum Vitamins A and
C According to Year Blood Samples Were
Taken[a]

Year	Serum vitamin A[b]	Serum vitamin C[b]
1975	43	7
1976	13	2
1979	0	0

[a] Kohrs (1982b).
[b] Low concentrations for vitamins A and C were
<20 μg/100 ml and <0.2 mg/100 ml, respectively.

scurvy for vitamin C) for serum vitamins A and C who participated
regularly than among the nonparticipants (Table X). Low serum values
for these vitamins indicate a risk for deficiency symptoms such as bleed-
ing gums and scurvy for vitamin C and impaired night vision and der-
matological problems for vitamin A. The authors of this evaluation indicated that their results document the need for registered dieticians and
nutritionists who have taken food and nutrition courses in an accredited
university program to be hired as managers at the regional, state, and
area levels of administration. The results from the Missouri evaluation
for vitamins A and C were strengthened with longitudinal data from the
nonparticipants. Thus, nonparticipants in 1975 who became participants
in 1976 had a lower incidence of low serum vitamin A and C values one
year later and no one had low values four years later (Kohrs, 1982b)
(Table X).

On the other hand, improvement in anemia, specifically anemia resulting from iron deficiency, was not documented by the results from
measurements of dietary intake and of hemoglobin and serum iron
(Kohrs, 1979; Kohrs et al., 1980). However, it should be emphasized that
there was no evidence of a concerted effort to improve iron intake or
provide iron-rich foods. Biochemical evaluation of iron deficiency anemia was reported for a small number of participants and nonparticipants
in Colorado (Harrill et al., 1981). Investigators there reported that iron
deficiency anemia was more common among participants than among
nonparticipants.

In view of the fact that energy, protein, and calcium were increased by
eating the program meal in Central Missouri, it has been suggested that
foods containing these nutrients would also have increased amounts of

saturated fats and cholesterol and thus be detrimental to the elderly participants. This assumes that increased intakes of saturated fat and cholesterol lead to an increase in serum cholesterol, which subsequently contributes to an increased risk of heart disease in the elderly. However, there is evidence that serum cholesterol is not a significant predictor of heart disease in the elderly (Whyte, 1975; Kohrs, 1982a). Nonetheless, analysis of the dietary intakes of total fat, saturated fat, and cholesterol according to participation in the congregate meal program in Central Missouri revealed no difference in intake of saturated fat and cholesterol for those who participated regularly in the program (two to five times per week) and those who were nonparticipants. The serum cholesterol concentrations were not different for regular participants and nonpartic-ipants (Kohrs et al., 1980; Kohrs, 1982b). Measures of obesity also indi-cated that there was no difference in the prevalence of obesity among regular participants and nonparticipants. In fact, regular participating women had a significantly greater incidence of underweight, indicating malnutrition and a definite need for the increased energy and nutrients. Malnutrition and underweight can lead to decreased immune function, which results in an increased susceptibility to disease and infection (Blackburn, 1977).

The Title III program is mandated to provide nutrition education as one of the services associated with the meal. The National Evaluation reported that the frequency of nutrition education at most sites was generally less than once a month (Opinion Research Corporation, 1983a). Site managers reported that nutrition education could be im-proved by increasing the frequency of the classes and by improving the qualifications of the personnel. Nutrition education is essential because it helps people to shop and prepare nutritional foods in an economical way. Also, it would not be financially feasible for the federal govern-ment to enroll every person over 59 years in the United States in the meal program. The cost-effectiveness of providing nutrition education by registered dieticians and trained nutritionists has not been evaluated and should be looked into further. A pilot study in Missouri did indicate that older persons were interested in participating in classes related to food for health and that those who attended a program regularly for five out of ten classes increased their nutrition knowledge (Kohrs, 1982b). The effect on dietary intake was not evaluated.

C. Adequacy of Food Delivery Systems

As mentioned previously, a study of the food delivery systems used in the Nutrition Program for Older Americans was commissioned by the

AOA (Administration on Aging, 1981). The evaluation looked at four factors which theoretically could influence the cost of the meals—delivery system, project size, urban/rural setting, and region. None of these factors influenced the cost of the meals despite the fact that the menus sampled at these sites for the most part contained more than one-third of the RDA for persons over 50. Statistical analyses were also used to determine possible relationships between cost and quality of the meals. The two were found to be unrelated.

Evaluations of meal safety were also performed by this study (Administration on Aging, 1981). The measures used in this assessment were sanitary inspections and microbiological analyses of meals. Wide differences in food safety were found among the meal sites, the findings indicating that some of the sites were deficient in this aspect. Overall, the results from the study of the food delivery systems indicate that the programs would benefit by utilizing dietitians in the food management aspect as well as for ensuring nutritional adequacy. Administrative dieticians are trained in food sanitation, food preparation to ensure optimum preservation of nutrients, and food management practices to ensure cost containment in addition to training in nutrient content of food. Although managers at the different sites were not evaluated, the results of the report suggest that use of trained dieticians would help to meet nutritional goals of the program while providing food in a safe manner. The contributions of the nutritionist-registered dietitian need to be demonstrated and evaluated further.

An additional evaluation has been reported on food delivery systems (Kincaid, 1981). This was a local study in Ohio of the acceptance of on-site prepared versus catered meals in the Title III program. Expert taste panels were used to assess the taste and aesthetic qualities of meals prepared by the two different methods of food delivery systems. Numerical ratings of the taste panel showed that the on-site prepared meals were of superior quality and larger in quantity. However, the evaluation also reported that the overall ratings for acceptance and food quality were low for both systems, indicating a need for careful assessment of recipes, production procedures, and storage practices and facilities. Only 36% of 501 respondents indicated they enjoyed the food at the meal sites. Analyses of the meals for microbial contamination also indicated that on-site preparation was more sanitary.

The Administration on Aging commissioned the American Dietetic Association to evaluate the food service systems and technologies provided by the Nutrition Program for Older Americans (McCool and Posner, 1982). It is not possible to assess whether state-of-the-art food service technologies are being utilized by the Title III nutrition programs. However, this report does present alternative food systems which are consistent with food safety, menu quality control, optimal nutrient value and participant acceptance of meals, and service cost-efficiency. One of the major findings from the report was that service regulations fail to designate the need for qualified nutrition personnel to plan, manage, and evaluate nutrition services. Among firms and individual technologists involved in services for the elderly, the major nutrition service problem identified was a lack of detailed federal specifications on food products, equipment, packaging, and food service systems for congregate and home-delivered meals. Other concerns of this group included: (1) maintenance of appropriate food temperatures during meal transportation, (2) a reliance on untrained volunteers to deliver meals and services, (3) variable food portion control, (4) limited space for food services operations, (5) safety and sanitation hazards, and (6) a limited number of certified management personnel in food service operations.

III. FOOD STAMP PROGRAM

A. Participation

Studies of the amount of participation and factors determining food stamp program participation have been conducted by two different groups (Blanchard *et al.*, 1982; Akin *et al.*, 1985). The evaluation of the food stamp program commissioned by the Human Nutrition Information Service of the USDA was based on subjects participating in the National Food Consumption Survey in 1977–1978 and in 1979–1980. The results for participation in the program in 1977–1978 differed from the results among the elderly sample interviewed in 1979–1980 (Akin *et al.*, 1985). Among those who were eligible for food stamps over twice as many participated in 1979–1980 as in 1977–1978. About 80 to 90% of those eligible in 1979–1980 participated as opposed to less than 40% of those eligible to participate in 1977–1978. The determinants of participation also differed depending on the year of interview. Income was a significant factor for participation in 1977–1978, lower incomes being more likely to participate than those with higher incomes. The very old are believed to be more nutritionally vulnerable because of progressing infirmities. In 1979–1980 this group participated at very high levels unlike in 1977–1978. Owning a home and living alone negatively influenced participation in the food stamp program in 1977–1978. Those who did not receive Supplemental Security Income (SSI) in 1977–1978 were less likely to participate in the food stamp program than those who received SSI. The food stamp program changes which occurred between 1977–1978 and 1979–1980 appeared to reduce these effects. Changes in the program included tightening of eligibility standards and elimination of the purchase requirement, i.e., the requirement to pay cash for food stamps. In 1979–1980 the factors relating to probability of participation differed for rural and urban persons. The important variables for those living in urban areas included age, education level, obtains sufficient food, retired, shops every week, owns own home, and participates in the SSI program. The rural subsample nonincome factors included age, health, shops every week, owns own home, and participates in the SSI program.

B. Nutritional Benefits

The Food Stamp SSI/Elderly Cashout Demonstration Evaluation looked at participation rates in the food stamp program (Blanchard *et al.*, 1982). These investigators reported that 50% of those eligible for food stamps use them. As in the other evaluation, SSI recipient households were more likely to use food stamps than those who did not receive SSI. This report also listed other factors relating to use of food stamps: lack of awareness, stigma, and distance to food stamp program offices. The following groups were less likely to participate in the food stamp program: households with male heads, those having at least some high

TABLE XI

Differences in Nutrient Intake as Determined by the Food Stamp SSI/Elderly Cashout Demonstration Evaluation[a]

Nutrient	Participant	Nonparticipant	Percentage difference
Kcal	1221	1160	6
Protein (g)	47	43	10[b]
Calcium (mg)	460	390	16[b]
Iron (mg)	8.0	7.6	7
Vitamin A (IU)	4270	3912	9
Vitamin C (mg)	80	64	21[b]
Thiamine, (mg)	0.92	0.87	11[b]
Riboflavin (mg)	1.15	1.06	9
Niacin (mg)	10.6	10.2	5

[a] Blanchard *et al.* (1982).
[b] $p < .05$.

school education, and those of older age. Analysis of effect of food stamp participation revealed that it increased food expenditures for those in the survey sample.

The Food Stamp SSI/Elderly Cashout Demonstration Evaluation also evaluated the effects of the food stamps and cashout on dietary intake of nutrients (Blanchard *et al.*, 1982). There were no significant differences for the intake of nine nutrients between food stamp participants and nonparticipants. However, those who received cash in place of stamps had a higher intake of four out of the nine nutrients—protein, calcium, vitamin C, and thiamine. The overall estimated (Table XI) effects of the food stamp program on dietary intake were positive for all nutrients, but significant for only one—calcium.

IV. OTHER PROGRAMS

A pilot program was recently initiated which provides commodity food supplements to the elderly who most need it (Opinion Research Corporation, 1983b). The supplementary foods provided by this Food for Seniors project provide over 100% of the monthly requirements for protein, calcium, iron, phosphorus, vitamin D, riboflavin, and vitamin B_{12}. The project has provided food items to 1900 persons and has a waiting list of over 8000.

V. CONCLUSION

The Title III congregate meal program of the Older Americans Act appears to be meeting the guidelines for nutrient intake for most nutrients. However, menus and meals have not been analyzed for some of the lesser known nutrients which may be inadequate such as zinc, folic acid, vitamin B_6, and copper. Recent surveys using biochemical assessments of status for these nutrients among the elderly suggest that a significant proportion of the elderly may be deficient in vitamin B_6, folic acid, and zinc (Bailey *et al.*, 1979; Grandjean *et al.*, 1981; Kohrs, 1982a; Wagner *et al.*, 1983). Lack of adequate information on the content of these nutrients in foods, geographical variation in nutrient content of foods, and variation in nutrient content of food due to food preparation is an important reason for chemically analyzing food aliquots of meals for these and other nutrients.

Only three of the reports—all were regional and/or local—have attempted to assess the impact of the meal program on nutritional status by utilizing the most objective measures of nutritional status: biochemical measurements of blood and urine, anthropometric measurements, and physical examinations. However, the subjects for these evaluations have been Caucasian. Evaluations of the impact of the congregate meal program using biochemical and clinical measures of the nutritional status of minorities and low-income residents in large urban areas are needed. These should include biochemical, anthropometric, and physical measurements.

One important potential benefit of the program needs to be assessed further—the impact of the congregate meal program and home-delivered meals on quality of life, both physiologically and psychologically, and on longevity. Several factors inherent in the program, including improvement of health through provision of nutrition and improvement of self-esteem through socialization, may have important consequences to morbidity and longevity. Another side benefit from improvement in these areas may be a reduction in health care costs. One-third of the national health care costs are related to provision of health care for the elderly (Kohrs, 1981).

Another nutritionally related mandate of the Title III program is to provide nutrition education to the elderly. The reports of the site managers suggest that this program needs to be offered on a more regular basis by trained personnel. The efficacy, cost-effectiveness, and cost-benefits of programs provided by registered dieticians need to be tested. As with the assessment of the impact of the meals on nutritional status, such an evaluation should include not only the subjective measures of success such as food records, attitudes, and reported benefits but also objective data such as anthropometric and biochemical measurements of nutritional status.

One of the major findings of a national evaluation of food delivery systems was that the policymakers indicated a lack of service regulations in that the regulations failed to designate the need for qualified nutrition personnel to plan, manage, and evaluate the nutrition services of the Title III programs (McCook and Posner, 1982). The findings from one of the studies commissioned by the AOA suggest that the type of delivery and/or setting does not affect the cost of the meal. This report also found that food safety was "woefully inadequate" at some sites. The positive effect of the Title III program on nutritional health in participants in Central Missouri was attributed to the use of qualified nutrition personnel. The results of the studies would indicate that such personnel are necessary to provide optimum nutrition quality and food safety in the meal program. The initial cost may be small compared to the savings from improved health and decreased morbidity.

The limited studies which have been conducted concerning the food stamp program suggest that 50% of the elderly persons who are eligible use it. Only one study is available on nutritional benefits of the food stamp program and it reports a positive effect of the program on nutrition of the elderly. Further evaluations of nutritional status using biochemical and anthropometric measures of participants in these and other programs for older Americans are needed, particularly of the homebound elderly.

REFERENCES

Administration on Aging (1981). "Nutrition Services Title III. Part C. Analyses of Food Service Delivery Systems Used in Providing Nutrition Services to the Elderly." Admin. Aging, U.S. Dep. Health Hum. Serv. (performed by Kirschner Assoc.), Washington, D.C.

Akin, J. S., Guilkey, D. K., and Popkin, B. M. (1985). *J. Nutr. Elderly* **4**, 25–51.

Bailey, L. B., Wagner, P. A., Christakis, G. J., Araujo, P. E., Appledorf, H., Davis, C. G., Masteryanni, J., and Dinning, J. S. (1979). *Am. J. Clin. Nutr.* **32**, 2346–2353.

Blackburn, G. L. (1977). *JPEN, J. Parenter. Enteral Nutr.* **1**, 11–22.

Blanchard, L., Butler, J. S., Doyle, P., Jackson, R., Ohis, J. C., and Posner, B. M. (1982). "Food Stamp SSI/Elderly Cashout Demonstration Evaluation," Final Report. Food Nutr. Serv., U.S. Dep. Agric., Washington, D.C.

Caliendo, M. E. (1980). *J. Nutr. Elderly* **1**, 23–40.

Caliendo, M. A. and Smith, J. (1981). *J. Nutr. Elderly* **3**, 21–39.

Cross, N., and Kohrs, M. B. (1986). *In* "Rehabilitation of the Elderly" (D. Olson and T. Byerts, eds.). Butterworth, London (in press).

Grandjean, A. C., Korth, L. L., Kara, G. C., Smith, J. L., and Schaefer, A. E. (1981). *J. Am. Diet. Assoc.* **78**, 324–329.

Harrill, I., Bowski, M., Kylen, A., and Wemple, R. R. (1981). *Aging* **311–312**, 36–41.

Kim, K., Kohrs, M. B., Twork, R., and Grier, M. R. (1984). *J. Am. Diet. Assoc.* **84**, 164–169.

Kincaid, J. W. (1981). *J. Nutr. Elderly* **1**, 27–38.

Kohrs, M. B. (1979). *J. Am. Diet. Assoc.* **75**, 543–546.

Kohrs, M. B. (1981). *Compr. Ther.* **7**, 39–46.

Kohrs, M. B. (1982a). *Am. J. Clin. Nutr.* **36**, Suppl. 4, 796–802.

Kohrs, M. B. (1982b). *Am. J. Clin. Nutr.* **36**, Suppl. 4, 812–818.

Kohrs, M. B. (1985). *Geriatr. Med. Today* **4**, 88–101.

Kohrs, M. B., O'Hanlon, P., and Eklund, D. (1978). *J. Am. Diet. Assoc.* **72**, 487–492.

Kohrs, M. B., O'Hanlon, P., Krause, G., and Nordstrom, J. (1979). *J. Am. Diet. Assoc.* **75**, 537–542.

Kohrs, M. B., Nordstrom, J., Plowman, E. L., O'Hanlon, P., Moore, C., Davis, C., Abrahams, O., and Eklund, D. (1980). *Am. J. Clin. Nutr.* **333**, 2643–2656.

Kohrs, M. B., Kapica-Cyborski, C., and Czajka-Nakins, P. (1984). *In* "Trace Substance in Environmental Health" (D. Hemphill, ed.), pp. 476–486. Univ. of Missouri Press, Columbia.

LeClerc, H. L., and Thornburg, M. E. (1983). *J. Am. Diet. Assoc.* **83**, 573–577.

McCool, A. C., and Posner, B. M. (1982). "Nutrition Services for Older Americans: Food Service Systems and Technologies. Administrative Guidelines," pp. 1–5. Am. Diet. Assoc., Chicago, Illinois.

O'Hanlon, P., and Kohrs, M. B. (1978). *Am. J. Clin. Nutr.* **31**, 1257–1269.

O'Hanlon, P., Kohrs, M. B., Hilderbrand, E., and Nordstrom, J. W. (1983). *J. Am. Diet. Assoc.* **82**, 646–653.

Opinion Research Corporation (1983a). "Analytic Report: An Evaluation of the Nutrition Services for the Elderly," Vol. 2. Admin. Aging, U.S. Dep. Health Hum. Serv., Washington, D.C.

Opinion Research Corporation (1983b). "An Evaluation of the Nutrition Services for the Elderly," Vol. 3. Admin. Aging, U.S. Dep. Health Hum. Serv., Washington, D.C.

Posner, B. M. (1979). "Nutrition and the Elderly," pp. 85–146. Lexington Books, Lexington, Massachusetts.

U. S. Congress, Office of Technological Assessment (1985). "*Technology and Aging in America*," OTA-BA-264, pp. 421–446. V. S. Off. Technol. Assess., Washington, D. C.

Wagner, P. A., Bailey, L. B., and Jernigan, J. A. (1983). *Fed. Proc., Fed. Am. Soc. Exp. Biol.* **42**, 579 (abstr.).

Whyte, A. M. (1975). *Lancet* **1**, 96–910.

12

The Elderly Alcoholic: Experience with Baltimore Veterans and Private Alcoholism Patients over Age 60

Frank L. Iber

*University of Maryland School of Medicine,
and Baltimore Veterans Administrative Medical Center
Baltimore, Maryland*

I. INTRODUCTION

The HANES Nationwide Food Consumption Survey Windham *et al.*, 1983) of the eating and drinking habits of a large sample of Americans from all regions and economic levels indicated that older Americans use alcohol less frequently than younger adults and alcoholic beverages make up fewer of the daily calories of elderly than of younger persons. Yet, despite these data it is clear that alcoholism is prominent among the elderly (Maletta, 1982; Mishara and Kastenbaum, 1980). This paper reports studies in Baltimore with alcoholic patients over age 60 to define some differences from a younger population. The groups of patients selected for each part of this study differed in their selection criteria and in the methods utilized. For clarification, these are included in the results.

II. PREVALENCE OF ALCOHOLISM

Male subjects seeking entry into the clinics or hospital at the Baltimore Veterans Administration Medical Center were evaluated for alcoholism contributing to their illness. The criteria used by the rating doctors were a history of alcohol use each day and at least one of the following: (a) alcoholic withdrawal syndrome within the past year; (b) a medical record of poor compliance with diet, medication, or physician appointments judged to be alcohol-related; and (c) diseases commonly associated with alcohol use including epilepsy, cirrhosis, pancreatitis, cerebral atrophy, or recurrent trauma.

Table I indicates the frequency of alcoholism in male patients seeking care for symptomatic illness at the Baltimore VA Medical Center. It was found that 13% of patients age 65–74 had alcoholism in contrast to 23% for all ages. Two independent groups of elderly persons had submitted blood specimens as part of a lipid screening project. Aliquots were analyzed for alcohol by a gas chromatographic method. One group resided in a wealthy retirement community in which each person maintained an individual apartment with access to alcohol if they chose. The other

TABLE I

Prevalence of Alcoholism in Male Veteran
Outpatients' First Visit

Age	Number	Percentage alcoholic
Under 45	88	37
45–54	71	23
55–64	54	22
65–74	57	13
Over 74	31	4
Total	301	23

TABLE II

Blood Levels of Alcohol in Elderly Free-Living Adults

Group	Under 60 years		60 to 70 years		Over 70 years	
	Men	Women	Men	Women	Men	Women
Affluent Retirement Community						
Number studied	12	10	51	61	19	35
Number with 5–1000 mg/liter ethanol	1	0	4	2	1	3
Number with over 1000 mg/liter	1	1	3	4	0	0
Senior Citizens Center						
Number studied	19	20	39	89	27	51
Number with 5–1000 mg/liter ethanol	2	2	4	10	3	6
Number with 1000 mg/liter	3	0	2	7	1	1

group was in a large community senior citizens center featuring "Eating Together" programs, entertainment, and many other services. Although alcohol was not served in this facility, persons were free to purchase supplies of alcohol for home consumption or patronize retail outlets on the way to and from the center. Table II indicates that 16% of the senior citizen center population had detectable alcohol levels; all samples were collected in the afternoon. Ten percent of the samples from the retirement community showed alcohol levels but these were taken as a fasting morning sample. For both groups 4–5% had levels over 1 g/liter, indicating very heavy drinking, with a higher percentage among men.

III. AMOUNT OF ALCOHOL INGESTED

The Veterans Administration Hospital operates an alcoholism detoxification unit which accepts acutely drinking patients on the basis of desire to be detoxified and available space. Patients with clear needs for alternative medical or surgical hospitalization are admitted to other services, but for the most part, this unit accepts alcoholics on a self-, family-, or employer-generated referral system. Similar data were accumulated from patients in private alcoholism treatment facilities. Although these facilities require payment or insurance reimbursement, they also operate

TABLE III

Alcohol Intake of Male Veterans[a]

Age	Number	Alcohol intake, mean ± SD (g/24 hr)	Mean percentage of daily calories as alcohol
Under 55	76	166 ± 104	64
55–64	44	118 ± 73	51
65–74	38	76 ± 42	32
Over 74	13	54 ± 35	27

[a] Estimates for period 2 weeks before admission to hospital from interview after hospitalization.

on a self-, family-, or employer-generated referral system. All patients in the private facilities require physician screening for substantial medical or surgical disease before admission is possible.

The VA unit, operating within a hospital with easy referral to other services, generally takes patients who may be more ill and less thoroughly screened than are the patients in the private facilities operated as freestanding units. Patients hospitalized for alcoholism treatment were interviewed for dietary recall retrospectively for their drinking period between the 5th and 15th day in the hospital. Approximately one-third of the eligible patients were excluded because they were unwilling to undergo such interviews or were unable to provide dietary and drinking data to the dieticians. A three-day recall was utilized for a period two weeks prior to the admission. From this the total caloric intake and the total alcohol intake were calculated. Table III outlines the data from the VA patients and Table IV outlines data from private hospitals. Two

TABLE IV

Alcohol Intake of Private Male Patients[a]

Age	Number	Alcohol intake, mean ± SD (g/24 hr)	Mean percentage of daily calories as alcohol
55–64	45	92 ± 84	48
65–74	45	56 ± 57	26
Over 74	20	55 ± 64	28

[a] Estimates for period 2 weeks before admission to hospital from interview after hospitalization.

trends were prominent. The older patients drank less alcohol in both absolute amount and as a percentage of the total calories ($p < .001$). The private patients of similar age consumed fewer alcohol calories than did the Veterans Administration patients at each age but this was not statistically significant.

IV. DURATION OF ALCOHOLISM

Alcoholics in both veterans and private patient facilities were classified on the basis of their drinking history and its relationship to the events of their lives regarding the time of onset of alcoholic drinking. New alcoholics were defined as those who had become alcoholic in the last 5 years and old alcoholics represented those were were alcoholics for more than 5 years. Table V indicates the number of alcoholics among the VA patients who were judged to be new alcoholics in the various decades of age. An increasing number of older patients were new alcoholics ($p < .01$), suggesting that factors in this population causing new alcoholism are at least as important as aging of former alcoholics. Table VI contrasts similar data for private and Veterans Administration patients. Although the trend of new alcoholics to increase with aging is present among private patients, at all ages a majority were old alcoholics.

V. DISEASES PRODUCED BY ALCOHOLISM

Mental impairment was considered present in alcoholics if after 5 days under hospital observation there were multiple statements in the chart concerning the orientation or thinking ability of the patient, if the patient's ability to care for himself was questioned by those planning dis-

TABLE V

New Alcoholics among Male Veterans
Hospitalized for Alcoholism

Age 55–64		Age 65–74		Age over 74	
New[a]	Old[b]	New	Old	New	Old
72	106	44	39	17	2

[a] New = less than 5 years.
[b] Old = more than 5 years.

TABLE VI

Comparison of 100 Consecutive Male Alcoholics over 60 Years of Age from Veterans and Private Hospital Populations

	Number	Percentage alcoholic more than 5 years	Percentage with major organ damage	
			Brain	Liver
Veterans				
Age 60–70	74	55	31	26
Age over 70	26	17	44	44
Private patients				
Age 60–70	56	81	38	8
Age over 70	44	58	56	10

position or a neurological-psychological assessment, or if a CT scan of the head indicated an ongoing abnormality. Liver disease was listed as present if the patient carried a historical diagnosis of cirrhosis, if liver tests were abnormal more than 10 days after admission, or if the chart indicated a verifiable diagnosis of liver disease. Table VI indicates the distribution of organ damage to the brain and to the liver in a sample of patients from the VA Hospital and a sample from several private alcoholism hospitals. It can be seen that both groups have a large number of patients with brain damage. The veterans group has similarly large numbers of patients with liver injury, but liver disease was not found extensively among the private patients.

Table VII indicates nutritional measurements in the VA patients at various ages encountered in a detoxification unit. Weight for height, skin-fold thickness for body fat, and muscle circumference were more often impaired in the older than the younger patients. Table VIII examines the time needed in a detoxification unit at the VA Hospital until the patient could be discharged into the community. Clearly, older patients are hospitalized longer. The reasons for very prolonged hospitalizations are noted in Table VIII.

During the two-year course of these studies, 16 patients were identified who were judged on initial assessment by an internist, neurologist, or psychiatrist to have permanent brain impairment. Further evaluation in each instance revealed moderate to substantial alcohol use and a great deal of functional recovery following detoxification. Review of these 16 patients is useful for understanding some of the manifestations of alcoholism in the elderly with regard to injury to the central nervous system.

TABLE VII

Nutritional Measurements on Male Veterans One Week after Entering an Alcoholism Program

	Percentage under indicated standard				
Age:	40–49	50–59	60–69	70–79	Over 79
Number:	45	40	40	25	7
Weight/height (<20%)[a]	2	2	23	60	58
Skin-fold thickness (10 mm)	6	12	16	32	72
Muscle circumference (26 cm)	8	14	32	40	72
Albumin (3.6 g/dl)	0	0	15	20	28
Hematocrit (35%)	0	5	15	20	14

[a] Laboratory standard value, Baltimore, V.A.M.C.

All 16 patients were over age 60 with one patient 82 and 6 aged 70 to 80. The *initial* history identified 5 that were heavy drinkers, 2 more used alcohol, and 2 were reputed to be nondrinkers, with no history recorded for the remainder. At a much later time, the actual drinking history was found to be as follows: 6 drank in excess of 100 g ethanol per day, 8 drank in the range of 50 to 100 g, and 2 drank less than 50 g per day. The initial diagnoses in these 16 patients were 6 with Alzheimer's disease, 5 with cerebral atrophy, 3 with multiple small strokes, and 2 with Korsakoff's psychosis. Table IX lists some of the clinical findings in the first week of hospitalization. All of these patients responded with improvement and were able eventually to return to their homes. Three demon-

TABLE VIII

Age and the Duration of Hospitalization in a Detoxification Unit

	Duration of hospitalization[a]		Reasons for delayed release		
Age (years)	Detoxification (days)	Percentage prolonged	Mental impairment	General health	Social problems
40–50	5.6	6	1	5	0
Over 51	11.9	28	15	9	4

[a] Time until allowed to resume community life.

TABLE IX

Initial Findings in 16 Alcoholics Diagnosed as Having
Permanent Brain Injury Who Recovered

Arousable not oriented	15/16 (1 unarousable)
Incontinent	9/16
Unable to feed or dress self	16/16
Focal signs	3/16
CT scan brain atrophy	11/16

strated improvement in the first 2 weeks, 9 improved by the end of the
fourth week, and 13 by the end of 6 weeks, but clear improvement in the
remaining 3 was not apparent until after 6 weeks. The improvement
continued for up to 2 months in 11 patients and up to 3 months in the
remaining 5. Table X provides early and late data on an additional 52
male veterans over age 60 who could not be discharged from an alcoholism unit due to brain injury. These data indicate that nearly all abnormalities improved in these patients but maximal improvement sometimes required 2 to 3 months.

VI. DISCUSSION

The data reported in this paper are not random samples since they do
include the major bias of self or family selection of alcoholics, yet they
reveal some information about the older alcoholic. These data confirm
that alcohol use is common in older people; our two samples of blood
from elderly free-living Baltimore citizens would place the intake of

TABLE X

Follow-up Data on 52 Male VA Patients with Alcohol-Related Brain Injury

Index of injury	Initial fraction abnormal (5 to 10 days)	Fraction abnormal (2 or more months)
Severe forgetfullness (short-term memory)	44/52	7/52
Impaired orientation[a]	28/52	2/52
Inability to feed self	11/52	0/52
CT scan	10/23	7/9

[a] By criteria of person, place, and time.

alcohol at a higher level than that found in the National Survey (Windham et al., 1983). Alcoholics are frequent users of health facilities (Gaitz and Baer, 1971), thus it is no surprise that 13% of the 65- to 75-year-olds entering the Veterans Administration outpatient department were believed to have an alcoholism problem. Our data show that self-identified alcoholics in alcoholism treatment programs consume less alcohol on the average as they get older; this is quite convincing for both private and Veterans Administration patients (Tables III and IV). This decrease in consumption has been noticed by others (Hartford and Samorajski, 1982; Comfort, 1981; Rix, 1982). The available studies of ethanol disappearance rates in older humans suggest that the metabolic rate is the same in the young and old (Vestal et al., 1977; Lieber and DeCarli, 1972), but in animals there is some support for a decrease in metabolic rate with aging (Thieden, 1971; Wiberg et al., 1970; McCourt et al., 1971). Vestal et al. (1977) showed clearly that intravenous alcohol given at a fixed dose per kilogram body weight results in higher blood levels in the elderly and they were able to relate this to the diminished total body water with aging. This information on normal tolerance to drinking from a metabolic point of view suggests increased "self-perception" of sensitivity to alcohol resulting in lowered intakes (Gaitz and Baer, 1971). Thus there is a great deal of support for the notion that there is increased CNS sensitivity to alcohol in the older person (Blusewicz et al., 1977; Parker and Noble, 1980; Leber and Parsons, 1982).

In our experience, alcohol in the elderly seems to produce more brain injury and nutritional damage than in younger patients despite an intake of less alcohol. The high incidence of liver disease in the VA patients may reflect a special interest in patients with liver problems that could reasonably account for the much higher prevalence of liver disease in contrast to patients in private facilities without such interest and advertised expertise. The demonstration of substantial occurrence of brain damage in our experience recorded here, even with relatively low intakes of alcohol, is important to note because nearly all of these patients showed improvement with alcohol abstinence.

Our observations of the responsiveness of the central nervous system damage in the elderly suggest that the prognosis is excellent with the majority returning to a more functional state, though the time of recovery may be as long as 3 months. The phenomenon of new alcoholics among the elderly has been observed previously (Rix, 1982; Rosin and Glatt, 1971; Comfort, 1981) and is associated with widowhood, loss of economic power, and loneliness. The treatment of alcoholism in the elderly is similar to that in younger persons (Schukit et al., 1980; Zimberg, 1978) with an excellent prognosis for recovery. Although the brain injury and peripheral neuritis of the elderly respond similarly to younger patients in treatment (Huang, 1981), the liver disease has a far higher mortality (Woodhouse and James, 1985).

These studies indicate that alcoholism in the elderly is more destructive to body function and nutrition than is alcoholism in the younger subject. Prominent brain injury is common in the elderly. The prognosis for recovery from the nutritional and organ damage is excellent and the prognosis for response to treatment for the alcoholism is good.

REFERENCES

Blusewicz, M. J., Dustman, R. E., Schenkenberg, T., and Beck, E. C. (1977). *J. Nerv. Ment. Dis.* **165,** 348–355.

Comfort, A. (1981). *Ala. J. Med. Sci.* **18,** 177–184.

Gaitz, C. M., and Baer, P. E. (1971). *Arch. Gen. Psychiatry* **24,** 372–378.

Hartford, J. T., and Samorajski, T. (1982). *J. Am. Geriatr. Soc.* **30,** 18–24.

Huang, C. Y. (1981). *J. Am. Geriatr. Soc.* **29,** 49–54.

Leber, W. R., and Parsons, O. A. (1982). *Int. J. Addict.* **17,** 61–68.

Lieber, C. S., and DeCarli, L. M. (1972). *J. Pharmacol. Exp. Ther.* **181,** 279–287.

McCourt, W. F., Williams, A. F., and Schneider, L. (1971). *Q. J. Stud. Alcohol* **32,** 310–317.

Maletta, G. J. (1982). *In* "Encyclopedic Handbook of Alcoholism" (E. M. Pattison and E. Kaufman, eds.), p. 779. Gardner Press, New York.

Mishara, B. L., and Kastenbaum, R. (1980). "Alcohol and Old Age." Grune & Stratton, New York.

Parker, E. S., and Noble, E. P. (1980). *J. Stud. Alcohol* **41,** 170.

Rix, K. J. B. (1982). *J. R. Soc. Med.* **75,** 177–180.

Rosin, A., and Glatt, M. (1971). *Q. J. Stud. Alcohol* **32,** 53–59.

Schuckit, M. A., Atkinson, J. H., Miller, P. L., and Berman, J. (1980). *J. Clin. Psychiatry* **41,** 412–416.

Thieden, H. I. D. (1971). *Acta Chem. Scand.* **25,** 3421–3427.

Vestal, R. E., McGuire, E. A., Tobin, J. D., Andres, R., Norris, A. H. and Mezey, E. (1977). *Clin. Pharmacol. Ther.* **21,** 343–347.

Wiberg, G. S., Trenholm, H. L., and Coldwell, B. B. (1970). *Toxicol. Appl. Pharmacol.* **16,** 718–727.

Windham, C. T., Wyse, B. W., and Hansen, R. G. (1983). *J. Am. Diet. Assoc.* **82,** 364–373.

Woodhouse, K. W., and James, O. F. W. (1985). *Age Ageing* **14,** 113–118.

Zimberg, S. (1978). *Alcoholism* **2,** 27–29.

Exercise and Muscle Metabolism in the Elderly

William J. Evans

USDA Human Nutrition Research Center on Aging at Tufts
Boston, Massachusetts

I. INTRODUCTION

Aging is associated with a slow but continual change in body composition. These changes can be characterized by an increasing amount of body fat and a concomitant decline in lean body mass. In an effort to define the body composition of a reference man aged 70, Fryer (1960) chose 26 men from a total sample size of 60 based on the criteria that they were within ±10% of a desirable weight for height (Metropolitan Life Tables). He then compared the body composition of this 70-year-old reference man to the 25-year-old reference man defined by Brozek (1954) (Fig. 1). Clearly the greatest percentage change is in skeletal muscle mass. Total body water has been shown to decrease as a percentage of body weight from early maturity through the seventh decade (Fryer, 1960). Associated with these changes are a decreased metabolic rate

179

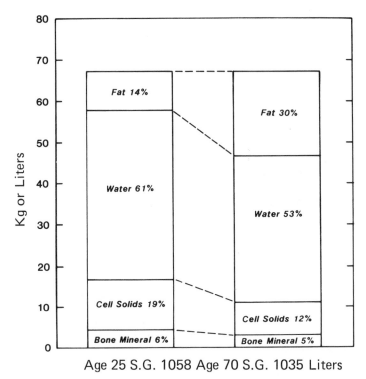

Age 25 S.G. 1058 Age 70 S.G. 1035 Liters

Fig. 1. A comparison of the body composition of a "reference man" aged 70 to that of a 25-year-old reference man described by Brozek (1954). Redrawn from Fryer (1960).

and lowered urinary creatinine levels (Tzankoff and Norris, 1977), reflecting losses in the skeletal muscle compartment of lean body mass. The decline in muscle mass is accompanied by a diminished functional capacity, strength, and bone mineral content (Asmussen, 1980). It has been argued that senescent changes in skeletal muscle are not only a result of the inevitable aging process, but are also a consequence of deconditioning (Bortz, 1982), as voluntary physical activity declines with age (McGandy et al., 1966; Mondon et al., 1983). This phenomenon is demonstrated by the rapid atrophy of skeletal muscle when muscular activity is reduced, as in bed rest, immobilization, or weightlessness during space flight. Muscle atrophy may be exacerbated in elderly individuals, who often have drastically reduced activity levels due to chronic or acute disease. The degree to which age-related changes in muscle function and metabolism may be reversed by physical activity will be explored in this review. Focus will be on the specific adaptations produced by regular training and how they alter senescent changes in skeletal muscle.

II. FACTORS AFFECTING SKELETAL MUSCLE MASS

Tzankoff and Norris (1977) examined the urinary creatinine and basal metabolic rate of a large number of subjects (956) from age 20 to 97 and found that in 50 years of aging there is a 33% loss in total muscle mass. The reduced urinary creatinine excretion with age was closely related to the reduced basal oxygen consumption which showed a similar age-related decline.

The cause of an age-related reduction in skeletal muscle mass has been ascribed to a number of factors, some of which cannot be modified while others are susceptible to change. It has been proposed that as a result of age-related changes in the nervous system, there is a long-term denervation process resulting in deficient neural input to the muscle (Larsson, 1982) as well as a decrease in the trophic influence of the neuron at the neuromuscular junction (Gutman and Hanzlekova, 1976). Other hypotheses include changes in the skeletal muscle, such as a decreased capacity to regenerate new muscle fibers (Gibson and Schultz, 1983) and a reduced oxygen diffusion to muscular mitochondria due to a loss in intracellular water (Ermini, 1976). Factors that can be altered by a modification of an individual's habits include diet and physical activity.

III. MORPHOLOGICAL CHANGES IN SKELETAL MUSCLE

It has been established in both human and animal studies that there is a decrease in the total number of muscle fibers with age (Gutman and Hanzlikova, 1966; Lexel et al., 1983). In one of the few studies examining total muscle fiber number in humans, Lexel et al. (1983) counted the number of fibers in the midsection of the vastus lateralis of autopsy specimens. These investigators found approximately 110,000 fewer fibers in elderly man (age 70–73) when compared to young men (age 19–37), representing a 23% difference. In vivo studies using the technique of computerized tomography (CT) have found a reduced cross-sectional area of the thigh as well as a decreased muscle density, which is associated with increased intramuscular fat (Imamura et al., 1983). Sato and Tauchi (1982) confirmed the reports of Lexel et al. (1983) by finding an

age-related reduction in the total fiber number and slight increase in
fiber diameter of the human m. vocalis muscle. These authors also observed a decrease in both Type I (red) and Type II (white) fibers, but
there was a disproportionate and earlier loss in Type II fibers with age.
In a cross-sectional study of 114 healthy male subjects between 11 and 70
years of age, Larsson *et al.* (1978) obtained muscle specimens from the
quadriceps using the percutaneous biopsy procedure. He found a decreased percentage of Type II muscle fibers with advancing age (Fig. 2)
and a diminished cross-sectional area of the Type II fibers, yet he found
no age-related change in Type I fiber area. Larsson also measured dynamic and isometric strength of the quadriceps in all 114 individuals. He
found dynamic and isometric strength to increase in the 20- to 29-year-
old group, remain unchanged in the 40- to 49-year-old group, and subsequently decline with increasing age thereafter. He speculates that reduced activity may preferentially affect Type II fibers by greatly reducing
recruitment. Type I fibers, on the other hand, are recruited daily during

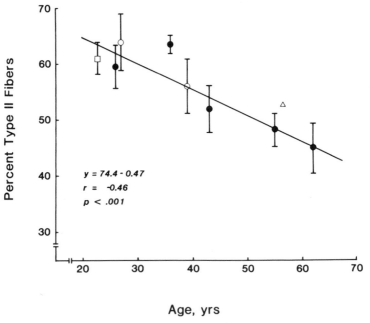

Fig. 2. Percentage of Type II fibers versus age. Included are data from Gollinck *et al.*
(1972; ○), Kiessling *et al.* (1974; △), and Saltin *et al.* (1976). Redrawn from Larsson *et al.*
(1978).

any submaximal activity. The age-related decrease in Type II fiber area was significantly correlated with decreasing muscle strength ($r = 0.54$, $p < .001$).

Aniansson and Gustafsson (1981) conducted a strength training study on 12 older men (age 69–74). Training consisted of stretching calisthenics and leg extension and flexion exercises using only the limb weight as resistance. Despite the fact that a more effective strength training program of progressive resistance or free weights was not used, these authors did observe a relative increase in the Type II muscle fiber area following a 3-month period of training. This observation led them to speculate that fiber atrophy due to an age-related reduction in physical activity can partially explain the morphological changes documented by Larsson.

Grimby *et al.* (1982) compared muscle biopsy specimens and body cell mass measurements from 24 elderly men and women to those of a young population. They found an age-related reduction in fiber area, with the most marked differences seen in Type II fibers. Fiber area changes did not adequately explain the differences in body cell mass, so these authors speculated that there was an age-related reduction in total number of fibers. They did not, however, see any differences in fiber composition (ratio of Type I/Type II) between old and young. Muscle "quality," including capillary density and muscle enzymne activities, did not differ between the elderly and young biopsy specimens. It was concluded that diminished functional capacity in older individuals is a result of a reduction in the quantity of muscle and not due to reductions in the "quality" of the muscle.

These authors (Grimby *et al.*, 1982) also found increased amount of type grouping (abnormal groupings of one fiber type) in the senile muscle, indicative of a denervation–renervation process. Tomonaga (1977) examined muscle biopsy samples from elderly men and women and found increased type grouping and evidence of selective Type II atrophy. Ultrastructural analysis revealed neuropathic and to a lesser extent myopathic changes. These changes included the appearance of "ragged red" fibers, nemaline rods, lipid storage including lipopigment and curvilinear bodies, various nuclear changes, thickening of the intramuscular capillary basement membrane, and deformity and reduction of the subsynaptic folds of the motor end plates. The extent to which these changes can be altered by exercise remains unclear, as few studies have systematically examined the effects of training on ultrastructural changes in senile skeletal muscle. Orlander and Aniansson (1980) found that 12 weeks of aerobic training did not alter the volume fractions of mitochondria or lipid droplets. They also found increased amounts of lipofuscin in the muscle with age that were not changed with training. In a study examining gastrocnemius biopsies from 40 marathon runners (ages 19–61), Warhol et al. (1984) found that, when compared to the younger runners, the older, veteran runners had increased intramuscular lipofuscin and intercellular collagen deposition suggestive of a fibrotic response to repetitive injury.

Moritani and DeVries (1980) conducted one of the few studies comparing in young and old subjects the effects of a progressive resistance strength training program. They examined the relationship between force production and muscle activation by measuring the integrated electromyographic activity (IEMG). By measuring changes in the IEMG with time, they could estimate approximately how much of the strength gain resulted from neurophysiological mechanisms and how much resulted from muscle hypertrophy. They calculated (Moritani and DeVries, 1979), in young people, that much of the initial gain in strength resulted from changes in neural factors, with muscle hypertrophy becoming the dominant factor after the first 3 to 5 weeks. They also determined that in the older subjects gains resulted almost totally from neural factors with muscle hypertrophy contributing very little.

Another possible mechanism for the age-related loss in total muscle cells is a reduced capacity to repair or replace damaged muscle cells. Most exercise will cause delayed muscle soreness to those who do not exercise regularly (Abraham, 1977; Friden et al., 1983). This delayed-onset muscle soreness is most likely due to damage to individual muscle fibers or muscle cell necrosis (Friden et al., 1981, 1983). The repair of damaged cells coupled with increased number of satellite cells is a normal phenomenon and is a part of the adaptive response to exercise. However, the capacity for muscle regeneration is reduced with age. Gibson and Schultz (1983) compared the absolute number of satellite cells in young and adult rat extensor digitorum longus (EDL), consisting of Type II muscle and soleus (Type I). They found an age-related reduction in the number of satellite cells in both muscles with the greatest reduction seen in the EDL. The numbers of satellite cells, the authors indicate, provide a crude indication of the regeneration potential of the muscle at various ages. They estimate that by 24 months the satellite cells in soleus retain the capability to regenerate 71% of the total myofibrillar nuclear population. The regenerative capability of the EDL declines to approximately 28% by 24 months. These data may also partially explain why aging affects Type II fibers to a greater extent than Type I muscle cells.

IV. EXERCISE AND PROTEIN METABOLISM
   IN MUSCLE

Exercise can lead to a delayed increase in the turnover of protein (Zackin *et al.*, 1986; Evans *et al.*, 1986). This is accomplished, in part, by an increase in the activities of acid hydrolases, which are responsible for muscle protein breakdown. Vihko *et al.* (1979) found that in untrained mice exhaustive exercise caused, 5 days later, muscle fiber necrosis and a marked increase in the activities of a number of acid hydrolases. They found that exercise training caused an apparent resistance to the damaging effects of exercise. They concluded that this increased hydrolase activity is reflective of an increase in muscle protein turnover. Salminen and Vihko (1981) found that exhaustive exercise caused a much greater delayed increase in the activities of cathepsin D, dipeptidyl aminopeptidase I, and β-glucuronidase in white and red muscle in young animals when compared to old. The authors state that this difference is probably caused by a partial loss in adaptive capacity of muscle cells during aging, which may in turn delay subcellular regeneration and "thus also the reattainment of the homeostasis of muscle fibers."

Golden and Waterlow (1977) showed that there is a significant reduction in whole body protein turnover with age. Uauy *et al.* (1978) found that skeletal muscle accounts for 30% of whole body protein turnover in young men compared to 20% in elderly men. Young *et al.* (1981) indicated that a reduced contribution by muscle to whole body protein metabolism might restrict the capacity of the elderly individual to respond successfully to an unfavorable dietary situation or to other stressful conditions that depend on adaptive changes in muscle protein and energy metabolism. This decline in protein turnover (Adelman, 1975; Blazejowski and Webster, 1983; Golden and Waterlow, 1977) and capacity of muscle for regeneration could lead to an age-related decrease in the response of skeletal and whole body protein metabolism to the stress of exercise.

Zackin *et al.* (1986) examined six active, middle-aged (52 ± 1.4 years) men to determine if increased activity altered protein turnover and dietary protein requirements. The men were well trained VO_2 max = 55.2 ± 11.7 ml O_2 kg^{-1} min^{-1}) and approximately 50% leaner (18.9 ± 2.8% fat) than average for middle-aged men. However, despite their fitness and time spend training per week (8.5 ± 1.4 hr), they had a reduced muscle mass (36.6 ± 0.6%) that is typical for their age. The authors determined that 0.98 g kg^{-1} day^{-1} of good quality protein was required to achieve nitrogen balance in these men. Using this figure for the amount of dietary protein to achieve nitrogen balance, the authors calculated a "safe" daily protein intake for active middle-aged men of 1.38 g of protein kg^{-1} day^{-1}, an intake that is more than the current recommended dietary allowance (RDA). They also measured urinary 3-methylhistidine levels and found that the 3-methylhistidine creatinine ration was higher than reported figures for young sedentary men (Young *et al.*, 1981), suggesting a high rate of protein turnover in skeletal muscle. These data indicate that despite a reduced muscle mass, chronic physical activity can increase protein turnover and affect dietary protein needs.

V. MUSCLE METABOLISM AND AGING

Along with a declining muscle mass, and most likely as a direct result, aging is associated with reduced work capacity. Performance in virtually every type of athletic event is reduced with age. Bottiger (1973) examined the relationship between age and performance in a 19-mile running race and a 54-mile skiing race. With a total population of almost 10,000 men, he found that performance is very closely matched with age with a decrease of 5–10% in performance (increased time to complete the event) every 10 years from the optimum age for the event (mid twenties).

Shephard (1966) summarized the results from a number of cross-sectional studies which included VO_2 max data from more than 5000 untrained men. He showed a 50% decline in VO_2 max between the ages of 20 and 70 years. Astrand *et al.* (1973), in one of the few truly longitudinal studies reporting changes in function with age, examined 44 female and 42 male physical education students in 1949 (ages 20–33 years) and again in 1970. Despite the fact that most of the subjects attempted to maintain their physical activity, maximal oxygen uptake was lower in 1970 when compared to the 1949 values, without exception. The decline in VO_2 max was 22% for the women and 20% for the men. These data correspond to the average rate of decline in VO_2 max estimated by Shephard.

Dill *et al.* (1967) remeasured VO_2 max in 16 athletes after a 20-year interval. Their data demonstrate a decline in maximum oxygen consumption of 30%, a more rapid decline than that seen by Astrand *et al.* (1973) and Shephard (1966), which was, no doubt, affected by both the aging process and decreased activity levels. The data of Dehn and Bruce (1972) showed that the subjects in their sample population who remained physically active demonstrated a much slower rate of decline in VO_2 max with age when compared with sedentary subjects. On the other hand, Suominen *et al.* (1977) examined a group of 22 men who exercised on a regular basis and a group of age-matched sedentary men. A regression was determined to predict the age-related changes in VO_2 max, which were found to be different in the active versus inactive men.

Active men: VO_2 max (ml kg^{-1} min^{-1}) = 91.0 − 0.70 (age in years)
Inactive men: VO_2 max (ml kg^{-1} min $^{-1}$) = 51.7 − 0.24 (age in years)

Their data thus suggest a greater loss in rate of maximal oxygen consumption in active than in inactive men.

In summary, these studies imply that increased physical activity will slow the rate of decline in functional capacity (VO_2 max) that accompanies the aging process. Those individuals who are very active in their early years and become inactive will demonstrate an accelerated loss in aerobic capacity. Only a lifetime of exercise will ensure a reduced loss of functional capacity during old age.

Both young and elderly men and women respond to endurance exercise training with similar relative increases in rate of maximal oxygen consumption capacity (Sidney and Shephard, 1977). As with young people, the magnitude of the increase in VO_2 max depends on the frequency, intensity, and duration of the exercise. Niinimaa and Shephard (1978) measured the responses of 16 older (60–76 years old) men and women to 11 weeks of endurance exercise training. They conclude that increases in VO_2 max in the elderly were due largely to a decrease in resting heart rate, with a resultant increase of cardiac reserve. They also state that, relative to younger subjects, metabolic needs were met to a larger extent by a widening of arteriovenous oxygen difference and a redistribution of blood flow, implying peripheral adaptations to the training. Seals *et al.* (1984a) examined the responses of 14 elderly (61–67 years old) to 6 months of low-intensity followed by 6 months of high-intensity endurance training and found an average increase of 12% of VO_2 max for the first 6 months and a further increase of 18% after the 6 months of high-intensity training for a combined increase of 30%. The range of responses, however, was quite variable (the increases ranged between 2 and 49%). They concluded that these increases in functional capacity resulted from an increase in maximal arteriovenous O_2 differences. Maximal cardiac output, measured using the CO_2-rebreathing method (Defares, 1985), remained unchanged following both training regimens.

Seals and co-workers (1984b) also found that blood lactic acid levels at a standard absolute exercise intensity were significantly reduced. They speculated that their results (1984a,b) indicated that the elderly can appreciably improve their aerobic capacity with very small changes in the

cardiovascular system and that most of the change results from peripheral adaptations. Fitts *et al.* (1984) examined regularly exercising and
sedentary 9-, and 18-, and 28-month-old rats. They observed that with
the same amount of contractile activity in skeletal muscle, aging results
in a higher rate of lactate production and higher glycogen use. These
age-related trends can be reversed with exercise. They also studied the
contractile characteristics and found that the isometric twitch duration is
prolonged with aging in both fast and slow twitch muscle fibers. They
found that skeletal muscle develops a prolonged $t_{1/2}$ for relaxation time
late in life that is even further increased with training. However, aging
and/or exercise had no effects on twitch tension, peak rate of tension
development, maximum shortening velocity, or calcium uptake by muscle homogenates.

Farrar *et al.* (1981) examined the oxidative capacity and mitochondrial
protein content in the gastrocnemius-plantaris muscle of 150-, 300-, and
720-day-old rats. They measured the subsarcolemmal and intermyofibrillar mitochondria concentration and found that they did not change
between 150 and 300 days. The muscle mitochondrial protein concentration was only 8% lower in the 720-day-old animals with a 15% increase
seen in the subsarcolemmal fraction and a 26% decrease measured in the
intermyofibrillar fraction. They found that aging did not cause significant changes in oxidative capacity of isolated mitochondria. Endurance
training increased the intermyofibrillar mitochondrial protein concentration by 38% in the 300-day-old rats and by 80% in the 720-day-old animals. They concluded that the decrease in oxidative capacity with age
was due to a decrease in mitochondrial protein. Exercise can increase the
oxidative capacity of senile skeletal muscle but it cannot reduce the
atrophy concomitant with age.

Beyer *et al.* (1984) also studied the effects of age and endurance exercise on oxidative capacity and mitochondrial protein content in old (25
months) and young (9 months) rats. They examined the ability of muscle
homogenates to catalyze the oxidation of succinate, pyruvate, palmitoyl-
coenzyme A, decanoylcarnitine, and palmitoylcarnitine in the presence
of ADP. The average loss in oxidative capacity was approximately 32%.
Following 21 weeks of treadmill running, the homogenates catalyzed
oxidations 55% more rapidly than those from 25-month-old sedentary
animals and 17% faster than those from 9-month-old sedentary rats,
with the greatest increase seen in the capacity to oxidize palmitoylcarnitine. The yield of mitochondrial protein from the quadriceps femoris
muscle decreased between 9 and 25 months but was restored to the 9-
month level by the training. The studies by Farrar *et al.* (1981) and Beyer
et al. (1984) indicate that although total muscle mass declines with age

the "quality" of the muscle need not change. Capacity to oxidize carbohydrates as well as fatty acids can be maintained into old age by adherence to a program of increased physical activity.

It has long been known that both aging and inactivity are associated with decreased glucose tolerance and increased incidence of maturity onset diabetes (Blotner, 1945; Fitzgerald *et al.*, 1960; Litwack and Whedon, 1959). Bjorntorp *et al.* (1972) examined a population of physically active, middle-aged men (mean age of 54 years) and found that they demonstrated an enhanced glucose tolerance with lower blood insulin levels (compared to sedentary controls) when given an oral glucose load. Similarly, Seals *et al.* (1984c) showed that master athletes, young athletes, and young untrained men had similar responses to an oral glucose load, whereas old, sedentary men had much higher glucose and insulin levels in response to the same glucose load. It is difficult to assess whether the effects of training enhance glucose tolerance by decreasing body fat content or by increasing insulin sensitivity by the contracting muscles. Both of these effects are known to occur with endurance training.

VI. SUMMARY

Aging is associated with a changing body composition that is characterized by decreasing skeletal muscle mass and increased body fat content. The declining muscle mass seems to be an inevitable consequence of aging and results from the loss of whole motor units, with Type II fibers being preferentially affected. Declining muscle mass and reduced cardiovascular function cause an age-related loss in functional capacity (VO_2 max) in both sedentary individuals and those who remain physically active. An increasingly sedentary life-style, also associated with aging, can lead to an accelerated decline in VO_2 max. Inactivity affects the quality of muscle by causing a decreased oxidative capacity and loss of insulin sensitivity. Chronic physical activity can slow the rate of decline of VO_2 max. Aerobic exercise can cause substantial increases in functional capacity in elderly men and women, even after a lifetime of sedentary living. Exercise can also decrease the accumulation of body fat and increase insulin sensitivity and glucose tolerance. Because such a large number of the elderly have a low enough aerobic capacity to limit everyday function, there is perhaps, no single group in our society that can benefit more from a moderate program of increased physical activity.

REFERENCES

Abraham, W. J. (1977). *Med. Sci. Sports* **9**, 11–20.

Adelman, R. C. (1975). *Fed. Proc., Fed. Am. Soc. Exp. Biol.* **34**, 179–182.

Aniansson, A., and Gustafsson, E. (1981). *Clin. Physiol.* **1**, 87–98.

Asmussen, E. (1980). In "Environmental Physiology: Aging, Heat and Altitude" (S. M. Horvath and M. K. Yousef, eds.), pp. 419–428. Elsevier/North-Holland Biomedical Press, Amsterdam.

Astrand, I., Astrand, P., Hallback, I., and Killbom, A. (1973). *J. Appl. Physiol.* **35**, 649–654.

Beyer, R. E., Starnes, J. W., Edington, D. W., Lipton, R. J., Compton, R. T., and Kusman, M. A. (1984). *Mech. Ageing Dev.* **24**, 309–323.

Bjorntorp, P., Fahlen, M., and Grimby, G. (1972). *Metab., Clin. Exp.* **21**, 1037–1044.

Blazejowski, C. A., and Webster, G. C. (1983). *Mech. Ageing Dev.* **21**, 345–346.

Blotner, H. (1945). *Arch. Intern. Med.* **75**, 39–44.

Bortz, W. M. (1982). *JAMA, J. Am. Med. Assoc.* **248**, 1203–1208.

Bottiger, L. E. (1973). *Br. Med. J.* **3**, 270–271.

Brozek, J. (1954). "Measurement of Body Composition in Nutritional Research" p. 265. Department of the Army, Office of the Quartermaster General, Washington, D.C.

Defares, J. G. (1958). *J. Appl. Physiol.* **13**, 159–164.

Dehn, M. M., and Bruce, R. A. (1972). *J. Appl. Physiol.* **33**, 805–807.

Dill, D. B., Robinson, S., and Ross, J. C. (1967). *J. Sports Med.* **7**, 1–32.

Ermini, M. (1976). *Gerontology* **22**, 301–316.

Evans, W. J., Meredith, C. M., Cannon, J. G., Dinarello, C. A., Frontera, W. R., Hughes, V. A., Jones, B. H., and Knuttgen, H. G. (1986). *J. Appl. Physiol.: Respir., Environ. Exercise Physiol.* (in press).

Farrar, R. P., Martin, T. P., and Ardies, C. (1981). *J. Gerontol.* **36**, 642–647.

Fitts, R. H., Troup, J. P., Witzmann, F. A., and Holloszy, J. O. (1984). *Mech. Ageing Dev.* **27**, 161–172.

Fitzgerald, M. G., Malins, J. M., and O'Sullivan, D. J. (1960). *Q. J. Med.* **30**, 57–70.

Friden, J., Sjöström, M., and Ekblom, B. (1981). *Experientia* **37**, 506–507.

Friden, J., Sjöström, M., and Ekblom, B. (1983). *Int. J. Sports Med.* **4**, 170–176.

Fryer, J. H. (1960). *Fed. Proc., Fed. Am. Soc. Exp. Biol.* **19**, 327–335.

Gibson, M. C., and Schultz, E. (1983). *Muscle Nerve* **6**, 574–580.

Golden, M. H. N., and Waterlow, J. C. (1977). *Clin. Sci. Mol. Med.* **53**, 227–288.

Gollnick, P. D., Armstrong, R. B., Saubert, C. W., IV, Piehl, K., and Saltin, B. (1972). *J. Appl. Physiol.* **33**, 312–319.

Grimby, G., Danneskiold-Samsoe, B., Hvid, K., and Saltin, B. (1982). *Acta Physiol. Scand.* **115**, 125–134.

Gutman, E., and Hanzlikova, V. (1966). *Nature (London)* **209**, 280–300.

Gutman, E., and Hanzlikova, V. (1976). *Gerontology* **22**, 290–300.

Imamura, K., Ashida, H., Ishikawa, T., and Fujii, M. (1983). *J. Gerontol.* **38**, 678–681.

Kiessling, K.-H., Pilström, L., Bylund, A.-C., Saltin, B., and Piehl, K. (1974). *Scand. J. Clin. Lab. Invest.* **33**, 63–69.

Larsson, L. (1982). In "The Aging Motor System" (F. J. Prozzolo and G. J. Malelte, eds.), pp. 60–97. Praeger, New York.

Larsson, L., Sjödin, B., and Karfsson, J. (1978). *Acta Physiol. Scand.* **103**, 31–39.

Lexel, J., Henriksson-Larsen, K., Wimblod, B., and Sjöström, M. (1983). *Muscle Nerve* **6**, 588–595.

Litwack, L., and Whedon, G. D. (1959). *Clin. Res.* **7**, 143–144.

McGandy, R. B., Barrow, C. H., Spanis, A., Meredith, A., Stone, J. L., and Norror, A. H. (1966). *J. Gerontol.* **21**, 581–587.

Mondon, C. E., Dolkas, C. B., Sims, C., and Reaven, G. M. (1983). *J. Appl. Physiol.* **58**, 1553–1557.

Moritani, T., and DeVries, H. A. (1979). *Am. J. Phys. Med.* **58**, 115–130.

Moritani, T., and DeVries, H. A. (1980). *J. Gerontol.* **35**, 672–682.

Niinimaa, V., and Shephard, R. J. (1978). *J. Gerontol.* **33**, 362–367.

Orlander, J., and Aniansson, A. (1980). *Acta Physiol. Scand.* **109**, 149–154.

Salminen, A., and Vihko, V. (1981). *Acta Physiol. Scand.* **112**, 89–95.

Saltin, B., Nazar, K., Costill, D. L., Stein, E., Jamsson, E., Essen, B., and Gollnick, P. D. (1976). *Acta Physiol. Scand.* **96**, 289–305.

Sato, T., and Tauchi, H. (1982). *Mech. Ageing Dev.* **18**, 67–74.

Seals, D. R., Hagberg, J. M., Allen, W. F., and Holloszy, J. O. (1984a). *J. Appl. Physiol.: Respir., Environ. Exercise Physiol.* **56**, 1521–1525.

Seals, D. R., Hagberg, J. M., Hurley, B. F., Ehsani, A. A., and Holloszy, J. O. (1984b). *J. Appl. Physiol.: Respir., Environ. Exercise Physiol.* **57**, 1024–1029.

Seals, D. R., Hurley, B. F., Schultz, J., and Hagbeg, J. M. (1984c). *J. Appl. Physiol.: Respir., Environ. Exercise Physiol.* **57**(4), 1030–1033.

Shephard, R. J. (1966). *Arch. Environ. Health* **13**, 664–672.

Sidney, K. H., and Shephard, R. J. (1977). *J. Appl. Physiol.: Respir., Environ. Exercise Physiol.* **43**, 280–287.

Suominen, H., Heikkinem, E., Liesen, H., Michel, D., and Hollimann, W. (1977). *Eur. J. Appl. Physiol.* **37**, 173–180.

Tomonaga, M. (1977). *J. Am. Geriatr. Soc.* **25**, 125–131.

Tzankoff, S. P., and Norris, A. H. (1977). *J. Appl. Physiol.: Respir., Environ. Exercise Physiol.* **43**, 1001–1006.

Uauy, R., Winterer, J. C., Bilmazes, C., Haverberg, L. N., Scrimshaw, N. S., Munro, H. N., and Young, V. R. (1978). *J. Gerontol.* **33**, 663–671.

Vihko, V., Salminen, A., and Rantamaki, J. (1979). *J. Appl. Physiol.: Respir., Environ. Exercise Physiol.* **47**, 43–50.

Warhol, M. J., Siegal, A. J., Evans, W. J., and Silverman, L. M. (1984). *Am. J. Pathol.* **118**, 331–339.

Young, V. R., Gersovitz, M., and Munro, H. N. (1981) In "Nutritional Approaches to Aging Research" (G. B. Moment, ed.), pp. 48–75. CRC Press, Boca Raton, Florida.

Zackin, M. J., Meredith, C. N., Frontera, W. R., and Evans, W. J. (1986). *Am. J. Clin. Nutr.* (submitted for publication).

14

Aging of Rats: The Roles of Food Restriction and Exercise

John O. Holloszy and E. Kaye Smith

Department of Medicine, and Office of Laboratory Animal Care
Washington University School of Medicine
St. Louis, Missouri

I. EFFECTS OF FOOD RESTRICTION IN RODENTS

Food restriction, i.e., chronic underfeeding, appears to be the only procedure that has clearly been proven effective in markedly prolonging life span in a species of mammal. This effect was first demonstrated in rats by McCay *et al.* (1935; McKay, 1952) and confirmed and extended in studies on rats by other investigators (Berg and Simms, 1960; Nolen, 1972; Ross, 1972, 1976; Masoro *et al.*, 1980; Yu *et al.*, 1982; Stuchlikova *et al.*, 1975) as well as on mice (Weindruch *et al.*, 1979; Good *et al.*, 1980; Weindruch and Walford, 1982). Severe caloric restriction, to 25–40% of voluntary consumption, from the age of 21 days increased mean length of life as much as

193

60%. Milder degrees of food restriction in the range of 60–75% of voluntary food intake have also been shown to increase life span, but not as markedly as more severe restriction (Nolen, 1972; Yu et al., 1982). Food restriction later in life, when rodents are full grown, also appears to increase life span, but not as markedly as food restriction begun very early in life (Nolen, 1972; Ross, 1972; Stuchlikova et al., 1975; Weindruch and Walford, 1982).

The effects of underfeeding in rodents appear to represent a true slowing of the rate of aging, with an increase in maximum life span, maintenance of immune system function at a "younger" level (Weindruch et al., 1979; Good et al., 1980), and a lower incidence of a wide variety of neoplasms (McCay et al., 1935; Berg and Simms, 1960; Weindruch et al., 1979; Good et al., 1980). One of the hypotheses that has been proposed to explain this slowing of aging is that underfeeding results in a persistence of "growth potential" in rodents (McCay et al., 1935; McCay, 1952). The body size of rats on food restriction early in life stabilizes far below that attained in rats fed ad libitum, and because the epiphyses close late in life in rats, they retain the ability to grow in response to increased food intake until late in life (McCay et al., 1935; McCay, 1952).

Certain reptiles and fish grow in proportion to their food supply and retain the capacity to grow as long as they live; their rate of aging appears to be inversely proportional to their rate of growth (Kohn, 1971). It has been postulated that a similar mechanism may be operative in food-restricted rats (McCay 1935; McCay, 1952). If growth retardation with maintenance of growth potential does play a role in the increase in longevity induced by food restriction, it is clearly not the only factor. This is evidenced by the finding that food restriction increases life span in rodents that have attained their adult size. A second mechanism that has been suggested to play a role in the greater longevity of food-restricted rats relates to their low body fat content (Young, 1979). According to this hypothesis, the prevention of obesity and the associated metabolic abnormalities, such as decreased glucose tolerance and insulin resistance, may account for the greater longevity of underfed animals (Young, 1979).

II. EFFECTS OF EXERCISE ON LONGEVITY

A. Background

Like food restriction, vigorous exercise causes growth retardation and prevents obesity in male rats (Crews et al., 1969; Oscai and Holloszy,

1969; Oscai *et al.*, 1971). Furthermore, some of the physiological adaptations to exercise run counter to the changes that occur with aging (Craig *et al.*, 1981; Spurgeon *et al.*, 1983; Starnes *et al.*, 1983; Mazzeo *et al.*, 1984). Laboratory rats are usually confined to cages that markedly restrict their physical activity and are provided with food *ad libitum*. This is an abnormal situation that generally results in development of obesity (Craig *et al.*, 1981; Mazzeo *et al.*, 1984). It therefore seemed possible that exercise might increase survival time in the laboratory rat either by (a) counteracting some of the deterioration in structure and function associated with aging, resulting in a true increase in longevity, or (b) countering deleterious effects of overeating combined with a sedentary life-style, thus improving survival without increasing maximum life span. On the other hand, it has been postulated that life span is inversely related to energy expenditure, and if this is correct exercise might, by increasing the "rate-of-living," shorten survival (Rubner, 1908; Pearl, 1928; Harman, 1962; Fridovich, 1976, Del Maestro, 1980).

B. The "Rate-of-Living" Theory

Rubner (1908) and Pearl (1928) noted an inverse relationship between life span and metabolic rate in mammals. Rubner (1908) estimated that total energy expenditure during an animal's lifetime is approximately 200 kilocalories per gram of body tissue, and postulated that each gram of tissue can do only a fixed amount of work in a lifetime. (The value of 200 kcal/g is roughly correct for some species, but is off by a factor of more than three for man.) An interspecies inverse relationship of life span to metabolic rate is well documented (Rubner, 1908; Pearl, 1928; Sacher, 1976). Reports that exercise and chronic cold exposure both shorten life span have been cited as supportive evidence of the rate-of-living theory (Slonaker, 1912; Benedict and Sherman, 1937; Johnson *et al.*, 1963; Everitt and Porter, 1976).

Stated in its most primitive form, i.e., that an organism is born with a certain amount of vital principle and dies when this principle is expended (Rubner, 1908; Pearl, 1928), the rate-of-living theory makes no sense in the context of current biological knowledge. However, the rate-of-living theory has been restated in a more modern form as the "free radical" theory of aging (Harman, 1962; 1968, 1969; Del Maestro, 1980; Fridovich, 1976). According to this theory, the slower the rate of O_2 consumption ($\dot{V}O_2$) the longer the life span. This theory may have some validity, as oxygen is toxic not only to obligate anaerobes but also to aerobic organisms. Although oxygen is rather unreactive in its ground state (i.e., molecular O_2), it gives rise to dangerously reactive free radicals and derivatives in the univalent pathway of oxygen reduction, i.e., the superoxide anion radical, hydrogen peroxide, and hydroxyl radical (Fridovich, 1976; Del Maestro, 1980).

Effective defenses against oxygen toxicity exist. One is avoidance of the univalent pathway of oxygen reduction by the reaction catalyzed by cytochrome oxidase in which electrons from the mithochondrial electron transport chain are transferred to oxygen in an apparent four electron reduction to H_2O, during which no intermediates of O_2 reduction are released from the enzyme. However, there appears to be a "leak current" or "univalent leak" in electron flow leading to formation of some free radicals (Fridovich, 1976; Del Maestro, 1980). At slow rates of O_2 utilization by mitochondria this univalent leak is probably controlled by the free radical scavenger mechanisms available (Del Maestro, 1980). However, when the rates of O_2 consumption and electron transport are greatly increased, the available scavenger mechanisms may not be able to keep pace with the rate of free radical formation, resulting in free radical injury to the tissues in which $\dot{V}o_2$ is increased.

A variety of enzymatic reactions and the spontaneous oxidation of hemoglobin, myoglobin, epinephrine, and other compounds also lead to production of superoxide radical and H_2O_2 (Fridovich, 1976; Del Maestro, 1980). Superoxide dismutase, catalases, and peroxidases function as defenses against free radicals and H_2O_2 (Fridovich, 1976; Del Maestro, 1980). However, no defense is perfect, and it appears that reactive oxygen radicals continually cause a low level of damage to cells of aerobic organisms. Free radical damage includes inactivation of enzymes, nicking of DNA, and peroxidation of lipids (Fridovich, 1976; Del Maestro, 1980). Nonmetabolizable products of lipid peroxidation accumulate in cells as age, or lipofuscin, pigments, which have been used as a marker for free radical damage (Tappel, 1973).

Davies *et al.* (1982) have reported that a bout of exercise can increase free radical concentration with damage to mitochondria in muscle. In a recent study, we investigated the possibility that muscle might adapt to endurance exercise training with an enhancement of enzymatic defenses against free radical damage (Higuchi *et al.*, 1985). A program of running that induced twofold increases in mitochondrial enzymes in leg muscles of rats resulted in no increase in catalase or cytoplasmic superoxide dismutase (SOD) activities. Mitochondrial SOD activity was increased 37% in fast-twitch red and slow-twitch red types of muscle and 14% in white muscle. Thus, despite an increase in mitochondrial SOD, the ratio of SOD to mitochondrial citrate cycle and respiratory chain enzymes was decreased. These findings make it seem unlikely that increased capacity for enzymatic scavenging of free radicals is a major protective adaptation against free radical damage in exercise-trained skeletal muscle.

Muscle pathology is not a significant contributor to mortality either in the rat or in humans. Therefore, it seems unlikely that increased free radical damage to muscle induced by exercise has a significant impact on longevity. It remains to be determined whether regularly performed exercise accelerates free radical-induced damage in other, more vital, tissues.

C. Previous Studies of the Effect of Exercise on Longevity

A large segment of the population of the United States participates in vigorous exercise. A likely motivating factor for much of this activity is the current perception among both health professionals and the public that exercise has health benefits. There is some evidence that exercise may have certain health benefits, particularly among populations of wealth Western nations in which consumption of calories, fat, cholesterol, and salt is excessive, and stress levels are often high (Thomas et al., 1981). In this context it seems important to determine whether or not exercise has the undesirable effect of accelerating the aging process. Such an effect would be extremely difficult to detect in humans, because (a) man is a long-lived species, (b) a detrimental effect on primary aging might be partly obscured by beneficial effects of exercise on certain of the disease processes, such as coronary atherosclerosis, essential hypertension, type II diabetes, and osteoporosis, that are largely responsible for secondary aging, and (c) there are large, genetically determined interindividual differences in longevity.

In this context, the rat seems to be a good model for studying the effects of exercise on life span because (a) rats are a short-lived species, (b) rats do not normally develop the diseases responsible for secondary aging in humans on which exercise may have a beneficial effect, (c) essentially all the experimental data that have been used to support the rate-of-living theory have come from studies on rats, and (d) the evidence that life span can be extended by food restriction has come from studies on rats and mice.

Information from early studies regarding the effect of exercise on longevity in rats is difficult to interpret and inconclusive (Slonaker, 1912; Benedict and Sherman, 1937; Retzlaff et al., 1966; Edington et al., 1972). Slonaker (1912) found that rats given access to exercise wheels were shorter-lived than those not allowed to exercise. Similarly, Benedict and

Sherman (1937) observed that previously sedentary middle-aged rats died prematurely when subjected to exercise. These studies were done before pathogen-free rats became available, i.e., on populations of rats with chronic endemic infections. We had a similar experience when we initially began our studies on the effects of exercise and used rats that were not pathogen-free. Rats subjected to moderately strenuous exercise would often lose weight rapidly, become febrile, develop a cough, and, frequently, die. At necropsy they usually had pneumonia and/or lung abscesses. We were not successful in bringing rats to a high level of training until we began to work with pathogen-free rats. We have not had problems with infections in our exercising animals since we began using pathogen-free rats in 1966. In this context, it seems likely that the rats in the early studies had chronic infections that were made worse by exercise.

In a later study, Retzlaff et al. (1966) reported that 10 minutes of daily running at 11.5 m/minute markedly increased mean survival and maximum life span in Sprague–Dawley rats. The results of this study are difficult to interpret because of the extremely short life span, only 474 days, of the sedentary control male rats compared to 605 days for the runners. Although the Sprague–Dawley strain is short-lived, their normal life expectancy when fed *ad libitum* is at least 2 years (Hoffman, 1978). Other unusual findings were that the runners were heavier than the sedentary controls and that the peak body weight of the sedentary *ad libitum*-fed male rats was only 401 g.

In another study, Edington et al. (1972) reported that 20 minutes of daily running at 10 m/minute increased the survival time of young rats but decreased the survival time of middle-aged and old rats. The results of this study are also difficult to interpret, because the apparent prolongation of survival time in the young rats appeared to be the result of a shortened survival of their sedentary controls, whereas the apparent reduction in survival time of the exercised older rats was due to prolonged survival of their sedentary controls. Thus, 50% of the sedentary controls for the rats that began to exercise at age 120 days were dead before age 650 days, while only 20% of the controls for the rats that began to exercise at age 600 days were dead at 960 days.

D. Our Findings on the Effect of Exercise on Longevity of Rats

Because the available information regarding the effect of exercise on longevity of rats was sparse and inconclusive, we performed a study to evaluate the effect of voluntary exercise on longevity of healthy rats (Holloszy *et al.*, 1985). We used male specific-pathogen-free Long Evans rats. A subgroup of these animals were necropsied; cultures were obtained and serum was examined for titers of antibodies against pathogenic viruses and mycoplasma. The necropsied rats were found to be pathogen-free, and the closed rat colony used for this study remained free of clinical and necropsy evidence of infectious disease. The rats were housed in a temperature- and light-controlled animal room with its own ventilation system with 15 air exchanges per hour, in a facility in which no other rats were housed. The people who entered the room to care for the animals did not work with other rodents or in areas where they were exposed to other rodents.

At 6 months of age rats were randomly assigned to a voluntary exercise group, a sedentary freely eating group, or a paired weight group whose food intake was restricted to keep their body weight the same as that of the runners. The sedentary rats were housed in individual stainless steel cages. The voluntary runners lived in stainless steel cages with attached running wheels, 112 cm in circumference, to which the rats had free access (Wahmann Co., Baltimore, Md.). The running wheels were fitted with counters that recorded the number of revolutions made by the wheels. The rats were fed a diet of Purina chow and water. After a few weeks, the runners were covering 2–7 miles/24 hours. However, after about 4–6 months they appeared to lose interest in running and abruptly would markedly reduce the distance they ran. We discovered that if we gave the runners slightly less food than they were eating *ad libitum*, so that there was a period during the day in which they were without food, this reversed the decrease in activity. Because it was essential to the purpose of the study that the rats continue to exercise, we made the decision to decrease each runner's food intake approximately 8% below its *ad libitum* intake at the time that the animal markedly reduced its running. By age 12 months all but one of the 32 runners were on the slightly restricted intake.

To control for the runners' slightly restricted food intake, a group of paired weight controls, i.e., rats that had been food-restricted to keep their weights in the same range as those of the runners from age 6 months on, was converted to pair-fed controls at age 12 months. These animals were given the same average amount of food as eaten by the runners. Since the animals reduced their running at different times, and as the decrease in running was reversed in 1 to 2 weeks, the abrupt, transient reduction is not evident in the graph of the average distances run per week by the voluntary runners in the longevity study (Fig. 1).

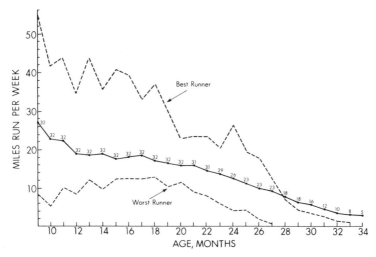

Fig. 1. Decline in the average distance run per week with aging. The number of rats per time point is shown above the line. From Holloszy *et al.*, 1985.

The distances that the rats ran during the last 3 months of their lives are not included in the averages in Fig. 1 to avoid including the terminal illness period.

Beginning at about 26 months of age, the sedentary freely eating animals began to lose weight, with a decline in average weight from roughly 600 to 500 g between 26 and 32 months of age (Fig. 2). The decline was due to loss of weight by the surviving animals rather than to a longer survival of smaller animals. There was no significant relationship between longevity and body weight in the freely eating sedentary group; the correlation coefficient between weight at age 12 months and age at death was −0.10 (*p* = .48) and for weight at age 18 months and age of death *r* = .14 (*p* = .32). The weight loss was gradual and occurred while the rats still appeared healthy; it did not appear to represent weight loss due to terminal illness. Weights during the last 2 months of life are not included in the averages in Fig. 2. The pair-fed sedentary controls showed a gradual increase in weight of about 80 g over the 12-month period after they were converted from paired weight to pair-fed; unlike the freely eating sedentary group, the pair-fed controls showed no decline in body weight after age 26 months.

The paired weight sedentary rats, whose food intake was restricted to keep their body weights in the same range as those of the runners, ate approximately two-thirds as much food as the freely eating sedentary controls during the first year of the study. Thereafter, the degree of food

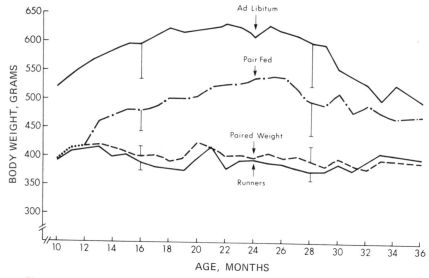

Fig. 2. Body weights of the rats in the four groups. From Holloszy *et al.*, 1985.

restriction relative to the freely eating animals decreased as the latter group voluntarily reduced their food intake; for the period of the study up to 32 months of age, the paired weight group ate approximately 28% less than the freely eating groups.

Figure 3 shows the survival curves for the four groups. As in many previous studies (Weindruch and Walford, 1982), reduced food intake was associated with an increase in life span. The sedentary paired weight rats had an average life span of 1113 ± 150 days (mean ± SD), 20% longer than that of the sedentary rats; freely eating rats had an average life span of 923 ± 160 days. The paired weight group's increased longevity was evidenced both in a later age of onset of mortality and in an extension of life span; the oldest three rats in the paired weight group (1317 ± 23 days) were more than 3 months older than the oldest rats in the other three groups. The degree of food restriction required to keep the body weight of the paired weight sedentary rats in the same range as that of the runners was relatively mild compared to that used in most previous studies of the life-prolonging effects of reduced food intake. The paired weight controls ate approximately 72% as much food as the freely eating controls, compared to 40–60% of *ad libitum* consumption in studies in which food restriction resulted in a more marked increase in longevity. Food restriction was also started later in life than usual, at 6 months as compared to 6–12 weeks.

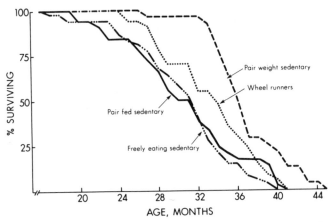

Fig. 3. Survival curves for the four groups of rats. From Holloszy *et al.*, 1985.

Although the runners' body weights were in the same range as those of the paired weight sedentary animals, their life span was significantly shorter (Fig. 3); the range of age at death was 735 to 1229 days for the runners and 801 to 1344 days for the paired weight controls. The runners had a significantly better survival than the freely eating sedentary controls; however, the difference in longevity was modest. Average length of life was 89 days (10%) longer than that of the freely eating sedentary controls (1012 ± 138 days versus 923 ± 160 days, $p < .01$). The runners also lived slightly longer (9%) than the pair-fed sedentary controls (1012 ± 138 days versus 928 ± 186 days, $p < .05$). Comparison of the longevity of the freely eating sedentary rats with that of the pair-fed sedentary controls (923 ± 160 days versus 928 ± 186 days) provides evidence that the slight food restriction required to keep the wheel runners running was not, in itself, sufficient to improve survival.

It appears from these findings that the wheel running improved survival without slowing the aging process or extending the life span. This interpretation is supported by the findings (a) that the three oldest runners were similar in age to the oldest pair-fed and freely eating sedentary controls (1220 ± 11 days versus 1212 ± 18 and 1209 ± 19 days) and (b) that there were no significant differences in the incidence of the pathological processes responsible for mortality in these three groups. This is in contrast to the food-restricted, paired weight sedentary rats, which had a significantly reduced incidence of malignancies. One possible interpretation of these results is that exercise may counteract deleterious effects of a sedentary life combined with overeating and thus allow a larger proportion of the animals to reach old age, but without slowing primary aging.

E. Discussion

The results of our study (Holloszy *et al.*, 1985), summarized above, appear to be in partial disagreement with the findings in a study by Goodrick (1980) published while our study was in progress. He found that male rats given access to running wheels lived, on the average, 4 months longer, while female runners lived 3 months longer than sedentary controls. While the absolute increase in survival was roughly similar to that seen in our rats, Goodrick's voluntary runners, in contrast to ours, appeared to have an increase in life span, as is seen with food restriction. This was evidenced by the finding that the oldest runners were roughly 3 months older than the oldest sedentary controls (Goodrick, 1980). As there was no necropsy data, it is not known whether the incidence of the pathological processes responsible for mortality was altered (Goodrick, 1980). It is not possible on the basis of the available information to explain the difference between our and Goodrick's results. However, there were major differences in study design and findings. One major difference is that Goodrick's sedentary freely eating male Wistar rats had an average survival of only 631 days, and half of his control rats were dead by age 21 months. This seems to be a short life span for *ad libitum*-fed male Wistar rats, which normally have an average life span of about 750 days (Hoffman, 1978). It is, therefore, difficult to accept the conclusion that the voluntary running retarded the aging process (Goodrick, 1980); instead it may have partially protected against disease processes that began to kill the rats at the relatively early age of 17–18 months. Possibly of relevance to this question is the finding by Goodrick *et al.* in other studies that rats housed in voluntary running wheels and fed every other day to reduce their food intake (Goodrick *et al.*, 1983) lived longer than *ad libitum*-fed rats (Goodrick, 1980) but did not live as long (14 weeks less) as sedentary rats fed every other day (Goodrick *et al.*, 1982). This finding would appear to argue against the interpretation that exercise slows the aging process.

As discussed in Section I, one of the hypotheses that has been proposed to explain the slowing of aging by food restriction in rodents is that underfeeding results in a persistence of "growth potential." A finding in our study that may have relevance to this hypothesis is that growth was retarded to the same extent in the runners and the paired weight sedentary rats that were food-restricted to keep their body weight the same as that of the runners. Thus, these two groups retained similar growth potential, yet the runners had a significantly shorter survival than the paired weight controls, and, in contrast to the paired weight group, had no extension of their life span or a reduction in the incidence of neoplasia. These findings may constitute evidence against the growth potential hypothesis.

Another mechanism that has been suggested to play a role in the greater longevity of food-restricted rats relates to their low body fat content (Young, 1979). According to this hypothesis, prevention of obesity and associated metabolic abnormalities, such as decreased glucose tolerance and insulin resistance, may account for the greater longevity of underfed animals. We have found that voluntary runners have a slightly lower body fat content than the paired weight sedentary controls, which argues against the hypothesis that reduced body fat stores are responsible for slowing aging in food-restricted animals. On the other hand, our findings are compatible with the hypothesis that exercise, by protecting against deleterious effects of obesity, improves survival and enables more rats to attain old age, but without an extension of life span. Food restriction apparently does something more.

An alternative possibility is that growth retardation with maintenance of growth potential and prevention of obesity do slow aging in rats but that these, and possibly other, beneficial effects are counteracted by a deleterious effect of exercise, possibly due to increased free radical damage associated with elevated rates of O_2 utilization. Therefore, although our results show that exercise slightly prolongs, instead of shortens (Slonaker, 1912; Benedict and Sherman, 1937), survival of healthy rats, they do not rule out the possibility, which requires further study, that exercise may also have deleterious effects due to an increased "rate-of-living" (Rubner, 1908; Pearl, 1928; Harman, 1962; Fridovich, 1976; Del Maestro, 1980).

In conclusion, our results provide evidence that exercise improves survival of rats (i.e., more attain old age) but, in contrast to food restriction, does not result in an extension of life span.

REFERENCES

Benedict, G., and Sherman, H. C. (1937). *J. Nutr.* **14,** 179–198.
Berg, B. N., and Simms, H. S. (1960). *J. Nutr.* **71,** 255–263.
Craig, B. W., Hammons, G. T., Garthwaite, S. M., Jarett, L., and Holloszy, J. O. (1981). *J. Appl. Physiol.* **51,** 1500–1506.
Crews, E. L., III, Fuge, K. W., Oscai, L. B., Holloszy, J. O., and Shank, R. E. (1969). *Am. J. Physiol.* **216,** 359–363.

Davies, K. J. A., Quintanilha, A. T., Brooks, G. A., and Packer, L. (1982). *Biochem. Biophys. Res. Commun.* **107,** 1198–1205.

Del Maestro, R. F. (1980). *Acta Physiol. Scand.* **492,** 153–168.

Edington, D. W., Cosmas, A. C., and McCafferty, W. B. (1972). *J. Gerontol.* **27,** 341–343.

Everitt, A. V., and Porter, B. (1976). *In* "Hypothalamus, Pituitary and Aging" (A. V. Everitt and J. A. Burgess, eds.), p. 570. Thomas, Springfield, Illinois.

Fridovich, I. (1976). *In* "Free Radicals in Biology" (W. A. Pryor, ed.), Vol. 1, p. 239. Academic Press, New York.

Good, R. A., West, A., and Fernandes, G. (1980). *Fed. Proc., Fed. Am. Soc. Exp. Biol.* **39,** 3098–3104.

Goodrick, C. L. (1980). *Gerontology* **26,** 22–33.

Goodrick, C. L., Ingram, D. K., Reynolds, M. A., Freeman, J. R., and Cider, N. L. (1982). *Gerontology* **28,** 233–241.

Goodrick, C. L., Ingram, D. K., Reynolds, M. A., Freeman, J. R., and Cider, N. L. (1983). *Exp. Aging Res.* **9,** 203–209.

Harman, D. (1962). *Radiat. Res.* **16,** 752–763.

Harman, D. (1983). *J. Gerontol.* **23,** 476–482.

Harman, D. (1969). *J. Am. Geriatr. Soc.* **17,** 721–735.

Higuchi, M., Cartier, L. J., Chen, M., and Holloszy, J. O. (1985). *J. Gerontol.* **40,** 281–286.

Hoffman, H. J. (1978). *In* "Development of the Rodent as a Model System of Aging, Book II" (D. C. Gibson, R. C. Adelman, and C. Finch, eds.), DHEW Publ. No. (NIH) 79-161, p. 19. U.S. Govt. Printing Office, Washington, D.C.

Holloszy, J. O., Smith, E. K., Vining, M., and Adams, S. (1985). *J. Appl. Physiol.* **59,** 826–831.

Johnson, H. D., Kintner, L. D., and Kibler, H. H. (1963). *J. Gerontol.* **18,** 29–36.

Kohn, R. R. (1971). "Principles of Mammalian Ageing." Prentice-Hall, Englewood Cliffs, New Jersey.

McCay, C. M. (1952). *In* "Cowdry's Problems of Aging" (A. I. Lansing, ed.), 3rd ed., p. 139. Williams & Wilkins, Baltimore, Maryland.

McCay, C. M., Crowell, M. F., and Maynard, L. A. (1935). *J. Nutr.* **10,** 63–79.

Masoro, E. J., Yu, B. P., Bertrand, H. A., and Lynd, F. T. (1980). *Fed. Proc., Fed. Am. Soc. Exp. Biol.* **39,** 3178–3182.

Mazzeo, R. S., Brooks, G. A., and Horvath, S. M. (1984). *J. Appl. Physiol.* **57,** 1369–1374.

Nolen, G. A. (1972). *J. Nutr.* **102,** 1477–1494.

Oscai, L. B., and Holloszy, J. O. (1969). *J. Clin. Invest.* **48,** 2124.

Oscai, L. B., Mole, P. A., Brei, B., and Holloszy, J. O. (1971). *Am. J. Physiol.* **220,** 1238–1241.

Pearl, R. (1928). "The Rate of Living." Knopf, New York.

Retzlaff, E., Fontaine, J., and Furuta, W. (1966). *Geriatrics* **21,** 171–177.

Ross, M. H. (1972). *Am. J. Clin. Nutr.* **25,** 834–838.

Ross, M. H. (1976). *In* "Nutrition and Aging" (M. Winick, ed.), p. 43. Wiley, New York.

Rubner, M. (1908). "Das Problem der Lebensdauer und seine Beziehungen zur Wachstum und Ernahrung." Oldenbourg, Munich.

Sacher, G. A. (1976). *Interdiscip. Top. Gerontol.* **9,** 69.

Slonaker, J. R. (1912). *J. Anim. Behav.* **2,** 20–42.

Spurgeon, H. A., Steinbach, M. F., and Lakatta, E. G. (1983). *Am. J. Physiol.* **244,** H513–H518.

Starnes, J. W., Beyer, R. E., and Edington, D. W. (1983). *Am. J. Physiol.* **245,** H560–H566.

Stuchlikova, E., Juricova-Horakova, M., and Deyl, Z. (1975). *Exp. Gerontol.* **10,** 141–144.

Tappel, A. L. (1973). *Fed. Proc., Fed. Am. Soc. Exp. Biol.* **32,** 1870–1874.

Thomas, G. S., Lee, P. R., Franks, P., and Paffenberger, R. S., Jr. (1981). *In* "Exercise and Health." Oelgeschlager, Gunn & Hair Publishers, Cambridge, Massachusetts.

Weindruch, R. H., and Walford, R. L. (1982). *Science* **215**, 1415–1418.

Weindruch, R. H., Kristie, J. A., Cheney, K. E., and Walford, R. L. (1979). *Fed. Proc., Fed. Am. Soc. Exp. Biol.* **38**, 2007–2016.

Young, V. R. (1979). *Fed. Proc., Fed. Am. Soc. Exp. Biol.* **38**, 1994–2000.

Yu, B. P., Masoro, E. J., Murata, I., Bertrand, H. A., and Lynd, F. T. (1982). *J. Gerontol.* **37**, 130–141.

15

Nutritional Factors in Age-Related Osteoporosis

B. Lawrence Riggs

Endocrine Research Unit
Mayo Clinic and Foundation
Rochester, Minnesota

I. THE PROBLEM OF OSTEOPOROSIS

Osteoporosis is defined pathologically as an absolute decrease in the amount of bone. The bone that is present is normal chemically and histologically. Fractures due to osteoporosis are mainly the result of bone loss. In the very elderly, however, an increased propensity to fall may be a contributory cause. More trabecular than cortical bone is lost with aging. This accounts for the characteristic locations of fractures associated with osteoporosis—the vertebrae, proximal femur, and distal radius.

Osteoporosis is an enormous public health problem (Melton and Riggs, 1983; Kelsey, 1984). About 1.3 million fractures in the United States each year are attributable to it.

207

Nutrition and Aging

Among women over the age of 65 years, 25% will have had one or more vertebral fractures. By extreme old age, one woman in three and one man in six will have had a hip fracture. These fractures are associated with a mortality of 15% and with long-term domiciliary care in 50% of the survivors. Indeed, falls are the leading cause of accidental death in the elderly, primarily because of hip fractures. The direct and indirect costs of osteoporosis have been estimated at $3.8 billion in the United States in 1983.

II. DETERMINANTS OF BONE MASS

The modern concept is that osteoporosis is caused by multiple factors (Riggs and Melton, 1986). The major determinants of bone mass are given in Table I. In any given individual, some factors may be more important than others. By far the most important determinant of bone mass is age. If chronological age is known, bone mass can be predicted for either sex with a standard deviation of only about 10%. Constitutional factors are also important, particularly in determining peak bone mass. At any age, blacks have denser bones than do whites and men have denser bones than women. Of hormonal factors, the most important is postmenopausal estrogen deficiency. In the decade following menopause, there is accelerated loss of both cortical and trabecular bone, amounting to about 10 to 15% over that predicted from the effect of age alone. Other hormonal abnormalities include abnormal vitamin D metabolism and both increases and decreases in parathyroid function in individuals. Various environmental risk factors for bone loss include decreased physical activity, high alcohol consumption, smoking, and excessive coffee consumption.

A number of investigators have suggested that nutritional factors may play a role in the pathogenesis of osteoporosis. These alleged factors include low calcium intake, increased calcium requirement with aging,

TABLE I

Determinants of Bone Mass

Aging
Constitutional factors
Hormonal factors
Environmental factors
Nutritional factors

excessive phosphate intake, increased protein intake, and insufficient vitamin D intake. In the remainder of this paper, I will review the evidence both for and against the importance of these nutritional factors.

III. CALCIUM

In contrast to requirements for other mineral nutrients, the requirement for calcium is relatively high because of obligatory fecal and urinary losses of about 150 to 250 mg/day (Heaney *et al.*, 1982). When the amount of dietary calcium absorbed is insufficient to offset these losses, calcium must be withdrawn from bone which contains 99% of total body stores. The desirable intake of calcium has not been rigorously established. Currently, the recommended dietary allowance is set at 800 mg/day for adults and 1200 mg/day for growing adolescents. A recent survey by the Public Health Service showed that, although American men have an average dietary intake that approximates this level, middle-aged and elderly women have an intake of only 550 mg/day (Abraham *et al.*, 1977). Osteoporotic women may have even a lower level of calcium intake (Riggs *et al.*, 1967). The recent NIH Consensus Conference on Osteoporosis (Peck, 1984) recommended an intake of 1000 mg/day for premenopausal women and 1500 mg/day for postmenopausal women. As a result of this and of increasing awareness of the problem of osteoporosis by the general public, there appears to have been an overall increase in calcium consumption in the last few years.

The dietary calcium requirement for adults is controversial, and different studies have reached conflicting conclusions (Gallagher and Riggs, 1978; Heaney *et al.*, 1982). The most detailed and widely quoted study was made by Heaney *et al.* (1978). These investigators performed metabolic balance studies on 168 normal perimenopausal women. For the premenopausal women, they found a positive relationship between calcium intake and calcium balance with a zero intercept (the theoretical level of calcium intake required to prevent negative calcium balance) of about 1000 mg/day. The findings were similar in postmenopausal women except that the slope of the regression was flatter with a zero intercept of 1500 mg/day (Fig. 1). This difference was due both to increased urinary losses and to decreased calcium absorption. These relationships suggest that both the recommended dietary allowance and the actual consumption of dietary calcium by perimenopausal women may be too low.

Both the menopause and aging impair calcium absorption, and thus increase calcium requirement. Although more calcium is needed after

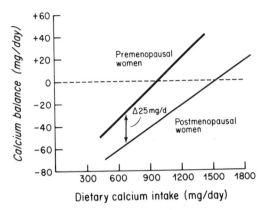

Fig. 1. Relationship between calcium intake and calcium balance in 130 normal women, aged 35–50 years, studied by Heaney *et al.* (1978). There was a direct and highly significant relationship between habitual dietary calcium intake and calcium balance. The zero intercept (the theoretical level of calcium intake that will prevent negative calcium balance) was 1000 mg for the premenopausal women but 1500 mg for the postmenopausal women. This suggests that menopause increases dietary calcium requirement.

midlife, Fig. 2 shows that less is consumed (Abraham *et al.*, 1977). Both aging and menopause are associated with an impaired metabolism of 25-hydroxyvitamin D (25-OH-D) to 1,25-dihydroxyvitamin D (1,25-(OH)$_2$D), the physiologically active metabolite (Gallagher *et al.*, 1979). In women with postmenopausal osteoporosis, the impaired absorption appears to be the secondary result of accelerated bone resorption due to estrogen deficiency; both serum 1,25-(OH)$_2$D and calcium absorption are normalized by estrogen replacement therapy (Gallagher *et al.*, 1980). By contrast, the impaired calcium absorption in the elderly appears to be related to a primary impairment in this conversion due to inadequate activity of 25-OH-D 1α-hydroxylase activity by the aging kidney (Tsai *et al.*, 1984).

There have been relatively few epidemiologic studies of the relationship of calcium intake to bone mass. Garn (1970), in several careful studies, could not find any appreciable relationship between calcium intake and metacarpal cortical area in either young or elderly subjects. Both significant (Hurxthal and Vose, 1969) and nonsignificant (Smith and Frame, 1965) relationships have been reported between calcium intake and radiographic density of the spine. However, Matkovic *et al.* (1979) found clear differences in bone mass in residents of two Yugoslavian districts, which had an approximately twofold difference in calcium intake. The residents from the district with the higher intake had higher values for bone mass (Fig. 3) and a lower incidence of hip fractures

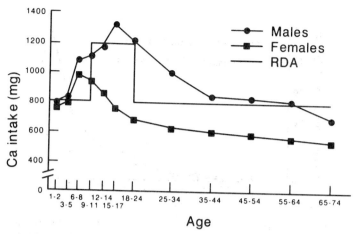

Fig. 2. Daily calcium intake for U.S. population, 1976–1980, as assessed by a U.S. Public Service survey. Note that women have a substantially lower calcium intake than do men, that calcium intake decreases with aging, and that levels in women are substantially below the recommended dietary allowance (RDA) for calcium.

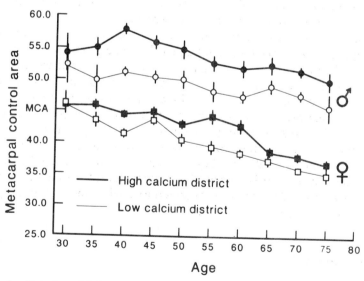

Fig. 3. Data from Matkovic *et al.* (1979) in which metacarpal width measurements were made in residents of two districts of Yugoslavia differing in calcium consumption. Note that for both men and women values were lower in the low-calcium than in the high-calcium district.

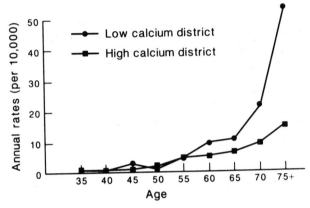

Fig. 4. Data from Matkovic *et al.* (1979) comparing rates of hip fracture in two districts of Yugoslavia differing in calcium consumption. The rates of hip fracture were significantly lower in the residents of the high-calcium district than in the residents of the low-calcium district.

(Fig. 4) than did the residents from the district with a lower calcium intake. The differences in bone mass, however, were apparent in young adulthood and did not diverge further as age progressed, suggesting that the major effect of calcium intake may have been on determining the level of peak bone mass that was achieved.

Prospective studies on the effect of calcium supplements on bone mass in postmenopausal women have indicated a protective effect if the dose of calcium is in excess of 1 g/day. Nordin *et al.* (1980) and Recker *et al.* (1977) found that calcium supplementation at 1200 and 1500 mg/day, respectively, decreased bone loss in postmenopausal patients as assessed by metacarpal radiogrammetry. In another study (Horsman *et al.*, 1977), supplements of 800 mg of elemental calcium per day slowed the rate of bone loss in postmenopausal women when assessed by measurements of the metacarpal bone, but the changes were of borderline significance statistically. Christiansen *et al.* (1980) found no effect on bone mineral density of the radius in postmenopausal women when only 500 mg/day were given.

IV. PHOSPHATE

Phosphate is so abundant in natural foods and renal conservation is so efficient that deficiency almost never occurs under conditions of normal life. Dietary consumption in the United States has remained relatively constant (1500 mg/day) during the past 70 years, despite marked shifts in the American diet during this period (Page and Friend, 1978). Acute administration of 1.5 g of orthophosphate stimulates the secretion of parathyroid hormone in human beings (Reiss *et al.*, 1970) and chronic administration of large doses increases bone resorption in experimental animals (Laflamme and Jowsey, 1972). Nonetheless, there is little evidence that phosphate intake in the range encountered in normal diets is deleterious to bone.

Two studies involving metabolic balance techniques found that varying phosphate intakes over a wide range had no adverse effect on calcium balance in normal adults (Spencer *et al.*, 1978; Heaney and Recker, 1982). Indeed, other studies suggest that increasing phosphate intake may have a beneficial effect on bone. Harris *et al.* (1976) showed that adult dogs receiving small phosphate supplements that reproduced normal alimentary phosphatemia several times a day markedly stimulated bone remodeling and more specifically converted the endosteal surface (which is normally dominated by resorption in adult dogs) into a bone-forming surface. Goldsmith *et al.* (1976) gave seven postmenopausal osteoporotic women supplements of 1.0 g/day of phosphate phosphorus for 3–20 months and noted improved calcium balance.

V. PROTEIN

The doubling of protein intake has been shown in many different studies to lead to a 50% increase in urinary calcium, and thereby decreases calcium retention (Heaney and Recker, 1982). The hypercalciuria results partly from an increase in the filtered load of calcium, due principally to a protein-induced increase in glomerular filtration rate, and partly due to increased acid load associated with catabolism of excess protein (Schuette *et al.*, 1980). Spencer *et al.* (1978) reported that when meat is the main dietary protein source, its high phosphorus content may offset, in part, the calciuric action of protein. Nonetheless, Eskimos of both sexes over 40 years of age who consume a high meat diet had 10–15% less bone than whites of the same age (Mazess and Mather, 1974). Thus, increased protein intake may increase bone loss, possibly by increasing the requirement for dietary calcium.

VI. VITAMIN D

Vitamin D is obtained either from the diet or from endogenous production in the skin after exposure to ultraviolet light. Deficiency in the adult produces characteristic bone changes called osteomalacia. About 30% of elderly women in Leeds, England, with fractures of the proximal femur were found to have histological osteomalacia and low serum 25-OH-D levels, with a peak incidence during the winter (Aaron et al., 1974). Residents from the United States are less likely to have nutritional vitamin D deficiency because of the more southern latitude and because of the fortification of dairy products with vitamin D. Although serum 25-OH-D levels decline with aging (Baker et al., 1980; K.-S. Tsai, H. W. Wahner, K. P. Offord, L. J. Melton, III, R. Kumar, and B. L. Riggs, unpublished data), this does not a support a role for inadequacy of vitamin D intake in age-related bone loss. Normal values for serum 25-OH-D have been found in American patients with vertebral fractures due to osteoporosis (Gallagher et al., 1979). In American patients with hip fractures, however, Sokoloff (1978) found histological evidence of osteomalacia, but Omdahl et al. (1982) were unable to find such evidence. Thus, if nutritional vitamin D deficiency occurs in American patients with osteoporosis, it is most likely to be found in elderly patients, particularly those requiring long-term domiciliary care.

VII. SUMMARY AND CONCLUSION

Although the importance of nutritional factors in the pathogenesis of osteoporosis is unclear, they are unlikely to be the major cause of the disorder. Nonetheless, a substantial amount of data suggests that the habitual dietary calcium intake of middle-aged and elderly American women (about 550 mg/day) is too low to contribute to calcium equilibrium. Until the requirement for dietary calcium in humans can be more accurately determined, it would seem reasonable to recommend that all adults increase their dietary calcium intake to at least 1000 mg daily. This level can be easily achieved by dietary means alone. Higher levels of calcium intake usually require use of supplementary medicinal calcium. This is probably indicated, however, in those individuals judged to be at increased risk for osteoporosis. A high protein intake may increase the requirement for dietary calcium by increasing urinary calcium excretion. Both beneficial and deleterious effects of a high phosphate intake on bone have been suggested. For levels of intake consumed by most Americans, however, the effect on bone is probably neutral. Except for elderly, house-bound individuals on inadequate dietary intake, vitamin D deficiency does not seem to play a role in the development of osteoporosis in America. Thus, although nutritional factors may not play a major role in the pathogenesis of osteoporosis, they are important because, in contrast to most other risk factors for osteoporosis, they can be safely and relatively easily corrected.

REFERENCES

Aaron, J. E., Gallagher, J. C., and Nordin, B. E. C. (1974). *Lancet* **2**, 84–85.

Abraham, S., Carroll, M. D., Dresser, C. M., and Johnson, C. L. (1977). "Dietary Intake Findings, United States 1971–1974," HEW Publ. No. HRA 77-1647. National Center for Health Statistics, Hyattsville, Maryland.

Baker, M. R., Peacock, M., and Nordin, B. E. C. (1980). *Age Ageing* **9**, 249–252.

Christiansen, C., Christensen, M. S., McNair, P., Hagen, C., Stocklund, K. E., and Transbol, I. B. (1980). *Eur. J. Clin. Invest.* **10**, 273–279.

Gallagher, J. C., and Riggs, B. L. (1978). *N. Engl. J. Med.* **298**, 193–195.

Gallagher, J. C., Riggs, B. L., Eisman, J., Hamstra, A., Arnaud, S. B., and DeLuca, H. F. (1979). *J. Clin. Invest.* **64**, 729–736.

Gallagher, J. C., Riggs, B. L., and DeLuca, H. F. (1980). *J. Clin. Endocrinol. Metab.* **51**, 1359–1364.

Garn, S. M. (1970). "The Earlier Gain and Later Loss of Cortical Bone." Thomas, Springfield, Illinois.

Goldsmith, R. S., Jowsey, J., Dube, W. J., Riggs, B. L., Arnaud, C. D., and Kelly, P. J. (1976). *J. Clin. Endocrinol. Metab.* **43**, 523–532.

Harris, W. H., Haney, R. P., Davis, L. A., Weinberg, E. H., Coutts, R. D., and Schiller, A. L. (1976). *Calcif. Tissue Res.* **22**, 85–98.

Heaney, R. P., and Recker, R. R. (1982). *J. Lab. Clin. Med.* **99**, 46–55.

Heaney, R. P., Recker, R. R., and Saville, P. D. (1978). *J. Lab. Clin. Med.* **92**, 953–963.

Heaney, R. P., Gallagher, J. C., Johnston, C. C., Neer, R., Parfitt, A. M., and Whedon, G. D. (1982). *Am. J. Clin. Nutr.* **36**, 986–1013.

Horsman, A., Gallagher, J. C., Simpson, M., and Nordin, B. E. C. (1977). *Br. Med. J.* **2**, 789–792.

Hurxthal, L. M., and Vose, G. P. (1969). *Calcif. Tissue Res.* **4**, 245–256.

Kelsey, J. F. (1984). *Proc. Natl. Inst. Health Consensus Dev. Conf., 1984*, pp. 25–28.

Laflamme, G. H., and Jowsey, J. (1972). *J. Clin. Invest.* **51**, 2834–2840.

Matkovic, V., Kostial, K., Simonovic, I., Buzina, R., Bordarec, A., and Nordin, B. E. C. (1979). *Am. J. Clin. Nutr.* **32**, 540–549.

Mazess, R. B., and Mather, W. (1974). *Am. J. Clin. Nutr.* **27**, 916–925.

Melton, L. J., and Riggs, B. L. (1983). *In* "The Osteoporotic Syndrome: Detection and Prevention" (L. V. Avioli, ed.). pp. 42–72. Grune & Stratton, New York.

Nordin, B. E. C., Horsman, A., Crilly, R. G., Marshall, D. H., and Simpson, M. (1980). *Br. Med. J.* **280**, 451–453.

Omdahl, J. L., Garry, P. J., Hunsaker, L. A., Hunt, W. C., and Goodwin, J. S. (1982). *Am. J. Clin. Nutr.* **36**, 1225–1233.

Page, L., and Friend, B. (1978). *BioScience* **28**, 192–197.

Peck, W. A. (1984). *JAMA, J. Am. Med. Assoc.* **252**, 799–802.

Recker, R. R., Saville, P. D., and Healey, R. P. (1977). *Ann. Intern. Med.* **87**, 649–655.

Reiss, E., Canterbury, J. M., Bercovitz, M. A., and Kaplan, E. L. (1970). *J. Clin. Invest.* **49**, 2146.

Riggs, B. L. and Melton, L. J. (1986). *N. Engl. J. Med.* **314**, 1676–1686.

Riggs, B. L., Kelly, P. J., Kinney, V. R., Scholz, D. A., and Bianco, A. J., Jr. (1967). *J. Bone Jt. Surg., Am. Vol.* **49A,** 915–924.

Schuette, S. A., Zemel, M. B., and Linkswiler, H. M. (1980). *J. Nutr.* **110,** 305–315.

Smith, R. W., and Frame, B. (1965). *N. Engl. J. Med.* **273,** 73–78.

Sokoloff, L. (1978). *Am. J. Surg. Pathol.* **2,** 21–30.

Spencer, H., Kramer, L., Osis, O., and Norris, C. (1978). *J. Nutr.* **108,** 447–457.

Tsai, K.-S., Heath, H., III, Kumar, R., and Riggs, B. L. (1984). *J. Clin. Invest.* **73,** 1668–1672.

16

Significance of Vitamin D in Age-Related Bone Disease

Hector F. DeLuca

Department of Biochemistry
College of Agricultural and Life Sciences
University of Wisconsin—Madison
Madison, Wisconsin

I. INTRODUCTION

There is little doubt that vitamin D is the most important hormone regulating the calcium content of bone. The existence of vitamin D became recognized primarily as a result of an epidemic of the deficiency disease rickets in Northern Europe, Northern Asia, and, to some extent, North America. A lack of mineralization of bone in this disease, especially evident in rapidly growing children elaborating large amounts of organic matrix, causes the overt symptoms of rickets, namely, grossly malformed skeletons. Sir Edward Mellanby, believing this widespread disease to be a nutritional problem,

217

Nutrition and Aging

was first able to produce it experimentally by feeding a diet of oatmeal to dogs maintained indoors (Mellanby, 1919). Since he was able to cure the disorder with cod liver oil, which contained the newly discovered fat-soluble vitamin A, he deduced that this must be another property of fat-soluble vitamin A. On the other hand, McCollum and his colleagues (1922) carried out a key experiment which demonstrated that the vitamin A activity could be destroyed by heating and oxidation, while anti-rachitic activity was not. He therefore deduced correctly the existence of a new vitamin called "fat-soluble vitamin D." At the same time, it was shown that rickets in children could be cured by means of ultraviolet irradiation (Huldshinsky, 1919). Steenbock (1924) demonstrated that ultraviolet irradiation of foods and skin converts a precursor to vitamin D. This discovery led to an elimination of rickets as a major medical problem and provided the basic physiologic information that resulted in the identification of vitamin D.

The failure of bone mineralization in the adult has been recognized as the vitamin D deficiency disease called osteomalacia (Hess, 1929). Thus in both the adult and growing children, vitamin D prevents bone diseases by eliciting mineralization of newly synthesized organic matrix. Two schools of thought have evolved in regard to how vitamin D brings about the mineralization of bone. One has been that vitamin D functions to elevate plasma calcium and phosphorus to levels that are required for mineralization and, therefore, does not function in either the elaboration of organic matrix or the mineralization process (DeLuca, 1967; Lamm and Neuman, 1958). Improvement of clinical bone disorders by the administration of vitamin D, allegedly without changing plasma calcium and phosphorus, has resulted in the implication that vitamin D might function directly on bone in one of these two processes (de Wardener and Eastwood, 1977; Rasmussen and Bordier, 1978). Similarly, some evidence that vitamin D might be involved in collagen synthesis of bone has been advanced (Hock et al., 1982). However, two key experiments have been carried out which essentially eliminate the possibility that any form of vitamin D functions either in the elaboration of organic matrix of bone or in the mineralization process itself. Vitamin D-deficient rats born to vitamin D-deficient mothers were continuously infused with calcium and phosphorus to maintain plasma calcium and phosphorus levels identical with those of animals of the same group given vitamin D (Underwood and DeLuca, 1984). Furthermore, other controls were carried out in which saline solutions were infused into identically treated rats given vitamin D. All animals were able to move about their cages and consume food and live otherwise normal lives for the period of 9 days of study. The results shown in Table I demonstrate that the femurs

TABLE I

Mineralization and Bone Growth Does Not Require Vitamin D if Bone Is Supplied with Calcium and Phosphorus

	Not infused		Infused	
	$-D^c$	$+D$	$-D$	$+D$
Serum Ca (mg/dl)	5.1^a	10.2	10.4	10.4
Serum P (mg/dl)	6.2^a	8.5^a	9.8	9.7
Femur length (nm)	22.2^a	24.5	25.1	25.8
Femur ash (%)	36.7	46.2	52.1^b	47.5
Femur ash (mg)	52.3^a	89.6	117.5^b	95.1

[a] Lower than others in group; $p < .001$.
[b] Higher than corresponding $+D$; $p < .001$.
[c] $-D$, vitamin D-deficient rats; $+D$, rats given 25 IU vitamin D_3 per day.

of rats infused with calcium and phosphorus accumulate at least as much mineral as do the femurs of animals given vitamin D either infused with saline or uninfused. Furthermore, bone histomorphometry was carried out to demonstrate that the mineralization was completely normal and that there was no evidence whatsoever of impaired synthesis of organic matrix in the vitamin D-deficient animals infused with calcium and phosphorus (Weinstein et al., 1984). These results and those of Holtrop et al. (1981) using high-calcium lactose-fortified diets provide a clear demonstration that vitamin D does not play a direct role in the synthesis of organic matrix or in the mineralization of bone. However, it is important to note from Table I that increased amounts of mineral are accumulated in the bones of animals not given vitamin D but given infusions of calcium and phosphorus. In this case, the trabeculae are much larger and do not show evidence of resorption (Weinstein et al., 1984). Since the active form of vitamin D has been shown in culture to cause bone resorption (Raisz et al., 1972; Stern et al., 1975), it is apparent that vitamin D does play an important role in bone by inducing resorption, which is followed by bone formation in the remodeling process. Thus, it is important to realize that vitamin D compounds do affect bones directly, but not by way of the bone formation mechanism.

Vitamin D increases blood calcium by at least three mechanisms. It markedly stimulates the enterocyte of the small intestine to absorb calcium against an electrochemical potential gradient (DeLuca, 1980). In the same cells, it stimulates active transport of phosphate. Another action of the vitamin is to permit the parathyroid hormone to mobilize calcium from bone (DeLuca, 1980). In vitamin D-deficient animals, injections of large amounts of parathyroid hormone will not cause the mobilization of calcium from bone (Rasmussen *et al.*, 1963). However, if the animals are primed with small amounts of vitamin D, the parathyroid hormone is then able to mobilize this calcium. Thus, the vitamin D compounds apparently provide the machinery which is then activated by the parathyroid hormone to mobilize calcium from bone to maintain blood calcium (Garabedian *et al.*, 1974). Finally, there is evidence that vitamin D stimulates renal absorption of calcium, a process that requires interaction with the parathyroid hormone in the distal renal tubule (Sutton and Dirks, 1978). By these mechanisms then, the vitamin D compounds bring about the necessary elevation of plasma calcium and phosphorus for mineralization of bone.

Vitamin D has other important functions. It is known that in osteomalacia the length of time required for bone remodeling is greatly increased (Frost, 1966). It is now clear that the active form of vitamin D stimulates the bone resorptive process, which is the precursor of both modeling and remodeling events of bone (Raisz *et al.*, 1972; Stern *et al.*, 1975). Thus, the repair and turnover of bone is dependent on the vitamin D hormone.

In addition to these sites, there is now increasing evidence that vitamin D may play an important role in such processes as differentiation of precursor stem cells to monocytes, which become precursors of osteoclasts (Tanaka *et al.*, 1982; Abe *et al.*, 1981). This is still in the realm of early investigation and should not yet be accepted as a physiologically significant finding. In addition, the receptor for the vitamin D hormone is found in a number of tissues not previously appreciated as being targets of vitamin D action. For example, it is found in the parathyroid glands, in the islet cells of the pancreas, in skin cells, and in mammary tissue (Link and DeLuca, 1985). Exactly what the function of vitamin D is, if any, in these organ is unknown.

II. THE VITAMIN D ENDOCRINE SYSTEM

Following the discovery of the nutritional forms of vitamin D and the form assumed to be produced in skin, it had been assumed that vitamin D was functional without metabolic modification (Kodicek, 1960). However, with the chemical synthesis of radiolabeled vitamin D of high specific activity and the subsequent series of investigations, it has become abundantly clear that vitamin D itself is biologically inactive and must be metabolized to its active hormonal form (DeLuca, 1974) (Fig. 1). Vitamin D is first converted in the liver to 25-hydroxyvitamin D_3 (25-OH-

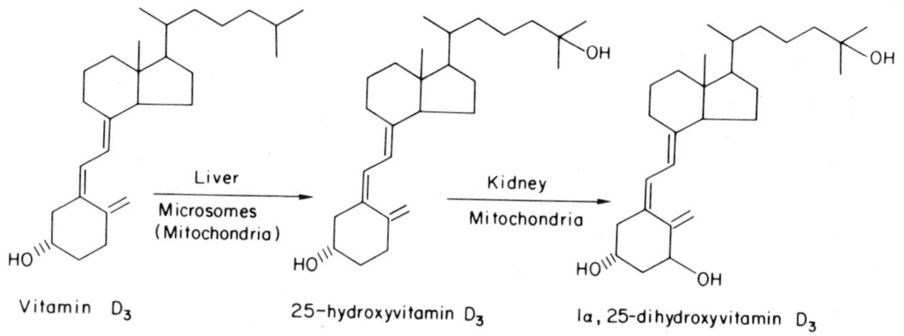

Fig. 1. Metabolism of vitamin D$_3$ required for function.

D$_3$). This is a process involving a microsomal cytochrome P-450 (Madhok and DeLuca, 1979) that has been purified (Anderson *et al.*, 1983). The 25-OH-D$_3$ is the circulating form of the vitamin and is transported to the kidney, where it is converted further to the vitamin D hormone 1,25-dihydroxyvitamin D$_3$ (1,25-(OH)$_2$D$_3$) (DeLuca, 1974). This conversion takes place in the mitochondria by a complex three-component cytochrome P-450 system that has been solubilized and reconstituted but not purified (Ghazarian *et al.*, 1974). This process occurs in the proximal convoluted tubule cells of the kidney, a site where there is abundant interaction with the parathyroid hormone (Brunette *et al.*, 1978). 1,25-(OH)$_2$D$_3$ is then transported to the intestine, to bone, and elsewhere in the kidney to initiate the events described in Section I.

There have been dramatic reports that bone cells, intestinal cells, and other cells in culture are able to produce 1,25-(OH)$_2$D$_3$ (Puzas *et al.*, 1983; Howard *et al.*, 1981). Activities of cells in culture do not necessarily represent activities *in vivo*. Nephrectomy of pregnant female rats does not prevent the synthesis of 1,25-(OH)$_2$D$_3$ (Weisman *et al.*, 1978; Gray *et al.*, 1979). However in nonpregnant rats in carefully done experiments, the removal of kidneys eliminates entirely the conversion of 25-OH-D$_3$ to 1,25-(OH)$_2$D$_3$ (Reeve *et al.*, 1983; Shultz *et al.*, 1983). Furthermore, in the hands of some investigators, plasma from anephric patients has no 1,25-(OH)$_2$D$_3$ (Shepard *et al.*, 1979). It is clear, however, that placenta, especially yolk sac and fetal renal tissue, is able to produce 1,25-(OH)$_2$D$_3$, accounting for the 1,25-(OH)$_2$D$_3$ found in the plasma of anephric pregnant mothers (Tanaka *et al.*, 1979; Gray *et al.*, 1981). For all practical purposes, therefore, in the normal physiologic state, the kidney is the exclusive site of synthesis of 1,25-(OH)$_2$D$_3$ except for the placenta. In a disease such as sarcoidosis, there is extrarenal or ectopic synthesis of 1,25-(OH)$_2$D$_3$ that causes hypercalcemia accounting for that disorder (Barbour *et al.*, 1981). This may also be true for lymphoma and other disease states but does not represent synthesis of 1,25-(OH)$_2$D$_3$ in the normal situation.

25-OH-D$_3$ is the central or intermediate form of vitamin D that is metabolized further. An abundant metabolism of vitamin D other than through 1α-hydroxylation occurs in the kidney and in target organs of 1,25-(OH)$_2$D$_3$ action (DeLuca and Schnoes, 1984). A summary of this metabolism appears in Fig. 2. As many as 33 metabolites of vitamin D have been identified from various *in vitro* and *in vivo* experiments involving large amounts of 25-OH-D$_3$ *in vitro* or large doses of vitamin D given to animals (DeLuca and Schnoes, 1984). Although these metabolites are of some interest, there is a strong question whether they exist under physiologic conditions. Figure 2, however, demonstrates the current physiologic pathways of vitamin D metabolism. The two most important pathways are 24R-hydroxylation to form 24R25-(OH)$_2$D$_3$, a process which occurs in target organs of intestine and bone as well as in the kidney (DeLuca and Schnoes, 1984), and 23S-hydroxylation followed by 26-oxidation, forming ultimately the 25-OH-D$_3$-26,23-lactone (DeLuca and Schnoes, 1984). Similar reactions can occur with 1,25-(OH)$_2$D$_3$ to form in small amounts 1α,24R,25-(OH)$_3$D$_3$ and 1α,25-(OH)$_2$D$_3$-26,23-lac-

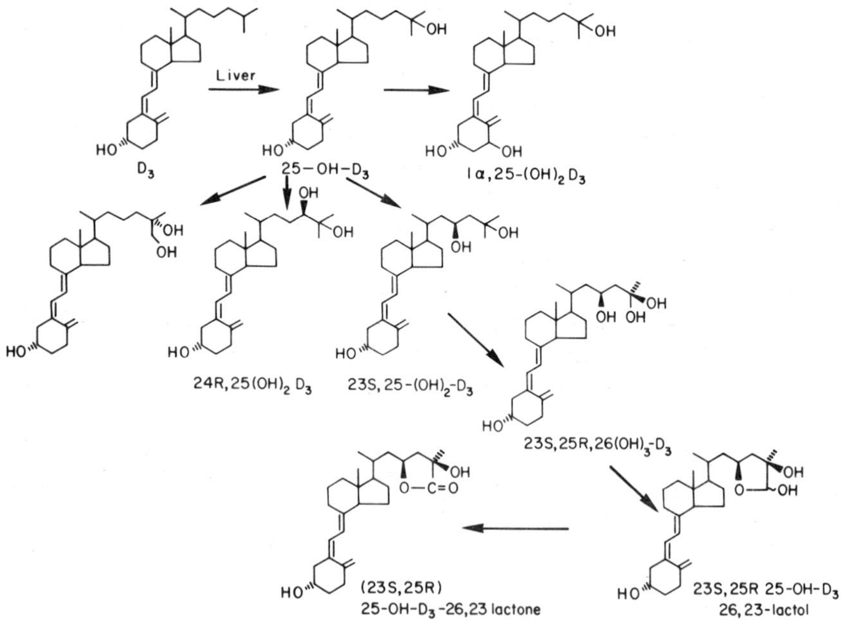

Fig. 2. The known physiologic metabolism of vitamin D. In addition to the reaction shown here, 1,25-(OH)$_2$D$_3$ is converted to C-23 carboxylic acid, known as calcitroic acid.

tone. Finally, it is important to realize that the vitamin D hormone itself, $1,25\text{-}(OH)_2D_3$, is oxidized in a series of reactions resulting in the side chain-cleaved metabolite called calcitroic acid (Esvelt *et al.*, 1979). This compound is biologically inert and clearly represents an inactivation form (Esvelt and DeLuca, 1981). However, $24R,25\text{-}(OH)_2D_3$ and to a lesser extent the other side chain modifications have received attention as possible metabolically active forms of the vitamin, especially $24R,25\text{-}(OH)_2D_3$. This compound has been claimed to be a hatching hormone (Henry and Norman, 1978), to be necessary for maintaining calcium homeostasis (Norman *et al.*, 1980), and to be an agent required for cartilage growth and maintenance (Garabedian *et al.*, 1978) and bone mineralization (Ornoy *et al.*, 1978), the latter two being outside the realm of function of vitamin D as described in Section I.

Chemically, synthesis of $25\text{-}OH\text{-}D_3$ with fluoro substitutions in key positions such as the 24,24-positions, the 23-23-positions, or the 26,27-positions has provided the means for investigating the functional role of modifications of the side chain at these sites. The C—F bond is stable and the fluoro group is less like hydroxyl than hydrogen and is ideal for testing for the importance of these modifications. The results of approximately 8 years of investigation with these compounds and with other experiments have demonstrated that none of the side chain-modified metabolites of $25\text{-}OH\text{-}D_3$ represent metabolically active forms and that the only activation of the vitamin D molecule is 25-hydroxylation followed by 1α-hydroxylation (DeLuca, 1985). A summary of this controversy has appeared in other reviews and in a review specifically devoted to this question (Brommage and DeLuca, 1985). The result of these investigations is that at the present time all attention must be focused on the 1α-hydroxylation pathway as the activation pathway.

Clear evidence that 1α-hydroxylation is required for function in man is provided by the existence of the disease vitamin D-dependency rickets Type I in which a defect in 1α-hydroxylation has been demonstrated (Fraser *et al.*, 1973; Scriver *et al.*, 1978). Finally, it has been shown that the intestine of both animals and man in the absence of kidneys does not respond to physiologic amounts of $25\text{-}OH\text{-}D_3$ while they do respond to physiologic amounts of $1\alpha,25\text{-}(OH)_2D_3$ (Boyle *et al.*, 1972b; Wong *et al.*, 1972). Since $1,25\text{-}(OH)_2D_3$ is made entirely in the kidney for all practical purposes and has its function elsewhere, it must be regarded as a hormone. As a true endocrine system, therefore, the kidney 1α-hydroxylase is regulated as described below.

The production of $1\alpha,25\text{-}(OH)_2D_3$ is feedback regulated by calcium through the parathyroid system (DeLuca, 1974). Thus, hypocalcemia causes a marked stimulation of $1\alpha,25\text{-}(OH)_2D_3$ synthesis, whereas hypercalcemia shuts down 1α-hydroxylation and turns on 24R-hydroxylation. This has been demonstrated both *in vivo* and *in vitro* many times. There is some question whether calcium can directly regulate 1α-hydroxylation or whether it functions entirely through the parathyroid system. The view of this author is that virtually all of this regulation is carried out by the parathyroid system under physiologic circumstances. Thus, hypocalcemia stimulates parathyroid secretion which in turn interacts with the proximal convoluted tubule cells to stimulate 1α-hydroxylation. The time course of this response is approximately 6 hours. It is blocked by RNA and protein synthesis inhibitors, suggesting that new protein synthesis is involved in this regulation.

In addition to regulation by parathyroid hormone 1α-hydroxylation is regulated by serum phosphorus as well (Tanaka and DeLuca, 1973). Hypophosphatemia causes increased production of $1\alpha,25\text{-}(OH)_2D_3$, and although there may be an additional effect on decreasing degradation (Baxter and DeLuca, 1976), this has not been completely verified or studied. Finally, $1,25\text{-}(OH)_2D_3$ itself can suppress 1α-hydroxylation and stimulate $24R,25\text{-}(OH)_2D_3$ production (Tanaka *et al.*, 1975). This also involves a nuclear activity and the mechanism is not entirely understood (Larkins *et al.*, 1974). Figure 3 demonstrates the calcium homeostatic

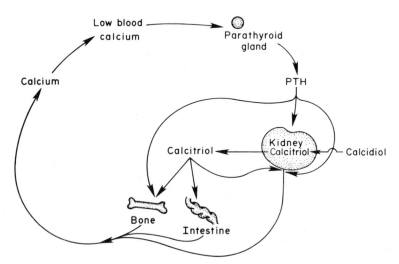

Fig. 3. Diagrammatic representation of the calcium homeostatic system involving the parathyroid gland and parathyroid hormone (PTH), which stimulates the conversion of $25\text{-}OH\text{-}D_3$ (calcidiol) to $1,25\text{-}(OH)_2D_3$ (calcitriol). Calcitriol acts on the target organs with or without parathyroid hormone to elevate plasma calcium, shutting off parathyroid secretion.

mechanism involving regulation by calcium and the parathyroid hormone.

Of considerable importance is the regulation of intestinal calcium absorption. Steenbock and his colleagues noted that animals on a low-calcium diet are able to better utilize calcium (Kletzien et al., 1932). Nicholaysen and his colleagues fully developed this investigation, demonstrating that an endogenous factor is responsible for providing a message to the intestine to stimulate intestinal calcium absorption when calcium is required by the skeleton (Nicolaysen et al., 1953). Thus, calcium-depleted skeletons in some way stimulate marked increases in intestinal calcium absorption (Nicolaysen et al., 1953). With the discovery of the vitamin D endocrine system, it became clear that this factor was merely the parathyroid system and the vitamin D endocrine system (Boyle et al., 1972a). Thus, under conditions in which calcium is needed or is being used by bone, the resulting slight hypocalcemia stimulates parathyroid secretion which in turn stimulates production of 1,25-$(OH)_2D_3$. 1,25-$(OH)_2D_3$ is the only hormone known that stimulates intestinal calcium absorption (DeLuca et al., 1982). By this mechanism, therefore, calcium from the environment is brought in when required by the skeleton (DeLuca, 1985). This mechanism of adjusting intestinal calcium absorption according to the needs of the organism is an important one for protection of the organism against excessive calcium absorption but more important is that it is a mechanism which protects the animal from loss of the skeleton. If intestinal calcium absorption is not increased when required by the skeleton, the parathyroid will continue to secrete parathyroid hormone and will mobilize calcium from bone to satisfy soft tissue needs (DeLuca, 1985). In this way, bone mass will be sacrificed for soft tissue needs. It is abundantly clear that interference with the metabolism of vitamin D to its active form will interfere with the ability to increase intestinal calcium absorption. It may also interfere with bone remodeling and, therefore, may play a role in predisposing the organism to loss of bone, a disease suffered by the aging population, and to poor bone quality.

III. OSTEOMALACIA AND OSTEOPOROSIS

Two diseases suffered by the aging population are osteomalacia and osteoporosis. Often, a senior citizen suffers a combination of both disorders—loss of bone mass and failure to mineralize newly synthesized matrix. The extent or distribution of these two can only be discerned by bone biopsy. However, there are markers of osteomalacia. If the patient presents with low circulating 25-OH-D levels, slight hypocalcemia and slight hypophosphatemia, and an elevated alkaline phosphatase of bone origin, the disease is likely to be osteomalacia (Habener and Mahaffey, 1978). Such a disorder would result from failure of cutaneous synthesis of the vitamin D compounds as described by Holick (see Chapter 5) or inadequate intakes of vitamin D or both. This disorder should be treated with vitamin D to bring the 25-OH-D_3 levels to normal. However, even if the patients have normal 25-OH-D_3 levels and still present with increased alkaline phosphatase, hypocalcemia, and hypophosphatemia, measurement of $1\alpha,25$-$(OH)_2D_3$ in the plasma is of considerable interest. Under conditions of hypocalcemia, hypophosphatemia, and high alkaline phosphatase, one would normally expect extremely high levels of $1\alpha,25$-$(OH)_2D_3$ (Papapoulos et al., 1980; Stanbury et al., 1981). If plasma levels of $1\alpha,25$-$(OH)_2D_3$ are found to be normal or low, a defect in vitamin D metabolism would be indicated. Thus, osteomalacia of aging may in part be a failure of 1α-hydroxylation of 25-OH-D_3

In the case of osteoporosis found in our aging population, the failure is not in vitamin D deficiency but is a failure in part in the vitamin D endocrine system. If there is a failure to synthesize adequate amounts of $1\alpha,25$-$(OH)_2D_3$ to meet the needs of the organism, there will be a response of the parathyroid system to secrete additional amounts of hormone to mobilize bone calcium. With the presence of some $1\alpha,25$-$(OH)_2D_3$, bone will be mobilized to provide for soft tissue needs. A continuation of this without stimulation of intestinal calcium transport will result in a bone loss. Similarly, such a bone loss can be brought about by inhibition of intestinal calcium absorption, for example, with glucocorticoids (Harrison and Harrison, 1960). Finally, the absence of adequate amounts of $1\alpha,25$-$(OH)_2D_3$ may retard bone remodeling, and a combination of these factors could lead to a loss of bone mass and a loss of bone quality, which could result in bone fracture.

IV. AGING AND VITAMIN D METABOLISM AND FUNCTION

In all species, it is clear that aging results in a decreased intestinal calcium absorption as shown in Fig. 4. This experiment was carried out in rats fed the various levels of calcium as shown in the figure (Horst et al., 1978). However, similar results have been obtained by Bullamore et al. (1970) and Gallagher et al. (1979) in humans. Thus, intestinal calcium absorption falls with age. In conjunction with Gallagher and his colleagues, we have demonstrated that this exactly correlates with plasma

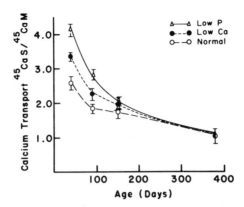

Fig. 4. Effect of age on intestinal calcium transport of rats maintained on either a low-phosphorus normal calcium diet, a low-calcium normal phosphorus diet, or a normal calcium, normal phosphorus diet and given adequate amounts of vitamin D. Injection of 1,25-$(OH)_2D_3$ at day 300 results in a marked increase in intestinal calcium transport.

1,25-$(OH)_2D_3$ levels, whereas 25-OH-D_3 levels are not changed (Gallagher et al., 1979). Similar results were obtained in our aging rat population (Horst et al., 1978). If 1,25-$(OH)_2D_3$ is given to older rats of patients, intestinal calcium absorption responds by increasing, although perhaps not to the same extent as in younger animals or subjects (Horst et al., 1978; Gallagher et al., 1979). Nevertheless, there is responsiveness present. Thus, failure of intestinal calcium absorption as the result of aging is at least in part failure to synthesize adequate amounts of 1,25-$(OH)_2D_3$. In an experiment carried out by Neer and his colleagues, it has been demonstrated that parathyroid injections into subjects over 65 do not bring about an increased plasma 1,25-$(OH)_2D_3$ levels, whereas injection into younger subjects brings about a marked increase in 1,25-$(OH)_2D_3$ levels, suggesting that the capacity of the 1α-hydroxylase to respond to parathyroid stimulation is lost with age (Slovik et al., 1981). Finally, as shown in Fig. 5, measurement of 1α-hydroxylase directly in renal tissue of old rats versus young rats demonstrates that the hydroxylase is absent or at very low levels as a result of age (Tanaka and DeLuca, 1984). Another critical experiment carried out by Gallagher et al. demonstrates that placing subjects on a low calcium diet will markedly stimulate fractional intestinal absorption of calcium when the patients are less than 65 years of age (Gallagher et al., 1979). If, however, in the over 65 age group the same study is done, calcium absorption is not increased by means of a low calcium diet, demonstrating that the capacity to adjust intestinal calcium absorption and thus presumably 1,25-$(OH)_2D_3$ level is absent. These results suggest that a deficiency of 1α-hydroxylase

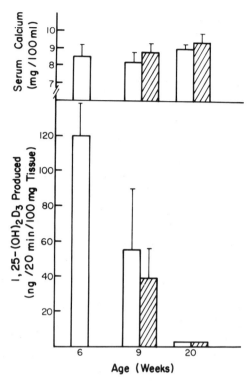

Fig. 5. Renal 25-OH-D$_3$-1α-hydroxylase of male (clear bars) and female (shaded bars) rats as a function of age. The corresponding serum calcium concentration is shown in the upper panel.

is an important factor in bringing about the calcium disorders of our aging population. It also suggests that treatment of these subjects with exogenous 1,25-(OH)$_2$D$_3$ may be beneficial in improving intestinal calcium absorption, increasing bone remodeling, and perhaps increasing bone mass.

V. POSTMENOPAUSAL OSTEOPOROSIS

It is well known that following the initiation of the menopause there is a rapid loss of bone (Meema and Meema, 1976). This bone loss can be prevented by administration of estrogen either together with progesterone or alone (Meema and Meema, 1976). This suggests that the primary disturbance in the rapid bone loss of this population is a withdrawal of the estrogen. However, it is clear that intestinal absorption of calcium is also diminished in this disorder (Gallagher *et al.*, 1980; Caniggia and Vattimo, 1979), and this loss of intestinal calcium absorption correlates with diminished level of plasma 1,25-$(OH)_2D_3$. Thus in studies carried out by Gallagher *et al.* (1979), in postmenopausal women with osteoporosis compared to their age and sex-matched controls, plasma 1,25-$(OH)_2D_3$ levels were decreased by 30% in the osteoporotic women compared with those not having osteoporosis but being of the same age. This is not the result of deficiency of vitamin D or failure to produce 25-OH-D_3, since the levels of this compound were either unchanged or increased in the osteoporotic female. Although there have been one or two reports failing to observe such a change, there now is an abundance of confirmations of this basic observation (Bishop *et al.*, 1980; Lawoyin *et al.*, 1980; Ohata and Fujita, 1979). Furthermore, it correlates with diminished intestinal calcium absorption and that postmenopausal women are unable to adjust their calcium absorption according to needs (Gallagher *et al.*, 1979). Therefore, it appears that in the postmenopausal woman, the sudden withdrawal of estrogen and other sex hormones as a result of this state brings about a flow of calcium from bone into the plasma that shuts off parathyroid secretion and in turn shuts off 1,25-$(OH)_2D_3$ production, resulting in diminished calcium absorption and an increased reliance on bone for soft tissue calcium needs. Therefore, the vitamin D endocrine system is indirectly involved in the bone loss of postmenopausal women. Furthermore, the diminished 1,25-$(OH)_2D_3$ levels would diminish bone remodeling, an essential event in maintaining a healthy skeleton.

Oophorectomy of rats as a model of the postmenopausal state results in a diminished bone density and a loss of bone mass as shown in Fig. 6 (Lindgren and DeLuca, 1982). Although it has been stated that rats do not get osteoporosis as found in the human population, the basic fundamental endocrine state can nevertheless be achieved and a bone loss can certainly be demonstrated. Rats, however, do not move in such a way as to put weight stress on the vertebral bodies, which is the primary site of fracture in the postmenopausal women suffering from osteoporosis. It is possible that oophorectomized rats could be a model of the bone disease suffered by the postmenopausal woman. Administration of 1,25-$(OH)_2D_3$ to oophorectomized rats largely prevents the bone loss and diminishes the decrease in bone density as shown in Fig. 7. It is, therefore, apparent that the vitamin D hormone may be of considerable use in the treatment of the postmenopausal osteoporotic condition.

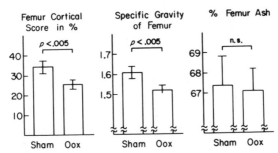

Fig. 6. The effect of oophorectomy of female rats on bone. Rats of 4 months of age were either sham-operated or oophorectomized and 6 weeks later they were sacrificed and femur cortical scores as well as specific gravity of the femur were measured. The same femurs were then used for determining total and percentage femur ash. Total ash changed with specific gravity and femur cortical score whereas percentage ash did not change significantly, illustrating that the disease suffered by these oophorectomized rats is an osteoporosis.

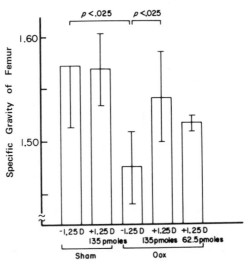

Fig. 7. Response of femur specific gravity of rats either sham-operated or oophorectomized as described in Fig. 6 and then treated with 1,25-(OH)$_2$D$_3$ at two dosage levels. The results show that 1,25-(OH)$_2$D$_3$ in the oophorectomized animals can improve the femur specific gravity.

VI. TREATMENT OF POSTMENOPAUSAL OSTEOPOROSIS WITH 1,25-(OH)$_2$D$_3$

Because of the above described experimental results, treatment with 1,25-(OH)$_2$D$_3$ of the postmenopausal woman with osteoporosis was initiated. One study by Christiansen used women on high-calcium diets but he was unable to give adequate amounts of 1,25-(OH)$_2$D$_3$ before hypercalcemia resulted (Christiansen *et al.*, 1981) from increased intestinal absorption of calcium. Thus, the dose of 1,25-(OH)$_2$D$_3$ was decreased to levels far below that manufactured in one day in normal humans, which is approximately 1–2 μg per day. This study cannot be regarded as an adequate test of whether 1,25-(OH)$_2$D$_3$ might be useful in the treatment of postmenopausal osteoporosis. 1,25-(OH)$_2$D$_3$ can be given by mouth only if the subjects are not given excessive calcium. Thus, treatment must be done in subjects with calcium intakes in the normal range between 500 and 800 mg per day (DeLuca, 1985; Gallagher *et al.*, 1982). Gallagher *et al.* (1982) carried out such a study in postmenopausal women and found that, in fact, one-half microgram a day of 1α,25-(OH)$_2$D$_3$ given by mouth increases bone mass, increases calcium absorption, improves calcium balance, and reduces bone resorption as shown by decreased urinary hydroxyproline (Table II). Most important, it markedly reduces the spinal fracture incidence (J. C. Gallagher, personal communication). Similar results have been obtained in a study by Recker and Gallagher at Creighton University. Large trials are currently under way in the United States at the Hoffmann–LaRoche Company to investigate the usefulness of this compound for treatment of postmenopausal osteoporosis. Furthermore, studies should be initiated on the use of this compound in the aging population over 65 years to determine whether their osteoporosis can be either prevented or corrected.

TABLE II

Postmenopausal Osteoporosis: Treatment with 1,25-(OH)$_2$D$_3$ (0.5 μg/day)

	Baseline	6–8 months	2 years
Ca absorption (%)	7	27[1]	27[1]
Ca balance (mg/day)	−59	2[2]	−27
Trabecular bone volume (%)	11.3	13.4	16.2[2]
Urinary hydroxyproline (mg/day)	26.3	21.1[2]	22.0[2]

[1] $p < .001$.
[2] $p < .01$.

VII. SUMMARY

The vitamin D endocrine system, a new arrival on the scene of calcium metabolism, has been described in general terms and its possible involvement in the disease process of osteoporosis of aging and osteoporosis of the postmenopausal woman is provided. Treatment of postmenopausal women with osteoporosis with one-half microgram of the vitamin D hormone a day is promising as a means of restoring bone mass and reducing fracture rate. Possible mechanisms of bone loss involving the vitamin D endocrine system have been presented. It therefore appears that no rational treatment or understanding of these disorders can take place without adequate consideration of the involvement of the vitamin D endocrine system.

REFERENCES

Abe, E., Miyaura, C., Sakagami, H., Takeda, M., Konno, K., Yamazaki, T., Yoshiki, S., and Suda, T. (1981). *Proc. Natl. Acad. Sci. U.S.A.* **78,** 4990–4994.

Andersson, S., Holmberg, I., and Wikvall, K. (1983). *J. Biol. Chem.* **258,** 6777–6781.

Barbour, G. L., Coburn, J. W., Slatopolsky, E., Norman, A. W., and Horst, R. L. (1981). *N. Engl. J. Med.* **305,** 440–443.

Baxter, L. A., and DeLuca, H. F. (1976). *J. Biol. Chem.* **251,** 3158–3161.

Bishop, J. E., Norman, A. W., Coburn, J. W., Roberts, P. A., and Henry, H. L. (1980). *Miner. Electrolyte Metab.* **3,** 181–189.

Boyle, I. T., Gray, R. W., Omdahl, J. L., and DeLuca, H. F. (1972a). *In* "Endocrinology 1971" (S. Taylor, ed.), pp. 468–476. Heinemann, London.

Boyle, I. T., Miravet, L., Gray, R. W., Holic, M. F., and DeLuca, H. F. (1972b). *Endocrinology (Baltimore)* **90,** 605–608.

Brommage, R., and DeLuca, H. F. (1985). *Endocr. Rev.* **6,** 491–511.

Brunette, M. G., Chan, M., Ferriere, C., and Roberts, K. D. (1978). *Nature (London)* **276,** 287–289.

Bullamore, J. R., Gallagher, J. C., Wilkinson, R., and Nordin, B. E. C. (1970). *Lancet* **2,** 535–537.

Caniggia, A., and Vattimo, A. (1979). *Clin. Endocrinol. (Oxford)* **11,** 99–103.

Christiansen, C., Christensen, M. S., Rodbro, P., Hagen, C., and Transbol, I. (1981). *Eur. J. Clin. Invest.* **11,** 305–308.

DeLuca, H. F. (1967). *Vitam. Horm. (N.Y.)* **25,** 315–367.

DeLuca, H. F. (1974). *Fed. Proc., Fed. Am. Soc. Exp. Biol.* **33,** 2211–2219.

DeLuca, H. F. (1980). *Ann. N.Y. Acad. Sci.* **355,** 1–17.

DeLuca, H. F. (1985). *In* "Calcium in Biological Systems" (R. P. Rubin, G. B. Weiss, and J. W. Putney, Jr., eds.), pp. 491–511. Plenum, New York.

DeLuca, H. F., and Schnoes, H. K. (1984). *Annu. Rep. Med. Chem.* **19,** 179–190.

DeLuca, H. F., Okamoto, S., Lindgren, U., and Halloran, B. (1981). *In* "Osteoporosis: Recent Advances in Pathogenesis" (H. F. DeLuca, H. M. Frost, W. S. S. Jee, C. C. Johnston, Jr., and A. M. Parfitt, eds.), pp. 203–214. University Park Press, Baltimore, Maryland.

DeLuca, H. F., Franceschi, R. T., Holloran, B. P., and Massaro, E. R. (1982). *Fed. Proc., Fed. Am. Soc. Exp. Biol.* **41,** 66–71.

de Wardener, H. E., and Eastwood, J. B. (1977). *In* "Phosphate Metabolism: Advances in Experimental Medicine and Biology" (S. G. Massry and E. Ritz, eds.), pp. 533–547. Plenum, New York.

Esvelt, R. P., and DeLuca, H. F. (1981). *Arch. Biochem. Biophys.* **206,** 403–413.

Esvelt, R. P., Schnoes, H. K., and DeLuca, H. F. (1979). *Biochemstry* **18,** 3977–3983.

Fraser, D., Kooh, S. W., Kind, H. P., Holick, M. F., Tanaka, Y., and DeLuca, H. F. (1973). *N. Engl. J. Med.* **289,** 817–822.

Frost, H. M. (1966). "Henry Ford Hospital Surgical Monograph Series." Thomas, Springfield, Illinois.

Gallagher, J. C., Riggs, B. L., Eisman, J., Hamstra, A., Arnaud, S. B., and DeLuca, H. F. (1979). *J. Clin. Invest.* **64,** 729–736.

Gallagher, J. C., Riggs, B. L., and DeLuca, H. F. (1980). *J. Clin. Endocrinol. Metab.* **51,** 1359–1364.

Gallagher, J. C., Jerpbak, C. M., Jee, W. S. S., Johnson, K. A., DeLuca, H. F., and Riggs, B. L. (1982). *Proc. Natl. Acad. Sci. U.S.A.* **79,** 3325–3329.

Garabedian, M., Tanaka, Y., Holick, M. F., and DeLuca, H. F. (1974). *Endocrinology (Baltimore)* **94,** 1022–1027.

Garabedian, M., Lieberherr, M., Nguyen, T. M., Corvol, M. T., Dubois, M. B., and Balsan, S. (1978). *Clin. Orthop. Relat. Res.* **135,** 241–248.

Ghazarian, J. G., Jefcoate, C. R., Knutson, J. C., Orme-Johnson, W. H., and DeLuca, H. F. (1974). *J. Biol. Chem.* **249,** 3026–3033.

Gray, T. K., Lester, G. E., and Lorenc, R. S. (1979). *Science* **204,** 1311–1313.

Gray, T. K., Lowe, W., and Lester, G. E. (1981). *Endocr. Rev.* **2,** 264–274.

Habener, J. F., and Mahaffey, J. E. (1978). *Annu. Rev. Med.* **29,** 327–340.

Harrison, H. E., and Harrison, H. E. (1960). *Am. J. Physiol.* **199,** 265–271.

Henry, H. L., and Norman, A. W. (1978). *Science* **201,** 835–837.

Hess, A. (1929). *In* "Rickets, Including Osteomalacia and Tetany" (A. Hess, ed.), pp. 22–37. Lea & Febiger, Philadelphia, Pennsylvania.

Hock, J. M., Kream, B. E., and Raisz, L. G. (1982). *Calcif. Tissue Int.* **34,** 347–349.

Holtrop, M. F., Cox, K. A., Clark, M. B., Holick, M. F., and Anast, C. S. (1981). *Endocrinology (Baltimore)* **108,** 2293–2295.

Horst, R. L., DeLuca, H. F., and Jorgensen, N. A. (1978). *Metab. Bone Dis. Relat. Res.* **1,** 29–33.

Howard, G. A., Turner, R. T., Sherrard, D. J., and Baylink, D. J. (1981). *J. Biol. Chem.* **256,** 7738–7740.

Huldshinsky, K. (1919). *Dtsch. Med. Wochenschr.* **45,** 712–713.

Kletzien, S. W. P., Templin, V. M., Steenbock, H., and Thomas, B. H. (1932). *J. Biol. Chem.* **97,** 265–280.

Kodicek, E. (1960). *Proc. Int. Congr. Biochem., 4th, 1958,* Vol. 11, pp. 198–208.

Lamm, M., and Neuman, W. F. (1958). *Arch. Pathol.* **66,** 204–209.

Larkins, R. G., MacAuley, S. J., and MacIntyre, I. (1974). *Nature (London)* **252,** 412–414.

Lawoyin, S., Jerwekh, J. E., Glass, K., and Pak, C. Y. C. (1980). *J. Clin. Endocrinol. Metab.* **50,** 593–596.

Lindgren, U., and DeLuca, H. F. (1982). *Calcif. Tissue Int.* **34,** 510–514.

Link, R., and DeLuca, H. F. (1985). *In* "The Receptors" (P. M. Conn, ed.), Vol. II, pp. 1–35. Academic Press, New York.

McCollum, E. V., Simonds, N., Becker, J. E., and Shipley, P. G. (1922). *Bull. Johns Hopkins Hosp.* **33,** 229–230.

Madhok, T. C., and DeLuca, H. F. (1979). *Biochem. J.* **184**, 491–499.

Meema, S., and Meema, H. E. (1976). *Isr. J. Med. Sci.* **12**, 601–606.

Mellanby, E. (1919). *Lancet* **1**, 407–412.

Nicolaysen, R., Eeg-Larsen, N., and Malm, O. J. (1953). *Physiol. Rev.* **33**, 424–444.

Norman, A. W., Henry, H. L., and Malluche, H. H. (1980). *Life Sci.* **27**, 229–237.

Ohata, M., and Fujita, M. (1979). *Endocrinol. Jpn.* **1**, 7.

Ornoy, A., Goodwin, D., Noff, D., and Edelstein, S. (1978). *Nature (London)* **276**, 517–519.

Papapoulos, S. E., Clemens, T. L., Fraher, L. J., Gleed, J., and O'Riordan, J. L. H. (1980). *Lancet* **2**, 612–615.

Puzas, J. E., Turner, R. T., Howard, G. A., and Baylink, D. J. (1983). *Endocrinology (Baltimore)* **112**, 378–380.

Raisz, L. G., Trummel, C. L., Holick, M. E., and DeLuca, H. F. (1972). *Science* **175**, 768–769.

Rasmussen, H., and Bordier, P. (1978). *Metab. Bone Dis. Relat. Res.* **1**, 7–13.

Rasmussen, H., DeLuca, H., Arnaud, C., Hawker, C., and von Stedingk, M. (1963). *J. Clin. Invest.* **42**, 1940–1946.

Reeve, L., Tanaka, Y., and DeLuca, H. F. (1983). *J. Biol. Chem.* **258**, 3615–3617.

Scriver, C. R., Reade, T. M., DeLuca, H. F., and Hamstra, A. J. (1978). *N. Engl. J. Med.* **299**, 976–979.

Shepard, R. M., Horst, R. L., Hamstra, A. J., and DeLuca, H. F. (1979). *Biochem. J.* **182**, 55–69.

Shultz, T. D., Fox, J., Health, H., III, and Kumar, R. (1983). *Proc. Natl. Acad. Sci. U.S.A.* **80**, 1746–1750.

Slovik, D. M., Adams, J. S., Neer, R. M., Holick, M. F., and Potts, J. T. (1981). *N. Engl. J. Med.* **305**, 372–375.

Stanbury, S. W., Taylor, C. M., Lumb, G. A., Mawer, E. B., Berry, J., Hann, J., and Wallace, J. (1981). *Miner. Electrolyte Metab.* **5**, 212–227.

Steenbock, H. (1924). *Science* **60**, 224–225.

Stern, P. H., Trummel, C. L., Schnoes, H. K., and DeLuca, H. F. (1975). *Endocrinology (Baltimore)* **97**, 1552–1558.

Sutton, R. A. L., and Dirks, J. H. (1978). *Fed. Proc., Fed. Am. Soc. Exp. Biol.* **37**, 2112–2119.

Tanaka, H., Abe, E., Miyaura, C., Kuribayashi, T., Konno, K., Nishii, Y., and Suda, T. (1982). *Biochem J.* **204**, 713–719.

Tanaka, Y., and DeLuca, H. R. (1973). *Arch. Biochem. Biophys.* **154**, 566–574.

Tanaka, Y., and DeLuca, H. F. (1984). *Am. J. Physiol.* **246**, E168–E173.

Tanaka, Y., Lorenc, R. S., and DeLuca, H. F. (1975). *Arch. Biochem. Biophys.* **171**, 521–526.

Tanaka, Y., Halloran, B., Schnoes, H. K., and DeLuca, H. F. (1979). *Proc. Natl. Acad. Sci. U.S.A.* **76**, 5033–5035.

Underwood, J. L., and DeLuca, H. F. (1984). *Am. J. Physiol.* **246**, E493–E498.

Weinstein, R. S., Underwood, J. L., Hutson, M. S., and DeLuca, H. F. (1984). *Am. J. Physiol.* **246**, E499–E505.

Weisman, Y., Vargas, A., Duckett, G., Reiter, E., and Root, A. (1978). *Endocrinology (Baltimore)* **103,**, 1992–1998.

Wong, R. G., Norman, A. W., Reddy, C. R., and Coburn, J. W. (1972). *J. Clin. Invest.* **51**, 1287–1291.

17

Diet, Immunity,
and Longevity

Robert A. Good and Amar J. Gajjar

University of South Florida
Department of Pediatrics/St. Petersburg
All Children's Hospital
St. Petersburg, Florida

I. INTRODUCTION

Since the late 1930s it has been known from the studies of Clive McCay (McCay *et al.*, 1935, 1939a,b) that the life span of rats can be significantly prolonged if the animals are fed a diet low in calories. Further, Tannenbaum (1945) showed that mammary adenocarcinomas can be prevented in mice and rats fed diets low in fat. Ross and Bras (1965, 1971) linked low dietary energy intake to inhibition of development of certain diseases that occur with aging in rats. Since these pioneering investigations were done, numerous studies including sev-

235

Nutrition and Aging

eral published in recent years have confirmed these observations (Masoro, 1985; Johnson et al., 1984; Kubo et al., 1984a,b). Walford (1969), who enunciated and has promulgated the immunologic theory of aging, showed in mice that not only does dietary restriction prolong life of these animals, but immunologic vigor is maintained much longer in mice fed a restricted calorie intake.

Our interest in the relation of diet to immune functions developed when we observed firsthand studies being conducted by Galal Aref et al. (1970) and Abassy et al. (1974a,b) and his colleagues in which they observed that so called protein-calorie malnutrition is regularly accompanied by deficiencies of both T-cell-mediated immune functions and the ability to produce antibodies to a variety of antigens. Antibody production was greatly deficient and even immunoglobulin levels reached hypogammaglobulinemic ranges in the children in whom protein-calorie malnutrition was imposed very early in life. Even after dietary rehabilitation was reestablished, defects caused by the protein-calorie malnutrition were still occurring.

This experience, together with several other opportunities to witness similar profound depression of both humoral and cell-mediated immunities and nutritional deprivation in forms which were dubbed protein-calorie malnutrition, allowed us to link protein-calorie malnutrition with profound deficiencies of both T-cell-mediated and B-cell-mediated immunities in Iran, Thailand, Indonesia, and Australia (R. Good, unpublished observations).

However, the studies of Jose et al. (1970a,b) suggested that the relationship between immunity and malnutrition might be somewhat complex. In studies of the relationship of immunity to malnutrition in the Australian aboriginals, Jose et al. (1970b) observed that protein and protein-calorie malnutrition in this population produced profound depression of certain immune functions and much lesser depression or actual increases in other immune functions. In reflecting on the nature of these relationships we concluded that it might be rather difficult from the field studies described above to sort out the influences of the variables involved in the complex picture that was emerging.

Consequently, over the past 16 years, we have been investigating in both human and animal systems the complexities of the profound influences of nutrition and dietary composition on immune functions (Good et al., 1976, 1980a,b). Our purpose here is to present some of the highlights of our observations which have been extensively documented in a series of scientific publications through the years. Emphasis is placed on our studies with animal systems because often it is not possible to draw firm conclusions from clinical observations. However, where possible the relations to observations with humans are considered. The animal studies seemed absolutely essential for appropriate interpretation because in the field multiple variables which are known to influence immunity are present and their contribution to the entire relationship cannot be sorted out.

II. INITIAL INVESTIGATIONS IN MICE, RATS, AND GUINEA PIGS OF PROTEIN AND CALORIE MALNUTRITION AND IMMUNE FUNCTIONS

Our initial investigations in collaboration with Jose, Cooper, and Mariani (Cooper *et al.*, 1974; Jose and Good, 1971, 1973a,b; Jose *et al.*, 1971, 1973) showed that moderate and more extreme protein and protein-calorie restriction inhibited the ability of mice to develop antibody-producing cells and to produce circulating antibody in a fashion unrelated to specific nutrients. In contrast, the immunologic functions of the thymus-dependent immune responses in mice or rats restricted in protein or protein and calories but receiving an adequate intake of vitamins and minerals were well maintained and even sometimes increased. We found also that specific restrictions of certain amino acids (Jose and Good, 1973a) could inhibit immune responses more profoundly than restrictions of other amino acids. Protein or protein-calorie restriction accelerated the tempo of allograft rejection, increased proliferative responses to phytomitogens, and permitted and/or enhanced delayed allergic responses. In guinea pigs, studies carried out with Kramer (Kramer and Good, 1978) showed clearly that delayed allergic reactions were at least as vigorous in guinea pigs fed 6 or 9% protein diets as those fed 26% protein. Even when an extremely low intake of protein (3 to 5%) was imposed (a highly lethal dietary restriction) that completely abrogated expression of skin sensitivity reactions of the delayed allergic type, we nevertheless found that the defects of cell-mediated immune reactions could not be attributed to defects of cell-mediated immunity but rather to defective inflammatory expressions of cell-mediated immunity. Indeed, such dietary restrictions actually enhanced the immune responsiveness of guinea pigs as reflected by the greater susceptibility of the protein-restricted animals to stimulation with very small doses of antigen. Thus, guinea pigs profoundly deficient in protein intake responded specifically after immunization with a sample protein antigen in Freund's adjuvant in dosages which could not be shown to produce cell-mediated immunity in well-fed controlled animals given an adequate intake of protein.

In mice, tumor immunities against autochthonous, syngeneic and allogeneic tumors, delayed allergic reactions, ability to initiate graft versus host reactions, and even ability to resist certain virus infections were actually found to be greatly enhanced by dietary protein or protein-calorie restriction (Good et al., 1977, 1980a; Good, 1981). In comparative studies when protein intake was restricted or both protein and calories were restricted, susceptibility of mice to lethal streptococcal infection was greatly enhanced, whereas susceptibility to lethal infection with the pseudorabies virus was substantially decreased.

Thus, the more these investigations were extended, the greater the paradox between field and clinical findings became. In the laboratory under well-controlled conditions, restriction of calorie intake, restriction of protein intake, or restriction of both dietary compounds over a wide range produced enhancement of many T-cell-mediated immune functions and decreases in ability to produce antibody. Under field conditions and from clinical observations, one might be tempted to conclude that protein or protein-calorie malnutrition inhibited both T-cell-mediated immunities as well as B-cell-mediated humoral immune functions. This puzzling paradox between experimental studies on animals and clinical data began to be resolved, at least in part, from consideration of the influence of certain micronutrients in both clinical and experimental perspectives.

III. ZINC AND IMMUNITY

Prasad (1976) discovered that dietary zinc deficiency produced stunting of growth, inhibition of sexual maturation, and increased susceptibility to infection. This was supported by the finding that the lethal A46 mutation in cattle inhibited thymus development and greatly abrogated T-cell immune functions. The immunologic abnormality was fully correctable by feeding or injecting extra zinc in adequate amounts (Brummerstedt et al., 1971, 1974; Andersen et al., 1976). Similarly, acrodermatitis enteropathica, which had been shown from our studies and those of many others to be accompanied by a form of severe combined immunodeficiency, was shown to be due to failure of normal absorption of zinc. This disease was completely cured by administration of adequate amounts of zinc (Moynahan and Barnes, 1973; Good et al., 1979a,b; Schloen et al., 1979). These findings led us to investigate zinc nutriture in relation to immunity functions. The results of these analyses were clear-cut and dramatic.

We, Fernandes et al. (1979a,b), and Fraker et al. (1986) independently found that restriction of zinc inhibited dramatically the development and expression of cell-mediated immunities in all animals studied. Thus, in mice, rats, guinea pigs, and monkeys, restriction of zinc as a single dietary variable led to profound thymic involution, plummeting of thymic hormone levels (Iwata *et al.*, 1978, 1979), profound deficiencies of all forms of T-cell-mediated immunologic function and deficiencies of T-dependent natural killer cells and natural killer cell functions, and decreased numbers of T lymphocytes (Tanaka *et al.*, 1978). When the zinc-restricted animals were fed zinc in sufficient quantity all these immunologic deficits were promptly restored to normal. T-cell-dependent antibody production, like all the other T-cell-mediated functions, was likewise deficient when zinc intake was restricted and was promptly restored when zinc was provided in adequate amounts.

Once the association of zinc as an essential element that is particularly crucial to immunologic function had been established, we and many others began to look into the clinical association of zinc deficiency and immune functions (Good *et al.*, 1982; Zanzonico *et al.*, 1981). In many different contexts, immunodeficiency can be associated with nutritional zinc deficiency and/or conditioned zinc deficiency. In our own work we found nutritional zinc deficiency to be associated with cancer of the head and neck region (Garofolo *et al.*, 1980a,b,c). Conditioned zinc deficiencies were particularly impressive in patients with Hodgkin's disease and certain other lymphomas and in patients with gastrointestinal cancers, especially when the latter were accompanied by intestinal fistulas (Schloen *et al.*, 1979). Similarly, in sickle-cell anemias and liver disease, zinc deficiencies were found to be commonplace. Before surgeons recognized the crucial role of zinc in immunity functions, zinc deficiency was frequently produced when total parenteral alimentation was given in which zinc had not been included in sufficient quantities. In an extensive review of zinc requirements with aging, we ascertained that borderline and clinically significant deficiencies of zinc occur with great frequency among the elderly (Sandstead *et al.*, 1982). Dietary zinc intakes are often borderline or deficient and when increased demands for zinc occur as a consequence of disease in the elderly, clinically significant zinc deficiencies often emerge. Indeed, most patients with advanced cancer have zinc intakes that are inadequate to meet their needs and the demands of their clinical disorders. Thus, in cancer patients some of the immunodeficiencies associated with the cancer process can actually be corrected by administration of adequate amounts of zinc (Gorafalo *et al.*, 1980a,b,c; Sandstead, 1982). In a similar vein, Golden *et al.* (1978) found that patients with deficient cell-mediated immunities associated with presumed protein-calorie malnutrition are restored immunologically by the administration of zinc without correction of the protein-calorie deficits, which had previously been presumed to be responsible for the deficiencies of the cell-mediated immune deficiencies in these patients (Golden *et al.*, 1978).

As it turns out, it is extremely difficult clinically to achieve a state of protein or protein-calorie malnutrition without also developing a deficiency of zinc nutriture and special attention to zinc nutritional needs is essential if the influences of protein-calorie malnutrition are to be corrected or averted. Zinc nutriture in protein-calorie malnutrition, however, represents one particularly poignant example of the complexities of protein and protein-calorie malnutrition and it seems to us that comparable consideration must be paid in this complex syndrome to deficiencies of vitamins (Beisel, 1982), trace metals (Schloen *et al.*, 1979), and other essential nutrients, as well as to the immunosuppressive influences of extreme deficiencies of protein and calories and the complex infestations and infections that regularly attend this complicated condition (Good *et al.*, 1981).

IV. INFLUENCE OF NUTRITION ON IMMUNOLOGIC INVOLUTION AND SUSCEPTIBILITY TO DISEASES OF AGING IN INBRED MICE

The influence of nutrition on susceptibility to diseases associated with aging requires particular attention. In the early 1970s we began to investigate as part of this same series of studies the influence of nutrition on the development of the several diseases we associate with aging in mice (Fernandes *et al.*, 1973, 1976a,b,c,d).

For genetically long-lived mice, the life span approximates 3 years. However, again on a genetically determined basis, certain inbred strains of mice, like members of certain human families, appear to be programmed for short lives. All or almost all of the genetically short-lived mice appear to be prone to develop diseases which are often associated in long-lived strains of mice as well as in all other animals with the aging process (Sigel and Good, 1972; Teague *et al.*, 1972; Yunis *et al.*, 1972). The diseases associated with aging in these strains of mice include autoimmunities, cancers (especially lymphoid cancers), renal diseases associated with glomerular hyalinization, hypertensive cardiovascular disease, cardiac diseases, and increased susceptibility to infection. We asked whether it was possible by nutritional manipulation to influence the life span of these autoimmune-prone short-lived strains of mice.

Might it be possible for mice genetically programmed to develop diseases associated with aging relatively early in life be able with appropriate nutritional management to live life spans comparable to those of the genetically long-lived mice?

Our studies began with efforts to alter disease expression in NZB or B/W mice by altering relative intake of fat and protein. Although these studies revealed only minimal influence on life span in these mice, differences in dietary composition did produce a significant small influence in the length of life and on expression of autoimmune disease (Fernandes et al., 1973, 1976a,b,c,d). In these initial investigations we used a diet relatively high in protein and low in fat when fed ad libitum. The animals fed the high-fat diet relatively low in protein developed autoimmunities in a more florid fashion and died earlier than those fed ad libitum on a diet that was higher in protein and lower in fat (Fernandes et al., 1973).

We then looked at the influence of a diet low in protein again fed ad libitum. In these studies we observed rather impressive and significant influences on the involution of immunologic functions, development of immunodeficiencies, and expression of manifestations of autoimmunity (Fernandes et al., 1976b). However, in spite of these influences on immunologic function and expression of certain manifestations of autoimmunity in the autoimmune-prone NZB strain of mice, the dietary change did not prolong life or completely prevent any of the changes in immunologic function that occur with aging in this autoimmune-prone strain of mice.

Studies were then begun to ascertain whether reduction of amount of food consumed could alter development of autoimmunity and prolong life span in mice of the autoimmune-prone short-lived strain. The first experiments were done with B/W mice, a strain that has been extensively studied as a model of lupus and lupus nephritis (Fernandes et al., 1976c). Female mice of this strain generally die of renal disease and vascular or cardiovascular disease before 1 year of age, the median survival being between 6 and 8 months in many studies. In our initial studies of the influence of caloric or total food intake with vitamins and minerals given in adequate amounts, the B/W female mice regularly survived two to three times as long as did mice fully fed a defined diet or fed ad libitum with a standard laboratory ration of rat chow (Fernandes et al., 1976c). This extraordinary influence of dietary restriction on length of life in the autoimmune-prone female B/W mice was accompanied by an equally dramatic reduction of development of autoimmune phenomena, decrease of circulating immune complex levels (Safai Kutti et al., 1980), delay of involution of thymus function (Tanaka et al., 1978), increases of T-cell immunity functions, and increases of T-dependent antibody production and levels of T-dependent antibodies. Thymus involution and development of the usual splenomegaly in mice of this strain were also inhibited by dietary choice restriction (Fernandes et al., 1976c,d). After it had been shown by several groups of investigators that interleukin-2 production is greatly reduced in mice of each of the autoimmune-prone strains, we found that dietary caloric restriction greatly enhanced interleukin-2 production in mice of this and other autoimmune-prone strains (Jung et al., 1982).

Izui et al. (1981) showed that GP70 production and GP70 anti-GP70 immune complex deposition in the kidneys of the autoimmune-prone B/ W mice are impressively correlated with the development of renal disease in these mice. In collaborative investigations with these scientists, we showed that dietary caloric restriction resulted in dramatic reduction of formation of GP70 antigen and GP70 and anti-GP70 antibody complexes and deposits in a capillary distribution in the glomeruli (Izui et al., 1981). We also discovered that the autoimmune-prone B/W mice produced antibodies with limited heterogeneity of affinities (Goidl et al., 1983, 1986). This immunologic abnormality in the B/W mice was also corrected by dietary restriction. In association with correction of these specific immunologic abnormalities in the autoimmune-prone B/W mice, we found that thymus involution and development of immunologic deficiency, as well as a variety of cell-mediated and humoral immunologic deficiencies characteristic of the aging autoimmune-prone mice, were dramatically reduced by dietary caloric restriction (Fernandes et al., 1976c). This set of investigations thus established for short-lived autoimmune-prone mice that restriction of calorie intake would greatly prolong life and inhibit development of immunologic perturbations thought to be associated with pathogenesis of the immunologically based renal and vascular diseases in mice of this strain. Further, the immunodeficiencies and extreme deviations from normal of immune functions that occur with aging in mice of this strain were dramatically inhibited by restriction of dietary calorie intake from the time of weaning (Fernandes et al., 1976c).

With Friend and associates (1978) at the University of Minnesota we then asked the question: Can dietary restriction be imposed *after* appearance of manifestations of autoimmune disease and progressive renal vascular disease and still influence the tempo of development of the renal vascular disease in mice of this autoimmune-prone strain? Again, the answer to this question was convincingly in the affirmative. We found it possible by dietary calorie restriction to slow very significantly, if not arrest, the development of renal vascular disease in the autoimmune-prone B/W mice.

V. DIETARY CONSTITUENTS CRUCIAL TO INHIBITION OF AUTOIMMUNITY AND NEPHRITIS

In collaboration with Kubo and with B. Connor Johnson, the distinguished nutritional biochemist at The University of Oklahoma, we set out to ask another set of questions concerning the influence of dietary manipulation on the development of diseases associated with aging in each of the known autoimmune-prone mice. Basically we were interested in determining whether the crucial variable in the dietary manipulation might be calories or whether some other variable or combinations of variables might be crucial in our experiments. We wanted to ascertain for certain whether calories alone were responsible for the dramatic prolongation of life and health we were witnessing or whether dietary composition could exert an important influence.

We also wanted to determine whether changes in dietary composition, when coupled with reduction of calorie intake, could alter the ultimate survival and disease expression in our several strains of mice (Johnson et al., 1986). With Kubo, Johnson, and Day we have carried out investigations of each of the known autoimmune-prone strains of mice. (Kubo et al., 1984b). Basically the results of each of these investigations have been similar. Thus, we can now describe what we believe to be a general case for inbred, autoimmune-prone mice. To ascertain this, we have used diets at the extremes of composition. For example, we have fed standard laboratory chow diets ad libitum, defined diets with conventional proportions of proteins, fats, and carbohydrate ad libitum, diets high in protein with low fat composition, diets very high in fat with no carbohydrate, and moderate protein diets very high in carbohydrate with a minimum of fat (2% safflower oil) to provide essential fatty acid intake. With each of these diets, protein intake on the fully fed diet was kept within a range where protein could be most efficiently utilized and not burned inefficiently as a source of calories (Hamilton, 1939). With each of the extremes of diet, vitamin and mineral content was adjusted to provide at least a minimal essential daily intake.

When fully fed to each of the known autoimmune-prone short-lived mice, each of these diets of extremely different content of major macronutrients permitted the development of the characteristic pattern of autoimmunity at a rate not significantly different from that observed with *ad libitum* feeding of a standard laboratory chow diet or *ad libitum* feeding of a conventional, defined diet. Thus, feeding diets at the extremes of composition of fat, carbohydrate, and protein did not influence significantly the development of autoimmunity, declining immunologic function, development of autoimmune diseases, and other diseases of aging or early death. By contrast, when each of these diets of widely different composition was fed in restricted amounts and the calorie intake but not vitamins or supplemental mineral intake was profoundly reduced, life span was considerably prolonged. Indeed with each of the diets, calorie reduction increased life span more than twofold. Mice of each of the short-lived autoimmune-prone strains fed a diet high in carbohydrate and low in fat with balanced vitamins and minerals at normal levels lived the longest of mice fed any diet. Thus, reduced calorie intake of a high-carbohydrate, low-fat diet provided the longest life and span of health (Johnson *et al.*, 1985a,b; 1986). A high-protein diet fed in restricted amount was almost as effective in prolonging life of these mice.

In the most extensively studied mice (the B/W short-lived autoimmune-prone strain), feeding a high-carbohydrate, very low fat diet increased survival as much as three to four times as long as occurred in mice fully fed a diet of similar composition or fully fed any of the extremes of diet which we investigated (Johnson *et al.*, 1986).

Dietary composition nevertheless clearly played a significant role when mice were fed restricted amounts of diets (Johnson *et al.*, 1986) of differing relative fat composition. When fed in restricted amount, diets low in fat but high in carbohydrates were associated with the longest life spans and longest span of vigorous good health. The mice fed the restricted caloric intake of a diet relatively high in carbohydrates were at every age at least as vigorous and for most of their lives far more vigorous than the mice fully fed on diets of the same composition or mice fully fed other diets of greatly differing composition.

Each of the known autoimmune-susceptible strains of mice showed a similar influence of caloric restriction and dietary composition. However, when fully fed, the pathologic characteristics of the autoimmune-prone mice provided a diet both high in calories and high in fat were quite different. In autoimmune-prone, but not in autoimmune-resistant long-lived, mice, *ad libitum* feeding of a diet high in fat composition and particularly diets high in saturated fats led to a high frequency of atherosclerotic lesions (Fernandes *et al.*, 1983). These lesions which involved coronary vessels, the aorta, and the large branches of the aorta, showed minimal endothelial proliferative lesions, and had marked thickening of the smooth muscular layer of the intima and cholesterol cleft deposits very similar to human atherosclerotic lesions. Such lesions were seen in mice of several of the autoimmune-prone strains fed *ad libitum* on high fat including high saturated fat diets. Recent studies by a group working initially with us in New York and later independently have confirmed this propensity of autoimmune-prone mice to develop waxy, lipid, vascular lesions as a function of diet (Mark *et al.*, 1984).

VI. BREAST CANCER IN MICE

In addition to these influences of caloric undernutrition without specific nutrient malnutrition, which we have shown to produce profound inhibition of progressive immunodeficiency, to promote longevity, and to greatly increase the span of life and span of health of each of the very different autoimmune-prone strains of mice, significant inhibition of cancer development has also been observed in our studies as well as those of several independent investigators. Our work has concentrated on breast cancer development in C3H/Bi mice (Dong *et al.*, 1982; Sarkar *et al.*, 1982; Day *et al.*, 1980). These mice develop mammary adenocarcinoma in association with infection with the Bittner retrovirus, which produces Type A and later Type B retroviral particles but not C-type retroviral particles. Calorie restriction and perhaps to some extent fat restriction can prevent the occurrence of mammary adenocarcinoma. The inhibition of tumor development cannot be attributed to inhibition or alteration of estrus cycles, TSH production, or other obvious hormonal changes. However, the development of precancerous minimal alveolar lesions and associated elevated circulating prolactin levels is greatly inhibited by the same diets that inhibit development of the mammary adenocarcinoma. The inhibition of the mammary adenocarcinoma appears to be associated with a very significant reduction in expression of recognizable A and B particles that reflect the extent of retrovirus infection in the mammary gland (Dong *et al.*, 1982; Sarkar *et al.*, 1982; Day *et al.*, 1980). While our studies have been in progress, others (e.g., Kritchevsky *et al.*, 1984) have reached similar conclusions with respect to other spontaneous or induced malignancies of the breast in rats (Day *et al.*, 1980; Klurfeld *et al.*, 1985). In their studies, calorie level seemed to be of paramount importance. However, whether or not calorie density of the diet is crucial needs futher study. In England, Tucker has shown that spontaneously developing tumors of a great variety in both mice and rats are significantly inhibited by a 25% reduction of food intake (Tucker *et al.*, 1979).

Weindruch and Walford (1982; Weindruch *et al.*, 1982) in the meantime have restudied the influence of dietary restriction in long-lived strains of mice and have found that a major influence of diet can be demonstrated in such animals even when the dietary restriction is delayed until after the animals are fully mature and have reached nearly the halfway point in their normal life span.

VII. CONCLUSIONS AND FUTURE STUDIES

Thus, profound influences of calorie undernutrition without malnutrition can be demonstrated in many different long-lived as well as short-lived autoimmune-prone mice, which for very different reasons appear to be genetically programmed to develop autoimmune diseases and other diseases associated with aging relatively early in life.

A major challenge remains, namely, to analyze in definitive and penetrating perspective the fundamental basis or bases of these extraordinary influences of diet on life span and expression of disturbed immunologic function associated with aging. This is no small challenge. However, today powerful tools are available for analyzing with increasing perception the mechanisms of control of cell replication, gene expression, neuroendocrinologic function, and immunologic function. Any or several of these approaches may yield penetrating understanding of these most challenging and still unique influences on life span and maintenance of health.

ACKNOWLEDGMENTS

Original work reported here has been supported by Grants AG05628 and AG05633 from the NIH of the HHS and the March of Dimes Birth Defects Foundation.

REFERENCES

Abassy, A. S., Badr El-din, M. K., Hassan, A. I., Aref, G. H., Hammand, S. A., El Araby, I. I., and Badr El-Din, A. A. (1974a). *J. Trop. Med. Hyg.* **77**, 13–17.
Abassy, A. S., Badr, El-din, M. K., Hassan, A. I., Anef, G. H., Hammad, S. A., El Araby, I. I., and Badr El-din, A. A. (1974b). *J. Trop. Med. Hyg.* **77**, 18–21.
Andersen, B., Basse, A., Brummerstedt, F., and Flagstad, T. (1976). *Nord. Veterinaer med.* **26**, 275–578.
Aref, G. H., Badr El-din, M. K., Hassan, A. I., and Araby, I. I. (1970). *J. Trop. Med. Hyg.* **73**, 186.

Beisel, W. (1982). *Am. J. Clin. Nutr.*, Suppl., February, pp. 417–468.

Brummerstedt, E., Flagstad, T., Basse, A., and Andersen, E. (1971). *Acta Pathol. Microbiol. Scand., Sect. A* **79A**, 686–687.

Brummerstedt, E., Andersen, E., Basse, A., and Flagstad, T. (1974). *Nord Veterinaer med.* **26**, 279–293.

Cooper, W. O., Good, R. A., and Mariani, T. (1974). *Am. J. Clin. Nutr.* **27**, 647–664.

Day, N. K., Fernandes, G., Witkin, S. S., Thomas, E. S., Sarkar, N. H., and Good, R. A. (1980). *Int. J. Cancer* **26**, 813–818.

Dong, Z. W., Witkin, S. S., Fernandes, G., Sarkar, N. H., Good, R. A., and Day, N. K. (1982). *J. Immunol.* **129**, 872–876.

Fernandes, G., Yunis, E. J., Jose, D. G., and Good, R. A. (1973). *Int. Arch. Allergy Appl. Immunol.* **44**, 770–782.

Fernandes, G., Yunis, E. J., Smith, J., and Good, R. A. (1976a). *Proc. Soc. Exp. Biol. Med.* **139**, 1189–1196.

Fernandes, G., Yunis, E. J., and Good, R. A. (1976b). *J. Immunol.* **116**, 782–790.

Fernandes, G., Yunis, E. J., and Good, R. A. (1976c). *Proc. Natl. Acad. Sci. U.S.A.* **74**(4), 1279–1283.

Fernandes, G., Friend, P. S., Good, R. A., and Yunis, E. J. (1976d). *Fed. Proc., Fed. Am. Soc. Exp. Biol.* **35**, 437.

Fernandes, G., West, A., and Good, R. A. (1979a). *Clin. Bull.* **9**(3).

Fernandes, G., Nair, M., Onoe, K., Tanaka, T., Floyd, R., and Good, R. A. (1979b). *Proc. Natl. Acad. Sci. U.S.A.* **76**, 457–461.

Fernandes, G., Alonso, D. R., Tanaka, T., Thaler, H. T., Yunis, E. J., and Good, R. A. (1983). *Proc. Natl. Acad. Sci. U.S.A.* **80**, 874–877.

Fraker, P. M., Gershwin, M. E., Good, R. A., and Prasad, A. S. (1986). *Fed. Proc., Fed. Am. Soc. Exp. Biol.* (In press).

Friend, P. S., Fernandes, G., Good, R. A., Michael A. F., and Yunis, E. J. (1978). *Lab. Invest.* **38**, 629–632.

Garofalo, J. A., Cunningham-Rundles, S., Braun, D. W., and Good, R. A. (1980a). *Int. J. Immunopharmacol.* **2**(1), 37–40.

Garofalo, J. A., Erlandson, F., Strong, E. W., Lesser, M., Gerold, F., Spiro, R., Schwartz, M., and Good, R. A. (1980b). *J. Surg. Oncol.* **15**, 381–386.

Garofalo, J. A., Ashikani, H., Lesser, K., Mendez-Botel, C., Cunningham-Rundles, S., Schwartz, M. K., and Good, R. A. (1980c). *Cancer* **46**, 2682–2685.

Goidl, E., Fernandes, G., Weksler, M., Siskind, G., and Good, R. A. (1983). *Cell. Immunol.* **80**, 20–30.

Goidl, E. A., Good, R. A., Siskind, G. W., Weksler, M. E., and Fernandez, G. (1986). *Cell. Immunol.* **107**(2), 281–286.

Golden, M. H. N., Golden, B. E., Harland, P. S. E. G., and Jackson, A. A. (1978). *Lancet* **1**, 1226–1227.

Good, R. A. (1981). *J. Clin. Immunol.* **1**, 3–11.

Good, R. A., Fernandes, G., Yunis, E. J., Cooper, M. C., Jose, D. C., Kramer, T. R., and Hansen, M. A. (1976). *Am. J. Pathol.* **84**, 599–614.

Good, R. A., Jose, D., Cooper, W. O., Fernandes, G., Kramer, T., and Yunis, P. (1977). *In* "Malnutrition and the Immune Response" (R. M. Suskind, ed.), pp. 169–184. Raven Press, New York.

Good, R. A., Fernandes, G., and West, A. (1979a). *Clin. Bull.* **9**(1).

Good, R. A., Fernandes, G., and West, A. (1979b). *In* "Aging and Immunity" (S. K. Singhal, N. R. Sinclair, and C. R. Stiller, eds.). Elsevier/North-Holland Biomedical Press, Amsterdam.

Good, R. A., West, A., and Fernandes, G. (1980a). *Fed. Proc., Fed. Am. Soc. Exp. Biol.* **39**, 3098–3104.

Good, R. A., West, A., and Fernandes, G. (1980b). *In* "Infections in the Immunocompromised Host—Pathogenesis: Prevention and Therapy" (J. Verhoef *et al.*, eds.), pp. 95–128.

Good, R. A., Jose, D. G., and Cooper, W. O. (1981). *In* "Microenvironmental Aspects of Immunity" (B. D. Jankovic and K. Isakovic, eds.), pp. 321–326. Plenum, New York.

Good, R. A., Fernandes, G., Garofalo, J. A., Cunningham-Rundles, C., Iwata, T., and West, A. (1982). *In* "Zinc and Immunity in Clinical, Biochemics, and Nutrition—Aspects of Trace Elements" (A. S. Prasad, ed.), pp. 189–202. Liss, New York.

Hamilton, T. S. (1939). *J. Nutr.* **17**, 565–582.

Iwata, T., Incefy, G. S., Tanaka, T., Fernandes, G., Mendez Botet, C. J., Pih, K., and Good, R. A. *Fed Proc., Fed Am. Soc. Exp. Biol.* **37**, 1827.

Iwata, T., Incefy, T., Tanaka, T., Fernandes, G., Mendez Botet, C. J., Pih, K., and Good, R. A. (1979). *Cell. Immunol.* **46**, 100–105.

Izui, S., Fernandes, G., Hara, I., McConahey, P. J., Jensen, F. C., Dixon, F. J., and Good, R. A. (1981). *J. Exp. Med.* **154**, 1116–1124.

Johnson, B. C., Kubo, C., Gajjar, A., and Good, R. A. (1985a). *Fed. Proc., Fed. Am. Soc. Exp. Biol.* **44**(4), 1152.

Johnson, B. C., Kubo, C., Day, N. K., and Good, R. A. (1985b). *In* "Nutrition: Immunity and Illness in the Elderly" (R. K. Chandra, ed.), pp. 177–191. Pergamon, New York.

Johnson, B. C., Gajjar, A., Kubo, C., and Good, R. A. (1986). *Proc. Natl. Acad. Sci. U.S.A.* (in press).

Jose, D. G., and Good, R. A. (1971). *Nature (London)* **231**, 323–325.

Jose, D. G., and Good, R. A. (1973a). *Cancer Res.* **33**, 807–812.

Jose, D. G., and Good, R. A. (1973b). *J. Exp. Med.* **137**, 1–9.

Jose, D. G., Welch, J. S., and Doherty, R. L. (1970a). *Aust. Pediatr. J.* **5**, 209–218.

Jose, D. G., Welch, J. S., and Doherty, R. L. (1970b). *Aust. Pediatr. J.* **6**, 192–202.

Jose, D. G., Cooper, W. C., and Good, R. A. (1971). *JAMA, J. Am. Med. Assoc.* **218**, 1428–1429.

Jose, D. G., Stutman, O., and Good, R. A. (1973). *Nature (London)* **241**, 57–58.

Jung, L. K. L., Palladino, M. A., Calvano, S., Mark, D. A., Good, R. A., and Fernandes, G. (1982). *Clin. Immunol. Immunopathol.* **25**, 295–301.

Klurfeld, D. M., Aglaw, E., Tepper, S. A., and Kritchevsky, D. (1985). *Nutr. Cancer* **5**(1), 16–25.

Kramer, T. R., and Good, R. A. (1978). *Clin. Immunol. Immunopathol.* **11**, 212–228.

Kritchevsky, D., Weber, M. M., and Klurfeld, D. M. (1984). *Cancer Res.* **44**, 3174–3177.

Kubo, C., Day, N. H., and Good, R. A. (1984a). *Proc. Natl. Acad. Sci. U.S.A.* **81**, 5831–5835.

Kubo, C., Johnson, B. C., Day, N. K., and Good, R. A. (1984b). *Am. J. Nutr.* **114**, 1884–1899.

Kubo, C., Johnson, B. C., Day, N. K., Gajjar, A., and Good, R. A. (1986). Submitted for publication.

McCay, C. M., Crowell, M. F., and Maynard, L. A. (1935). *J. Nutr.* **10**, 63–79.

McCay, C. M., Maynard, L. A., Sperling, G., and Barnes, L. L. (1939a). *J. Nutr.* **18**, 15–25.

McCay, C. M., Ellis, G. H., Barnes, L. D., Smith, C. A. H., and Sperling, G. (1939b). *J. Nutr.* **18**, 15–25.

Mark, D. A., Alonso, D. R., Quimby, F., Thaler, F., Kim, Y. T., Fernandes, G., Good, R. A., and Weksler, M. E. (1984). *Am. J. Pathol.* **117**(1), 110–124.

Masoro, E. J. (1985). *J. Nutr.* **115**, 842–848.

Moynahan, E. J., and Barnes, P. M. (1973). *Lancet* **1**, 676.

Prasad, A. S. (1976). *In* "Trace Elements in Human Health and Disease" (A. S. Prasad, eds.), Vol. 1, pp. 1–20. Academic Press, New York.

Ross, M. H., and Bras, S. (1965). *J. Nutr.* **87**, 245–260.

Ross, M. H., and Bras, S. (1971). *J. Natl Cancer Inst.* **47**, 1095–1113.

Safai Kutti, S., Fernandes, G., Wang, Y., Safai, B., Good, R. A., and Day, N. K. (1980). *Clin Immunol. Immunopathol.* **15**, 293–300.

Sandstead, H. H., Henniksen, L. K., Greger, J. L., Prasad, A. S., and Good, R. A. (1982). *Am. J. Clin. Nutr.* **36**, 1046–1059.

Sarkar, N. H., Fernandes, G., Telang, N. T., Kourides, I. A., and Good, R. A. (1982). *Proc. Natl. Acad. Sci. U.S.A.* **79**, 7758–7762.

Schloen, L. R., Fernandes, G., Garofalo, J. A., and Good, R. A. (1979). *Clin. Bull.* **9**(2).

Sigel, M. M., and Good, R. A., eds. (1972). "Tolerance, Autoimmunity and Aging." Thomas, Springfield, Illinois.

Tanaka, T., Fernandes, G., Tsao, C., Pih, K., and Good, R. A. (1978). *Fed. Proc., Fed. Am. Soc. Exp. Biol.* **37**, 931.

Tannenbaum, A. (1945). *Cancer Res.* **5**, 609–615.

Teague, P. O., Friou, C. J., Yunis, E. J., and Good, R. A. (1972). *In* "Tolerance, Autoimmunity and Aging" (M. M. Sigel and R. A. Good, eds.), Chapter 3. Thomas, Springfield, Illinois.

Tucker, S. M., Mason, R. L., and Beauchire, R. E. (1979). *Int. J. Cancer* **23**, 803.

Walford, R. L. (1969). "The Immunological Theory of Aging". Munksgaard, Copenhagen.

Weindruch, R., and Walford, R. L. (1982). *Science* **215**, 1415–1418.

Weindruch, R., Gottesman, S. R. S., and Walford, R. L. (1982). *Proc. Natl. Acad. Sci. U.S.A.* **79**, 898–902.

Yunis, L. J., Fernandes, G., Teague, R. O., Stutman, O., and Good, R. A. (1972). *In* "Tolerance, Autoimmunity and Aging" (M. M. Sigel and R. A. Good, eds.), Chapter 4.

Zanzonico, P., Fernandes, G., and Good, R. A. (1981). *Cell. Immunol.* **60**, 203–211.

18

Nutrition and the Aging Hematopoietic System

David A. Lipschitz

Division of Hematology/Oncology and Division on Aging
University of Arkansas for Medical Sciences
and John L. McClellan Veterans Administration Hospital
Little Rock, Arkansas

I. INTRODUCTION

The hematopoietic system plays a critical role in physiologic homeostasis. Each day billions of hematopoietic cells are produced. These enter the peripheral blood and function in oxygen transport, hemostasis, and host defense. Because of its high proliferative activity the bone marrow is particularly susceptible to nutritional deficiencies. In addition there is some evidence that aging adversely affects the ability of the hematopoietic system to respond to increased stimulation.

251

This review will discuss the effects of age on the normal hematopoietic system, describe the presentation of nutrition-related hematopoietic diseases, and discuss the possibility that nutritional variables participate in the physiologic decline in hematopoietic function usually ascribed to normal aging.

II. EFFECT OF AGE ON NORMAL BONE MARROW FUNCTION

Normal bone marrow function represents a complex interaction between hematopoietic cells, their microenvironment, and a series of diffusible molecules which are involved in the modulation of cellular proliferation (Wintrobe, 1981). Morphologically recognizable (differentiated) bone marrow precursors of the erythroid, myeloid, and megakaryocytic lines are derived from a small pool of totipotential stem cells which have the capacity to differentiate into pluripotent stem cells that are committed either to hematopoietic or lymphoid cell differentiation (Schofield, 1979). This small totipotent and pluripotent stem cell compartment is characterized by a self-renewal capacity which allows a small number of stem cells to amplify into a large number of differentiated hematopoietic cells while maintaining a very small pluripotent stem cell compartment. The pluripotent hematopoietic stem cell is termed CFU-S (colony-forming unit-spleen) by virtue of its ability to produce colonies in spleens of lethally irradiated mice (Till and McCulloch, 1961). CFU-S is also capable of repopulating the marrow of irradiated recipients and preventing marrow failure. The pluripotent stem cells can divide into committed hematopoietic cells of the myeloid, macrophage, erythroid, or megakaryocytic lines. These committed progenitor cells differentiate into the morphologically recognizable cells of the various hematopoietic lineages (Table I). They have no morphologic characteristics and can only be recognized by their ability to form clonal colonies *in vitro* in the appropriate culture environment. A high proliferative activity of this organ system is continually required to maintain normal levels of the formed elements of peripheral blood.

A finite replicative capacity of normal cells is one of the major theories of cellular aging (Hayflick, 1965). When this replicative capacity has been reached, the cell's ability to divide is lost and death occurs. The evidence that the pluripotential hematopoietic stem cell has a limited self-renewal capacity is controversial. There is evidence that CFU-S has a heterogeneous self-renewal capacity and an age structure in which young CFU-S with high self-renewal capacity produce older CFU-S with

TABLE I

The Hierarchy and Production of Hematopoietic Precursors

from Primitive Pluripotent Stem Cells

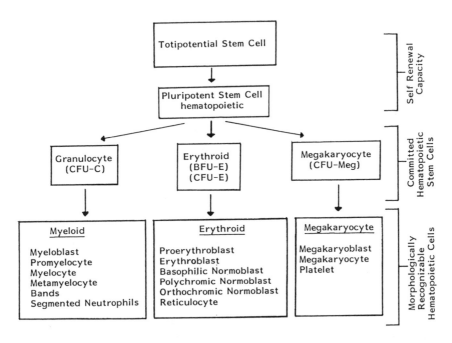

decreasing self-renewal capacity thus increasing differentiation potential (Phillips, 1978; Schofield and Lajtha, 1974; Schofield *et al.*, 1980). The hypothesis has been strengthened by studies of long-term bone marrow culture which show that CFU-S with a high replicative history are likely to be recruited into committed progenitor cells more readily than CFU-S that divided a fewer number of times (Hellman *et al.* 1978; Mauch *et al.*, 1980). We have shown that maintenance of hematopoiesis in long-term bone marrow culture varies inversely with the age of the donor from which the culture was initiated (Lipschitz *et al.*, 1982). Additional evidence for a finite replicative capacity for stem cells has been obtained in a series of elegant studies in which stem cell kinetics and myeloid cell production were examined in long-term bone marrow subjected to varying degrees of irradiation (Reincke *et al.*, 1982; Mauch *et al.*, 1982). Results from *in vivo* serial transplantation studies suggest a limited life span and proliferative capacity of these cells (Albright and Makinodan, 1976). However, there is evidence that the pluripotent stem cell compartment can maintain hematopoiesis for a period which extends far beyond the maximum expectancy of the animal being studied (Harrison, 1975a). Furthermore, CFU-S decline minimally or not at all with age (Chen, 1971) and there is evidence that earlier transplantation, suggesting a finite replicative capacity, may be related to methodologic artifact (Harrison et al., 1978; Ross et al., 1982).

It must be emphasized that the hematopoietic system is particularly sensitive to physiologic and pathologic variables which affect its function. Thus the interpretation of age on hematopoiesis is made difficult by the fact that even healthy elderly individuals frequently have coexisting diseases or nutritional deficiencies or have been exposed to drugs and toxicants that have a profound effect on the bone marrow. Because of this, information obtained from the studies of animal models is important. In the mouse, red cell mass is unaffected by aging. The apparent anemia is caused by an expansion of plasma volume (Boggs and Patrene, 1985; Wiliams et al., 1985). A careful evaluation of the effect of age on hematopoiesis in the mouse has failed to demonstrate any age-related alteration in the number of formed elements in the peripheral blood or in the number of differentiated precursors in the marrow of these animals. Furthermore, measurement of the committed myeloid stem cell (colony-forming unit-culture, CFU-C) or erythroid stem cells (burst-forming unit-erythroid, BFU-E, or colony-forming unit-erythroid, CFU-E) have shown no age-related reduction as healthy aged animals approach their maximum life expectancy. Evaluation of the kinetics of erythropoiesis has demonstrated that plasma iron turnover and erythron iron turnover are unchanged with aging and red cell survival is not altered. It is apparent from the study of animal models that minimal if any change in basal hematopoiesis occurs with age. There is, however, good evidence that hematopoietic reserve capacity is compromised. The rate of return of hematocrit to normal following phlebotomy is decreased in aged mice (Harrison, 1975b) and in vivo and in vitro studies have shown that the erythropoietic cells from aged animals respond less well to increased stimulation than do erythroid cells from young animals (Udupa and Lipschitz, 1984). Similarly, compromise in granulocyte production following increased stimulation has been demonstrated in the aged mouse.

III. EFFECT OF AGE ON HEMATOPOIESIS IN MAN

Biologically, the effect of age on hematopoiesis in man should be similar to that in animal models. Thus basal hematopoiesis should be unchanged. There is good evidence that a reduction in cellularity of the bone marrow occurs in the elderly, but the functional significance of this observation is unknown (Hartsock *et al.*, 1965). Epidemiologic studies have shown that a reduction in hematocrit is common even in healthy elderly subjects. This observation is primarily derived from epidemiologic studies in the United States, Canada, and Europe [U.S. Department of Health, Education and Welfare (USDHEW), 1981; Nutrition Canada, 1973; Parsons *et al.*, 1965]. The prevalence of anemia in females above aged 59 is approximately equal to that found in females of childbearing age. In men, a definite increase in the prevalence of anemia is found in the older age groups. Studies from Great Britain are important as they have determined the incidence of anemia in large numbers of subjects above age 60 (Hill, 1967; Myers *et al.*, 1968; McLennan *et al.*, 1973). In both males and females the prevalence of anemia increases significantly with each successive decade. Although anemia in healthy elderly subjects is common, the cause is usually not obvious (Lipschitz *et al.*, 1981). Careful hematologic evaluation of these subjects show that iron deficiency, the anemia of chronic disease, folate deficiency, hemolysis, and other rarer causes of anemia are uncommon. The elderly males and females with the unexplained anemia have significantly lower leukocyte and neutrophil counts than nonanemic subjects, suggesting mild marrow failure. A careful assessment of hematopoiesis in these individuals reveals significant decreases in differentiated bone marrow hematopoietic cells of myeloid, erythroid, and megakaryocytic lines (Lipschitz *et al.*, 1984). When the committed hematopoietic progenitor cells are measured, a significant reduction in CFU-C and CFU-E precursors is found. In contrast, the level of the most primitive hematopoietic precursors (BFU-E) is not decreased. This finding suggests that rather than an absolute decrease in stem cell number an abnormality in cellular proliferation exists in elderly subjects with anemia. A major unanswered question is whether or not these alterations result from the aging process or some other related abnormalities. Since animal studies indicate that aging does not alter basal hematopoiesis, other causes for these changes must be considered. Likely possibilities include chronic exposure to a factor or factors resulting in suppression of hematopoiesis, the presence of a chronic inflammatory disorder, or nutritional deficiencies.

IV. EPIDEMIOLOGIC EVIDENCE IMPLICATING NUTRITION IN THE ANEMIA OF THE ELDERLY

There is suggestive evidence from epidemiologic studies that nutritional factors may be important in the prevalence of anemia in the elderly. In every large-scale study anemia has been shown to be more common in subjects of low socioeconomic status (USDHEW, 1981; Nutrition Canada, 1973). Of particular importance is the recent finding that anemia is extremely rare in an affluent, very healthy elderly population examined in New Mexico (Garry et al., 1985). The number of elderly males and females at risk for anemia in this group was dramatically less than that reported in other populations. Furthermore, longitudinal monitoring of these patients over a five-year period failed to demonstrate an increased prevalence of anemia. A nutritional evaluation of these subjects showed that no nutritional deficiencies existed that would likely contribute to the anemia. This contrasts with a higher prevalence of nutritional deficiencies in low socioeconomic populations. Recently we performed a comprehensive nutritional and hematologic evaluation on a group of 73 elderly veterans living in a domiciliary facility in Hampton, Virginia. A high prevalence of anemia was present in this population. A close evaluation demonstrated that iron deficiency, folate deficiency, or other usually described causes of anemia were quite rare. We then performed a multivariate analysis of the data using age, hematopoietic, and nutritional factors as covariants. We demonstrated that while age appeared to be the major variable accounting for the decline in immunologic measurements observed in this elderly population, age did not appear to be an important factor in the prevalence of anemia. In contrast, serum albumin, transferrin, and prealbumin, which assess nutritional status, appeared to be excellent predictors of anemia.

These studies taken together generally indicate an interrelationship between parameters of nutritional status, affluence, and anemia. They thus provide indirect support for a role of nutrition in the anemia seen in the elderly individuals.

V. ROLE OF NUTRITION IN AGE-RELATED CHANGES IN HEMATOPOIESIS IN ANIMALS

Preliminary data from out laboratory have shown that protein depletion in aged animals aggravates the anemia, causes reductions in neutrophil count, and adversely affects neutrophil function. The degree of suppression is similar to that found in young animals. The potential role of nutritional factors in age-related changes in hematopoiesis is highlighted by studies on mice and their maximal life expectancy (Williams et al., 1985). The median life span of C57BL/6 mice is 24 months but the maximum reported life expectancy is 48 months. Provided 48-month-old mice are housed in individual cages (1 animal per cage), no change in hematopoiesis is seen. If, however, they are housed in groups of 5

animals per cage, a significant alteration in bone marrow function occurs. The animals become more anemic and the number of stem cells in their bone marrow decreases. Significant decreases also occur in the morphologically recognizable erythroid precursors. These findings are identical to hematopoietic changes previously described with overcrowding of animals (Boranic and Poljak-Blazi, 1983). The effects of overcrowding, however, are only seen when young, or even 24-month-old, animals are housed in groups of 10 mice per cage. This finding indicates that a minor stress, which does not affect hematopoiesis in young cases, causes significant abnormalities in aged animals. The mechanism whereby overcrowding affects hematopoiesis is also unclear. Aggressive behavior, competition for food, or infection are likely possibilities.

VI. HEMATOPOIETIC MANIFESTATIONS OF PROTEIN-CALORIE MALNUTRITION IN THE ELDERLY

The classic description of changes in immune and hematopoietic systems with protein-energy malnutrition was initially and elegantly described in children with kwashiorkor and marasmus (Viteri et al., 1968). More recently a high incidence of protein-energy malnutrition has been demonstrated in hospitalized subjects and in elderly with an array of medical disorders (Bistrian et al., 1976). There is a marked similarity between alterations in immune and hematopoietic functions which occur with apparent normal aging and those which occur with protein deprivation. This raises the possibility that protein deprivation in some form may contribute to alterations in hematopoietic changes normally ascribed to aging. Thus, to more closely examine the role nutritional factors play in age-related changes in hematopoiesis, we performed a careful analysis of the hematologic status of hospitalized elderly subjects with protein-energy malnutrition (Lipschitz and Mitchell, 1982). It is clear that anemia is invariably present in these individuals. An evaluation of the mechanism demonstrates that the features are identical to those normally ascribed to the "anemia of chronic disease." Thus the transferrin saturation is reduced as is the serum iron and the total iron binding capacity. Red blood cell protoporphyrin to heme ratios (which measure iron-deficient erythropoiesis) are decreased and serum ferritin levels, which measure tissue iron stores, are elevated. It is unclear whether this hematopoietic pattern reflects the presence of an acute or chronic disease process in these subjects or whether nutritional deprivation per se gives rise to an identical erythropoietic picture. Of particular interest in this regard is the prompt rise in the serum iron levels which occur within 48 hours of commencing a nutritional rehabilitation program (Fig. 1). This finding suggests a role of a nutritional factor in iron supply for erythropoiesis in these patients. In addition to anemia, relative neutropenia is frequent in elderly individuals with protein-calorie malnutrition. Quantitation of their home bone marrow precursors demonstrates reductions in the number of morphologically recognizable bone marrow precursors of the erythroid, myeloid, and megakaryocytic lines. The myeloid stem cell number (CFU-C) level is markedly reduced. These hematopoietic findings represent an aggravation of the age-related changes in hematopoiesis present in healthy subjects.

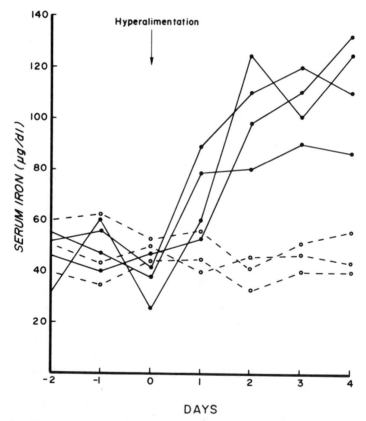

Fig. 1.   Change in serum iron following commencement of nutritional rehabilitation in four elderly subjects with protein-calorie malnutrition (●——●). No increase in serum iron was seen in three subjects followed for 5 days prior to commencing nutritional support (○------○).

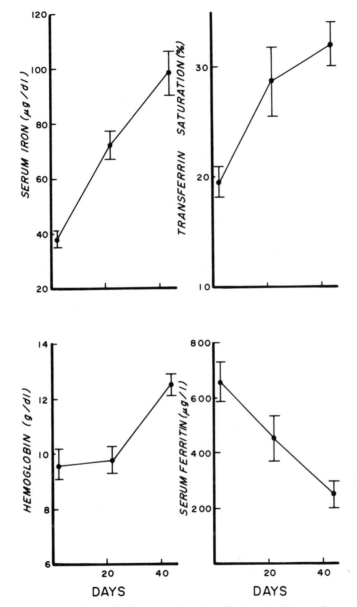

Fig. 2. Changes in hemoglobin, serum iron, transferrin saturation, and serum ferritin prior to and following repletion. The transferrin saturation is the ratio of serum iron to TIBC as a percentage.

Of particular interest is the effect of nutritional rehabilitation on bone marrow function. As shown in Fig. 2, correction of nutritional deficiencies in malnourished older individuals markedly improved their hematologic status. After 42 days highly significant elevations in hemoglobin levels occur. This is associated with significant increases in the serum iron and transferrin levels (presumably reflecting improved nutritional status). Because of redistribution of tissue iron from stores to circulating red cells, serum ferritin levels fell. Examination of bone marrow cell number in these subjects shows that nutritional rehabilitation increases bone marrow precursors toward the normal range. CFU-C levels increase significantly from a mean of 0.21 (± 0.11) $\times$ 10^7 cells/kg to 0.64 (± 0.21) $\times$ 10^7 cells/kg following nutritional rehabilitation. This contrasts to a CFU-C level of 0.88 (± 0.04) $\times$ 10^7 cells/kg in healthy elderly controls and 0.94 (± 0.06) $\times$ 10^7 cells/kg in young controls.

The interpretation of improvements in the hematologic status of malnourished, hospitalized aged subjects is extremely difficult. Any hospitalized elderly individual has coexisting diseases (including infection, dehydration, and metabolic changes) which effect hematopoietic function and thus the overall improvement of the medical status of the patient. To evaluate this possibility more closely, the effect of increased feeding on immune and hematopoietic status was examined in relatively healthy elderly who lived at home, who were ambulatory but were underweight, and who had marginal evidence of protein-energy deprivation (Lipschitz et al., 1985). By providing polymeric dietary supplements to these subjects between meals it is possible to maintain a 50% increase in total protein and caloric intake for a 16-week period. Weight gain and significant increases in nutritional parmeters indicate that the nutritional status of these subjects can be substantially improved. Thus increases in serum albumin and total iron binding capacity occur and highly significant elevations in selected vitamin measurements are seen. Despite a positive impact on nutritional status, immune function and hemoglobin levels do not improve. Thus no anergic subjects convert their skin test from negative to positive and alterations of T- and B-cell function persist.

VII. POTENTIAL AGE–NUTRITION–HEMATOPOIETIC INTERACTIONS

From these two studies some conclusions can be made with regard to the role of malnutrition in immune and hematopoietic function in the elderly. It is clear that significant nutritional deficiencies reversibly aggravate host defense abnormalities in the elderly. Nutritional deprivation is not, however, a major cause of hematopoietic changes seen predictably with aging in healthy subjects. It is possible that nutritional factors contribute to the reported hematopoietic changes with age but alternative mechanisms other than simple nutritional deficiencies must be considered. Marginal reductions of one or more nutrients acting alone or in combination over a prolonged period of time may modulate the hemtopoietic change usually ascribed to aging. Alternatively, nutrient delivery to the target organ may be altered with aging or changes in nutrient–target interactions may occur. These possibilities could account for the higher prevalence of anemia reported in epidemiologic studies. They remain untested hypotheses that provide opportunities for clinical research.

VIII. CONCLUSION

There is evidence from both animal models and humans that basal hematopoiesis is either unchanged or only minimally altered with aging. There is suggestive evidence in man that changes in hematopoiesis that occur with aging may have a nutritional etiology. The mechanism of nutrition-related alteration in hematopoiesis cannot be explained by simple deficiencies, which are quite rare in the elderly. Because of compromised reserve capacity, hematopoietic alterations are likely to occur with more subtle stresses in the elderly than in young individuals. This reduced reserve capacity makes the elderly particularly susceptible to nutritional deprivation and may contribute to the increased susceptibility to infection in the elderly. Aging and nutritional deficiencies are likely to severely compromise an elderly individual's potential to recover from a relatively minor stress.

ACKNOWLEDGMENTS

Supported by Grant R01 AG02603 from the National Institutes of Health (NIA) and funds from the Veterans Administration.

REFERENCES

Albright, J. A., and Makinodan, T. (1976). *J. Exp. Med.* **144,** 1204–1213.
Bistrian, B. R., Blackburn, G. L., Vitale, J., Cohran, D., and Walor, J. (1976). *JAMA, J. Am. Med. Assoc.* **235,** 1567–1570.
Boggs, D. R., and Patrene, K. D. (1985). *Am. J. Hematol.* **19,** 327–338.

Boranic, M., and Poljak-Blazi, M. (1983). *Exp. Hematol.* **11**, 873–878.

Chen, M. G. (1971). *J. Cell. Physiol.* **78**, 225–232.

Garry, P. J., Goodwin, J. S., and Hunt, W. C. (1985). *In* "Nutrition, Immunity and Illness in the Elderly" (R. J. Chandra, ed.), pp. 77–83. Pergamon, Oxford.

Harrison, D. E. (1975a). *J. Gerontol.* **30**, 279–285.

Harrison, D. E. (1975b). *J. Gerontol.* **30**, 286–291.

Harrison, D. E., Astle, C. M., and Delaittre, J. A. (1978). *J. Exp. Med.* **147**, 1526–1531.

Hartsock, R. J., Smith, E. B., and Kettan, C. S. (1965). *Am. J. Clin. Pathol.* **43**, 325–331.

Hayflick, L. (1965). *Exp. Cell Res.* **37**, 614–636.

Hellman, S., Botnick, L., Hannon, E. C., and Vignuelle, R. H. (1978). *Proc. Natl. Acad. Sci. U.S.A.* **75**, 490–494.

Hill, R. D. (1967). *Practitioner* **217**, 963–967.

Lipschitz, D. A., and Mitchell, C. O. (1982). *J. Am. Coll. Nutr.* **1**, 17–25.

Lipschitz, D. A., Mitchell, C. O., and Thompson, C. (1981). *Am. J. Hematol.* **11**, 47–54.

Lipschitz, D. A., McGinnis, S. K., and Udupa, K. B. (1982). *Age* **6**, 122–127.

Lipschitz, D. A., Udupa, K. B., Milton, K. Y., and Thompson, C. O. (1984). *Blood* **63**, 502–509.

Lipschitz, D. A., Mitchell, C. O., Steel, R. W., and Milton, K. Y. (1985). *JPEN, J. Parenter. Enteral Nutr.* **9**, 343–347.

McLennan, W. J., Andrews, G. R., MacLeod, C., and Caird, F. I. (1973). *Q. J. Med.* **52**, 1–13.

Mauch, P., Greenberger, J. S., Botnick, L., Hannon, E. C., and Hellman, S. (1980). *Proc. Natl. Acad. Sci. U.S.A.* **77**, 2927–2930.

Mauch, P., Botnick, L. E., Hannon, E. C., Obbagy, J., and Hellman, S. (1982). *Blood* **60**, 245–252.

Myers, M. A., Saunders, C. R. G., and Chalmers, D. G. (1968). *Lancet* **2**, 261–263.

Nutrition Canada (1973). Information Canada, Ottawa.

Parsons, P. L., Whithey, J. L., and Kilpatrick, G. S. (1965). *Practitioner* **195**, 656–660.

Phillips, R. A. (1978). *In* "Differentiation of Normal and Neoplastic Hematopoietic Cells" (B. Clarkson *et al.*, eds.), pp. 109–120. Cold Spring Harbor Lab., Cold Spring Harbor, New York.

Reincke, U., Hannon, E. C., Rosenblatt, M., and Hellman, S. (1982). *Science* **215**, 1619–1622.

Ross, E. A. M., Anderson, H., and Micklem, H. S. (1982). *J. Exp. Med.* **155**, 432–444.

Schofield, R. (1979). *Clin. Haematol.* **8**, 221–237.

Schofield, R., and Lajtha, L. G. (1974). *Br. J. Haematol.* **25**, 195–202.

Schofield, R., Lord, B. !., Kyffin, S., and Gilbert, C. W. (1980). *J. Cell. Physiol.* **103**, 355–362.

Till, J. E., and McCulloch, E. A. (1961). *Radiat. Res.* **13**, 213–222.

Udupa, K. B., and Lipschitz, D. A. (1984). *J. Lab. Clin. Med.* **103**, 574–580.

U.S. Department of Health, Education and Welfare (USDHEW) (1981). "Ten State Nutrition Survey—1968–1970," *DHEW* 72–8132. USDHEW, Washington, D.C.

Viteri, R. E., Alvarado, J., Luthinger, D. Y., and Wood, R. P., II (1968). *Vitam. Horm.* (N.Y.) **26**, 573–581.

Williams, L. H., Udupa, K. B., and Lipschitz, D. A. (1985). *Exp. Hematol.* (in press).

Wintrobe, M. (1981). *In* "Clinical Hematology" (M. M. Wintrobe *et al.*, eds.), pp. 35–47. Lea & Fibiger, Philadelphia, Pennsylvania.

19

Nutrition and the Aging Cardiovascular System

Robert B. McGandy

*Tufts University Schools of Medicine and Nutrition,
and USDA Human Nutrition Research Center on Aging at Tufts
Boston, Massachusetts*

I. INTRODUCTION

One of the major physical impairments associated with aging from middle adult life onward is a decline in cardiovascular function. The continuing loss of reserve capacity can be described by the decrements in left ventricular function and maximum oxygen consumption during exercise (Weisfeldt, 1980). The proportions of functional loss ascribable to true age changes in the cardiovascular system, to physical deconditioning associated with increasingly sedentary life-style, or to the cardiovascular effects of age-associated atherosclerotic disease are difficult to determine in studies of subjects from Western societies in whom the latter process is inevitably present.

263

Comparative quantitative studies of atherosclerosis in coronary and other major arteries have shown the universality of this disease in U.S. adult population groups (Eggen and Solberg, 1968). As illustrated in Fig. 1, the age-related increase in the surface area of coronary arteries involved with fatty streaks (lesions thought to be readily reversible) increases in males during the second and third decades of life and remains constant thereafter. But the extent of raised lesions, the lesions which gradually lead to functional impairment of blood flow, increases steadily throughout adult life. Among females, the picture is different and is consistent with their relative protection from coronary heart disease during the reproductive years. The extent of fatty streaks increases to age 50, but the progression of raised lesions is retarded by almost 20 years as compared to males. Since the raised lesions are thought to develop in the setting of a disruption of endothelial cell continuity overlying fatty streaks (Faggiotto and Ross, 1984), the major focus for clinical trials to examine the potential primary preventability of clinical complications of the raised, atherosclerotic lesions has been on male adults in the fourth and fifth decades of life.

An important reason for not studying older individuals in these clinical trials is a consideration of the natural history of the atheromatous

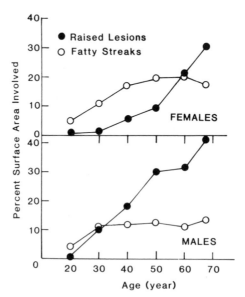

Fig. 1. Mean percentage of intimal surface area of coronary arteries involved with fatty streaks or raised lesions in New Orleans whites. Redrawn from Eggen and Solberg (1968).

lesions at various stages of development. The greatest likelihood of reversal occurs only with the smaller, less mature plaques. The larger, fibrous, and calcified lesions may be prevented from further progression, but they probably do not regress (Hennerici *et al.*, 1985).

The progression of the surface area involved by raised lesions continues beyond the age of 70 years. Waller and Roberts (1983) examined the coronary arteries of 40 subjects over 90 years of age. They found severe, calcified raised lesions in 39; in 28 of these cases at least one of the four major branches was narrowed by 76 to 100% in cross-sectional area.

The clinical complications of coronary atherosclerosis account for a very large share of both morbidity and mortality among older segments of the population. Throughout adult life, the coronary heart disease (CHD) mortality rates rise logarithmically with age. Among all adults, CHD accounts for 38% of all deaths; at ages 65 years and above, the proportion is 44% (U.S. Congress, Office of Technology Assessment, 1985). Thus the elderly, who contribute 68% of all U.S. deaths annually, account for 78% of all U.S. deaths ascribed to CHD. In terms of morbidity, the prevalence of chronic circulatory conditions reported by surveys of the elderly is extraordinarily high. Twenty-eight percent reported significant health impairments owing to heart conditions (angina pectoris, congestive heart failure, disturbances of rhythm) in 1981 (U.S. Congress, Office of Technology Assessment, 1985).

During the 1950s, epidemiological, clinical, and experimental animal studies demonstrated that several nutritionally modulated risk factors were important determinants of CHD incidence and mortality and of the development and progression of the underlying atherosclerosis. Of particular interest in terms of delaying or preventing CHD is the role of dietary fats in regulating levels of circulating lipoproteins and the importance of energy balance and obesity in regulating levels of both blood lipoproteins and blood pressure. Almost coincidentally with the increasing publicity about CHD risk factors, it became known that CHD mortality rates in the United States (which had increased throughout the 1940s and 1950s) were beginning to decline. Between the period 1968 to 1976, CHD death rates in the adult population decreased by 20%. In the age groups over age 65 years, the decline ranged from 13 to 27%. Even among males and females aged 85 years and above the decrements were 17 and 21%, respectively (Rosenberg and Klebba, 1979).

While there is agreement that the decline in CHD mortality is not just an artifact of vital statistics classification, the reasons for it have been more elusive and speculative. Several studies suggest that the decline in deaths is actually the result of a decline in CHD incidence rates over this period of time (and not merely secondary to better medical management with a resultant improved case fatality rate). Pell and Fayerweather (1985), reporting on studies of a large industrial population of males aged 25 to 64 years, have documented secular declines in age-specific incidence rates of myocardial infarction between the early 1960s and mid 1970s. Even in their oldest age group (55–64 years), the decline in incidence was 22%. Were the decreases in morbidity and mortality the result of a secular decrease in coronary atherosclerosis? Comparing autopsy studies of males living in New Orleans over this same time span (1960s and 1970s), Strong and Guzman (1980) have shown a decrease in the percentage surface area of coronary arteries involved in both fatty streaks and raised lesions. Their oldest age group was the mid forties, however, thus leaving unanswered the question of possible declines in raised lesions among older men and in women of all ages.

Among the factors thought to be causally associated with this substantial reversal of a major cause of mortality are favorable changes in the distributions of several CHD risk factors in the U.S. population in the 1960s and 1970s. Among these are changes in the U.S. diet and lipoprotein levels, in control of blood pressure, and in smoking habits (Walker, 1983). In this context, the role of CHD risk factors in older adults will be reviewed. Particular attention will be paid to the potential benefits and risks of dietary programs involving fat modification and of weight reduction in elderly individuals.

II.   RISK FACTORS AND AGING

A.   Changes in Risk Prediction with Age

As shown by the risk factor analyses from the Framingham Study (Kannel and Gordon, 1971) in Table I, the relative predictive power of the major CHD risk factors declines over adult life in both sexes. Data from the same publication allow a closer examination of the age trends in the risk of CHD predicted by each of these factors alone, after standardizing for the others. As can be seen in Table II, the factors showing the greatest loss in predictive power, particularly among males, is serum total cholesterol level. The risk ratios for total cholesterol levels of 310 versus 185 mg/dl are 5.2 at age 35 and only 1.1 at 65 years. Among females, the comparable ratios are 2.5 at age 45 and 1.5 at age 65 years. In this type of analysis, the age-related declines in the relative predictive power of smoking or of having a positive glucose tolerance test (G.T.T.)

TABLE I

Probability (per thousand) of Developing Coronary Heart
Disease in 8 Years at Specified Age

Age	Males High/low[a]	Ratio	Females High/low	Ratio
35	169/3	56	—	—
45	358/15	24	89/4	22
55	463/37	13	180/13	11
65	428/53	8	257/25	10

[a] High means that a person has a systolic blood pressure of
180 mm Hg, a serum cholesterol of 310 mg/dl, smokes cigarettes, has a left ventricular hypertrophy by electrocardiogram,
and has a positive glucose tolerance test (G.T.T.). Low means a
systolic pressure of 105, a serum cholesterol of 185, a nonsmoker of cigarettes, has no left ventricular hypertrophy, and a
negative G.T.T.

are less apparent. Blood pressure, on the other hand, loses almost no
discriminatory power over the adult years in either sex.

Subsequent examination of the strength of the association between
blood lipid levels and CHD incidence by Gordon et al. (1977) has led to a
reinterpretation of the separate effects of low- and high-density lipoproteins (LDL and HDL) over mid to late adult life. Multivariate analysis
has shown that LDL cholesterol level is only marginally associated with
CHD incidence in males aged 70 to 79 years and not at all among women
of this oldest age group. HDL cholesterol level, in contrast, remains
strongly and inversely related to CHD risk over the 50- to 79-year age
range in both sexes. But here too the predictive power of HDL cholesterol is diminished below statistical significance in both males and females over age 70.

One of the few studies showing a significant effect of cholesterol level
on CHD risk in the elderly is the mortality experience reported by Barrett-Connor et al. (1984). This group found a significant predictive effect
of total cholesterol (but not of systolic blood pressure or smoking) in
groups of men and women aged 65–79 years who were observed for a
nine-year follow-up period. Thus in the elderly years, when practically
all Americans have substantially advanced coronary artery atheromata,
the predictive power of lipoprotein levels is less impressive than among
younger adults. One cannot conclude from this, however, that the po-

TABLE II

Probability (per thousand) of Developing Coronary Heart Disease in 8 Years at Specified Age

Risk factor	Males			Females	
	35	55	65	45	65
Total cholesterol (mg/dl)[a]					
185	6	72	96	10	61
210	8	81	99	12	66
235	12	91	102	15	72
260	16	103	104	18	78
285	23	116	107	21	85
310	31	130	110	25	92
Ratio high/low	**5.2**	**1.8**	**1.1**	**2.5**	**1.5**
S.B.P. (mm/Hg)[b]					
105	8	64	71	10	50
120	10	76	85	12	60
135	12	91	102	15	72
150	14	109	121	18	86
165	17	130	143	21	102
180	21	153	169	26	120
Ratio high/low	**2.6**	**2.4**	**2.4**	**2.6**	**2.4**
Nonsmoker/smoker[c]					
Nonsmoker	12	91	102	15	72
Smoker	19	141	155	15	74
Ratio	**1.6**	**1.5**	**1.5**	**1.0**	**1.0**
neg G.T.T./pos G.T.T.[d]					
neg. G.T.T.	12	91	102	15	72
pos. G.T.T.	15	112	125	25	119
Ratio	**1.3**	**1.2**	**1.2**	**1.7**	**1.7**

[a] S.B.P. 135 mm Hg, nonsmoker, negative G.T.T.
[b] Cholesterol 235 mg/dl, nonsmoker, negative G.T.T.
[c] Cholesterol 235 mg/dl, S.B.P. 135 mm Hg, negative G.T.T.
[d] Cholesterol 235 mg/dl, S.B.P. 135 mm Hg, nonsmoker.

tential for preventing further progression of these lesions through favorable modification of lipoprotein levels is lost among the elderly. The secular decline in CHD mortality suggests that it is not.

B. Age Trends in Risk Factors and Their Interrelationships

Cross-sectional studies of the United States population (Lipid Research Clinics Program, 1980) show the age trends in blood lipoproteins, blood pressure, and in indices of obesity in adults from 20 to over 70 years of age. In both sexes, mean total and LDL cholesterol levels increase throughout the third to fifth decades of life, plateau in the sixth and seventh decades, and then decline. The decline in persons over the age of 70 years is a real one and is not simply the result of selective mortality, since it has been observed in cohorts examined longitudinally (Hershcopf et al., 1982). In contrast, mean levels of HDL cholesterol are relatively stable throughout the entire span of adult life. The well-known age-related increase in systolic blood pressure is observed in both males and females and shows no indication of a leveling off in the oldest age groups. Diastolic blood pressure, however, reaches a plateau in the sixth to seventh decades. The Lipid Research Clinics data on blood pressure are quite similar to the age trends from the Framingham Study (Kannel and Gordon, 1973). This latter paper has also shown that the age-related changes in blood pressure estimated by longitudinal cohort observations are almost identical to the counterpart slopes inferred from cross-sectional studies.

Since obesity is one of the characteristics associated with both lipoproteins and blood pressure, it is of interest to examine age trends in anthropological indices of relative adiposity. Cross-sectional and longitudinal studies (Kannel et al., 1979; Elahi et al., 1983) show that mean relative body weight increases in young adult life and then begins to decline in the 50- to 59-year age group and older. Between the mid 50s and age 70, the decline in relative body weight in both sexes is approximately 4%. The contribution of the loss of adipose tissue to this overall negative energy balance is suggested by the cross-sectional values for triceps skin-fold thickness. Between age 50 and 70 years, mean triceps thickness decreases by about 4 mm in both men and women.

Just as the distributions of blood lipids, blood pressure, and adiposity show different age trends over adult life, so too do the strengths of the associations between obesity and these two risk factors change with age. In the Framingham Study (Kannel and Gordon, 1968) the correlation coefficients between relative body weight and either systolic or diastolic pressure decline steadily over adult life. In the 35- to 39-year age group, the systolic coefficients are 0.35 and 0.41 for males and females, respectively; at ages 60 to 64 years, the values are 0.09 and 0.28. Havlik, et al. (1983) have reported similar age decrements in the correlations between another estimator of obesity (body mass index) and blood pressure over the 30- to 70-year age range in males. Using United States population survey data, Harlan et al. (1984) have also shown a reduction of the association between weight relative to height (body mass index) and systolic blood pressure in older men and women. The weaker association in older males (55 to 74 years) still remains statistically significant, but not among the females of this age group.

The report from Framingham (Kannel *et al.*, 1979) has documented the age-related decline in the association (as measured by the correlation coefficient) between relative body weight and total plasma cholesterol. The coefficient in males aged 30–34 years is 0.27; at ages 60 to 64 years, the value is −0.01, and none of the coefficients in age groups over 50 years are statistically significant. Among females, this association was insignificant over the entire age range, with the exception of the 35- to 39-year age groups for which the correlation was 0.10.

Utilizing lipoprotein cholesterol levels measured in the Framingham Study, Wilson *et al.* (1983) have produced a picture slightly different from the earlier study. Over the age of 50 years, body mass index is no longer significantly associated with LDL cholesterol levels in either sex. In contrast, the strong inverse relationship between this measure of obesity and HDL cholesterol is undiminished in size and is statistically significant over the adult life span of both males and females—including the 70- to 79-year-old age group. Thus the benefits of HDL cholesterol in preventing CHD are best obtained by maintaining optimal weight for height.

There is evidence that recent changes in relative body weight are more strongly associated with changes in blood lipids and blood pressure than is a static weight with either risk factor. Ashley and Kannel (1974) have analyzed the Framingham Study data from the point of view of relating relative change in weight over two consecutive examinations to the simultaneous changes in these two risk factors. They reported quite substantial, dynamic effects of weight change: a 10 unit change in body weight relative to height is associated with a change in serum total cholesterol of 11 mg/dl in men and 6.3 mg/dl in women and with changes in systolic blood pressure of 6.6 and 4.5 mm Hg, respectively, in men and women. Furthermore, these authors found no diminution in these relationships in older age groups. The importance of regulating relative obesity in the conservative, nutritional management of elevated blood pressure cannot be overestimated (Kaplan, 1985). The association between change in weight and total serum cholesterol described by Ashley and Kannel has been clarified by Wolf and Grundy (1983) and Zimmerman *et al.* (1984). In short-term metabolic studies, both of these groups have documented that the decline in LDL cholesterol is the major basis for the decreases in total serum cholesterol occurring with weight loss. In addition, and in partial confirmation of the previously described inverse relationship between obesity and HDL cholesterol, these latter studies have found modest increases in the HDL fraction accompanying the weight reduction.

III.   SECULAR TRENDS IN NUTRITION-RELATED RISK FACTORS

The decline in CHD mortality which began in the 1960s occurred contemporaneously with some remarkable changes in the American diet. Stamler (1978) and Walker (1983) have reported on some of the past trends in per capita food consumption patterns. Between 1960 and 1974, egg consumption decreased by 14%, milk and cream by 25%, butter by 50%, and animal fats by 39%. Over this same time period, the per capita use of margarine increased by 33%, poultry by 50%, and fish by 30%. Thus, the national trends have been toward less total and saturated fat, less cholesterol, and more polyunsaturated fats. A comparative analysis of dietary data from epidemiological studies of middle-aged Americans over the past 20 years or so (Goor et al., 1985) shows the impact of these altered food habits on fat intake. As a proportion of total daily calories, energy from total and saturated fat declined by 2 to 3%. The intake of dietary cholesterol decreased by 100 to 200 mg per day. The decline in saturated fatty acids and the increase in polyunsaturated fatty acids have been sufficient to raise the dietary P : S ratio from 0.25 to 0.30 in the early 1960s to close to 0.50 in the mid 1970s. There are few data regarding recent trends in patterns of food consumption among older individuals. But analyses of the current intakes of dietary fat by elderly persons in the Boston area (McGandy et al., 1986) show that men and women in their eighties and nineties have diets providing about 35% of calories from fat. The dietary P : S ratio is 0.40 and average daily intake of cholesterol is 300 to 400 mg. These values are quite similar to the data from the oldest age groups (up to age 70 years) in the Lipid Research Clinics Study (Goor et al., 1985).

Have these dietary changes affected levels of blood lipids in the American population? Over the age span 20 to 74 years, there is ample documentation of a significant secular decline in serum total cholesterol between the late 1950s and the mid 1970s. Data from the large national health surveys and from the Framingham Study have shown substantial decreases among both males and females of all age groups (Beaglehole et al., 1979). An analysis of secular trends in serum cholesterol levels among the male participants of the Baltimore Longitudinal Aging Study by Hershcopf et al. (1982) has demonstrated that this phenomenon has also affected males in their seventies and eighties. Thus the declines in blood total (and presumably in LDL cholesterol) observed over the past 25 years are consistent with the simultaneous changes in the American diet. It is not unreasonable to assume that the lower levels of blood cholesterol were, at least in part, causally associated with the simultaneous decline in CHD mortality.

Since the levels of both blood lipids and blood pressure are also responsive to the degree of obesity, it may be of interest to review the secular trends in the relative weights of our population. As summarized by Abraham and Carroll (1979) and by Kannel et al. (1979), relative weights of U.S. males actually increased between the 1950s and the mid 1970s. Furthermore, this increase in fatness was also observed in the 65- to 74-year-old age groups included in the national surveys. The secular trends observed among females have been more complicated. Among women of young and middle ages, relative weights decreased, whereas there have been no real trends among females in the 65- to 74-year age group over this time period. The trend in relative weights suggest that this is not a factor contributing to the decline in blood cholesterol levels in males. On the contrary, the increased fatness may have blunted the observed secular change in this lipid. But among women, the "weight consciousness" of the 1960s and 1970s may indeed have been a factor in the simultaneous decline of serum cholesterol.

Similar conclusions apply to the effects of relative weight trends on the secular changes in blood pressure. Dannenberg et al. (1985) have shown a small but significant decline in age-specific average blood pressures of Americans studied in the national health surveys of the past 25 years. Kannel and Schatzkin (1983) have commented on similar secular differences in the blood pressure levels of the original Framingham cohort as compared to their offspring studied at comparable ages. The increased relative body weights of males would appear to have mitigated the secular decreases in blood pressure. Without doubt, more effective control of obesity and, in particular, the prevention of weight gain throughout middle adult life would offer a substantial potential of further reducing CHD mortality.

The consensus conference on blood cholesterol level (Office of Medical Applications of Research, 1985) has affirmed the recommendations for a fat-modified diet and for maintenance of a desirable body weight. These guidelines, aimed at the prevention of CHD, are specifically stated in this report to be applicable to the elderly. On the other hand, consideration of the long time course of atherosclerosis—from adolescence onward—would argue persuasively for attention to these dietary goals from the second decade of life. There are no known risks in their continuance into the elderly years providing that the requirements for protein, vitamins, and minerals are met.

In this context, a consistent observation in recent surveys of the nutritional status of elderly American population groups has been the extraordinarily low levels of energy intake (McGandy *et al.*, 1986; Garry *et al.*, 1982). Since the intake of essential nutrients is closely related to overall energy consumption, there is an increased risk of nutrient deficiencies in older age groups. This is shown in Table III, in which the prevalence of potential nutrient deficiencies in a healthy population group of 70 to 98 years of age is examined. For each sex, the energy intakes per unit body weight are expressed as the lowest and the highest tertiles. This shows the potential risks involved in restricting calories among the elderly. The observations suggest that weight reduction diets in these age groups should be carefully supervised and monitored to assure that dietary quality is maintained. The observations also point to the potential value of emphasizing increased energy expenditure— rather than just caloric restriction—in the control of obesity among the elderly.

TABLE III

Percentage of Elderly Subjects Receiving Less Than Two-thirds of RDAs from Diet Alone at Low and High Energy Intakes[a]

| | Daily energy intake (cal/kg) | | | |
| | Males | | Females | |
Nutrient	<21.5	>27.5	<20.0	>25.5
Vitamin A	32	8	13	6
Ascorbic acid	12	4	9	3
Thiamine	10	0	11	1
Riboflavin	6	0	6	0
Niacin	8	0	2	0
Folic acid	75	27	85	55
Vitamin B_6	83	48	85	62
Vitamin B_{12}	27	12	45	19
Iron	1	0	8	0
Calcium	39	4	60	14
Zinc	65	18	77	56

[a] From McGandy *et al.* (1986).

IV. SUMMARY

Nutrition has an important role to play in maintaining the functional integrity of the aging cardiovascular system. Prevention, or at least the retardation, of age-related atherosclerotic vascular disease has already begun to occur. Along with more effective pharmacological management of hypertension and the control of cigarette smoking, continued modification of dietary fats and better regulation of energy balance can be expected to lead to further reductions in CHD morbidity and mortality. Even though the strength of the associations between blood lipids and CHD risk apparently decline in older age groups, there is good reason to believe that continued attention to dietary fats and to energy balance in the elderly makes sound preventive and therapeutic sense. That the oldest age groups have shared in the contemporary secular decline in CHD mortality provides compelling evidence of benefit.

REFERENCES

Abraham, S., and Carroll, M. D. (1979). In "Proceedings of the Conference on the Decline in Coronary Heart Disease Mortality" (R. J. Havlik and M. Feinleib, eds.), DHEW Publ. No. (NIH) 79-1610, pp. 253–281. U.S. Department of Health, Education, and Welfare, Washington, D.C.
Ashley, F. W., and Kannel, W. B. (1974). *J. Chronic Dis.* **27,** 103–114.
Barrett-Connor, E., Suarez, L., Khaw, K., Criqui, H., and Wingard, D. L. (1984). *J. Chronic Dis.* **37,** 903–908.
Beaglehole, R., LaRosa, J. C., Heiss, G. E., Davis, C. E., Rifkind, B. M., Muesing, R. M., and Williams, O. D. (1979). In "Proceedings of the Conference on the Decline in Coronary Heart Disease Mortality" (R. J. Havlik and M. Feinleib, eds.), DHEW Publ. No. (NIH) 79-1610. pp. 282–295. U.S. Dep. Health, Education and Welfare, Washington, D.C.
Dannenberg, A., Drizd, T., Horan, M., Leaverton, P. E., and Feinleib, M. (1985). *CVD Epidemiol. Newsl.,* January, p. 68 (abstr).
Eggen, D. A., and Solberg, L. A. (1968). In "The Geographic Pathology of Atherosclerosis" (H. C. McGill, ed.), pp. 111–119. Williams & Wilkins, Baltimore, Maryland.
Elahi, V. K., Elahi, D., Andres, R., Tobin, J. D., Butler, M. G., and Norris, A. H. (1983). *J. Gerontol.* **38,** 162–180.
Faggiotto, A., and Ross, R. (1984). *Arteriosclerosis (Dallas)* **4,** 341–356.
Garry, P. J., Goodwin, J. S., Hunt, W. C., Hooper, E. M., and Leonard, A. G. (1982). *Am. J. Clin. Nutr.* **36,** 319–331.
Goor, R., Hosking, J. D., Dennis, B. H., Graves, K. L., Waldman, G. T., and Haynes, S. G. (1985). *Am. J. Clin. Nutr.* **41,** 299–311.
Gordon, T., Castelli, W. P., Hjortland, M. C., Kannel, W. B., and Dawber, T. R. (1977). *Am. J. Med.* **62,** 707–714.
Harlan, W. R., Hull, A. L., Schmouder, R. L., Landis, J. R., Larkin, F. A., and Thompson, F. E. (1984). *Hypertension* **6,** 802–809.

Havlik, R. J., Hubert, H. B., Fabsitz, R. R., and Feinleib, M. (1983). *Ann. Intern. Med.* **98,** Part 2, 855–859.

Hennerici, M., Rautenberg, W., Trockel, U., and Kladetzky, R. G. (1985). *Lancet* **1,** 1415–1419.

Hershcopf, R. J., Elahi, D., Andres, R., Baldwin, H. L., Raizes, G. S., Shocken, D. D., and Tobin, J. D. (1982). *J. Chronic Dis.* **35,** 101–114.

Kannel, W. B., and Gordon, T. (1968). "An Epidemiological Investigation of Cardiovascular Disease," Sect. 5. U.S. Department of Health, Education and Welfare, Public Health Serv. Nat. Inst. Health, U.S. Gov. Printing Office, Washington, D.C.

Kannel, W. B., and Gordon, T. (1971). "The Framingham Study. An Epidemiological Investigation of Cardiovascular Disease," Sect. 27, Publ. No. 1740–0320. U.S. Department Health, Education and Welfare, Public Health Serv., Nat. Inst. Health, U.S. Gov. Printing Office, Washington, D.C.

Kannel, W. B., and Gordon, T. (1973). "The Framingham Study," Publ. No. 74–478. U.S. Dep. Health, Education and Welfare, Public Health Serv., Nat. Inst. Health, U.S. Gov. Printing Office, Washington, D.C.

Kannel, W. B., and Schatzkin, A. (1983). *Prog. Cardiovasc. Dis.* **16,** 309–332.

Kannel, W. B., Gordon, T., and Castelli, W. P. (1979). *Am. J. Clin. Nutr.* **32,** 1238–1245.

Kaplan, N. M. (1985). *Ann. Intern. Med.* **102,** 359–373.

Lipid Research Clinics Program (1980). "The LRC Population Studies Data Book," Vol. 1, DHHS Publ. No. (NIH) 80-1527. Nat. Inst. Health, Bethesda, Maryland.

McGandy, R. B., Russell, R. M., Hartz, S. C., Jacob, R. A., Tannenbaum, S., Peters, H., Sahyoun, N., and Otradovec, C. L. (1986). *Nutr. Res.* (in press).

Office of Medical Application of Research, N.I.H. (1985). *JAMA, J. Am. Med. Assoc.* **253,** 2080–2086.

Pell, S., and Fayerweather, W. E. (1985). *N. Engl. J. Med.* **312,** 1005–1011.

Rosenberg, H. M., and Klebba, A. J. (1979). *In* "Proceedings of the Conference on the Decline in Coronary Heart Disease Mortality" (R. J. Havlik and M. Feinleib, eds.), DHEW Publ. No. (NIH) 79-1610, pp. 11–39. U.S. Department of Health, Education and Welfare, Washington, D.C.

Stamler, J. (1978). *Ann. N.Y. Acad. Sci.* **304,** 333–358.

Strong, J. P., and Guzman, M. A. (1980). *Lab. Invest.* **43,** 297–301.

U.S. Congress, Office of Technology Assessment (1985). "Technology and Aging in America," OTA-BA-264, pp. 369–412. U.S. Off. Technol. Assess., Washington, D.C.

Walker, W. J. (1983). *N. Engl. J. Med.* **308,** 649–651.

Waller, B. F., and Roberts, W. C. (1983). *Am. J. Cardiol.* **51,** 403–421.

Weisfeldt, M. L. (1980). *N. Engl. J. Med.* **303,** 1133–1137.

Wilson, P. W. F., Garrison, R. J., Abbott, R. D., and Castelli, W. P. (1983). *Arteriosclerosis (Dallas)* **3,** 273–281.

Wolf, R. N., and Grundy, S. M. (1983). *Arteriosclerosis (Dallas)* **3,** 160–169.

Zimmerman, J., Kaufman, N. A., Fainaru, M., Eisenberg, S., Oschry, Y., Friedlander, Y., and Stein, Y. (1984). *Arteriosclerosis (Dallas)* **4,** 115–123.

Index